COLOR DOPPLER IMAGING IN OBSTETRICS AND GYNECOLOGY

COLOR DOPPLER IMAGING IN OBSTETRICS AND GYNECOLOGY

Editors

RICHARD JAFFE, M.D.

Assistant Professor
Division of Maternal-Fetal Medicine
Department of Obstetrics and Gynecology
University of Illinois at Chicago
Chicago, Illinois

STEVEN L. WARSOF, M.D.

Associate Professor, Director
Division of Maternal-Fetal Medicine
Department of Obstetrics and Gynecology
University of Illinois at Chicago
Chicago, Illinois

McGRAW-HILL, INC.

Health Professions Division

New York   St. Louis   San Francisco   Auckland   Bogotá   Caracas   Lisbon
London   Madrid   Mexico   Milan   Montreal   New Delhi   Paris   San Juan
Singapore   Sydney   Tokyo   Toronto

COLOR DOPPLER IMAGING
IN OBSTETRICS AND GYNECOLOGY

1 2 3 4 5 6 7 8 9 0   KGPKGP   9 8 7 6 5 4 3 2

ISBN 0–07–105420–0

This book was set in Times Roman by Arcata Graphics/Kingsport.
The editors were Edward M. Bolger and Muza Navrozov;
the production supervisor was Richard Ruzycka;
the cover was designed by José Fonfrias;
the index was prepared by Philip James.
Arcata Graphics/Kingsport was printer and binder

Library of Congress Cataloging-in-Publication Data

Color Doppler imaging in obstetrics and gynecology/editors,
  Richard Jaffe, Steven L. Warsof.
      p.   cm.
    Includes bibliographical references and index.
    ISBN 0–07–105420–0
    1. Doppler ultrasonography.   2. Ultrasonics in obstetrics.
3. Fetus—Ultrasonic imaging.   4. Generative organs, Female—
Ultrasonic imaging.   I. Jaffe, Richard.   II. Warsof, Steven L.
[DNLM: 1. Echocardiography, Doppler.   2. Genital Diseases, Female—
ultrasonography.   3. Pregnancy Complications—ultrasonography.
4. Ultrasonography, Prenatal. WQ 202 C719]
RG527.5.U48C65
618′.047543—dc20
DNLM/DLC
for Library of Congress

92–6257
CIP

*To our wives, Jaffa and Valerie,
and our children, Adi, Shirley,
Beth, Alison, and Elliot,
for their love and understanding.*

Contents

Contributors*

Jacques Abramowicz, M.D. [12]
Assistant Professor of Obstetrics
    and Gynecology
Director Perinatal Ultrasound
Department of Obstetrics and Gynecology
Strong Memorial Hospital
The University of Rochester School
    of Medicine and Dentistry
Rochester, New York

Domenico Arduini, M.D. [11]
Deputy Director, Perinatal Unit
    Department of Obstetrics and
    Gynecology
Catholic University of S. Cuore
Rome, Italy

Joseph G. Bell, M.D. [13]
Fellow
Division of Maternal-Fetal Medicine
Department of Obstetrics and Gynecology
Pennsylvania Hospital
Philadelphia, Pennsylvania

Carolyn B. Coulam, M.D. [16]
Director of Reproductive Immunology
Genetics and IVF Institute
Fairfax, Virginia

Greggory R. DeVore, M.D. [8]
Fetal Diagnostic Center
Salt Lake City, Utah

Tjeerd W. A. Huisman, M.D. [9]
Division of Prenatal Diagnosis
Department of Obstetrics and Gynecology
Academic Hospital Dijkzigt
Erasmus University Rotterdam
Rotterdam, The Netherlands

Richard Jaffe, M.D. [1, 2, 4, 5, 12]
Assistant Professor
Division of Maternal-Fetal Medicine
Department of Obstetrics and Gynecology
University of Illinois at Chicago
Chicago, Illinois

Sanja Kupesic-Urek, M.D. [14]
Ultrasonic Institute
University of Zagreb
Zagreb, Yugoslavia

Asim Kurjak, M.D. [6, 14, 15]
Professor
Ultrasonic Institute
University of Zagreb
Zagreb, Yugoslavia

---

* The numbers in brackets following the contributor name refer to chapter(s) authored or co-authored by the contributor.

Abraham Ludomirski, M.D. [13]
Director of Research
Department of Obstetrics and Gynecology
Pennsylvania Hospital
Philadelphia, Pennsylvania

William J. Meyer, M.D. [1]
Assistant Professor
Division of Maternal-Fetal Medicine
Department of Obstetrics and Gynecology
University of Illinois at Chicago
Chicago, Illinois

Albert J. Peters, D.O. [16]
Fellow in Reproductive Immunology
Methodist Center for Reproduction
    and Transplantation Immunology
Indianapolis, Indiana

Roger A. Pierson, M.D. [3]
Associate Professor
Reproductive Biology Research Unit
Department of Obstetrics and Gynecology
Royal University Hospital
Saskatoon, Saskatchewan
Canada

Kathryn L. Reed, M.D. [10]
Associate Professor
Head, Obstetrical Ultrasound
Department of Obstetrics and Gynecology
Arizona Health Sciences Center
Tuscon, Arizona

Giuseppe Rizzo, M.D. [11]
Perinatal Unit
Department of Obstetrics and Gynecology
Catholic University of S. Cuore
Rome, Italy

**Joaquin Santolaya-Forgas, M.D.,
    Ph.D.** [7]
Assistant Professor
Division of Maternal-Fetal Medicine
Department of Obstetrics and Gynecology
University of Illinois at Chicago
Chicago, Illinois

J. Jaroslav Stern, M.D. [16]
Fellow in Reproductive Immunology
Methodist Center for Reproduction
    and Transplantation Immunology
Indianapolis, Indiana

Patricia A. Stewart, Ph.D. [9]
Division of Prenatal Diagnosis
Department of Obstetrics and Gynecology
Academic Hospital Dijkzigt
Erasmus University Rotterdam
Rotterdam, The Netherlands

**Juriy W. Wladimiroff, M.D.,
    Ph.D.** [9]
Professor of Obstetrics and Gynecology
Head, Division of Prenatal Diagnosis
Department of Obstetrics and Gynecology
Academic Hospital Dijkzigt
Erasmus University Rotterdam
Rotterdam, The Netherlands

Ivica Zalud, M.D. [6, 15]
Ultrasonic Institute
University of Zagreb
Zagreb, Yugoslavia

Preface

The purpose of this book is to expose the reader to the many potential areas in which color Doppler imaging can expand the clinical and research arenas for the obstetrician and gynecologist.

This book is a culmination of many years of combined experience by the authors in the use of diagnostic ultrasound. Most of the authors were introduced to ultrasound in its infancy as an A-mode curiosity of limited practical use. The contact B-mode scanner introduced in the late 1960s and gray scaling of the early 1970s raised the potential of fetal biometry. With the advent of real time imaging in the mid-1970s, the ease of imaging was greatly improved and, when combined with Doppler waveform analysis of the 1980s, biophysical assessment of the fetus became a reality. Vaginal scanning enhanced the role of the ultrasound in gynecology, gynecologic oncology, and reproductive endocrinology. Each advance in technology was heralded by a brief text designed to capture the imagination of the reader and to spur on the clinical and research community for further investigations.

We hope that after studying this text the reader will be similarly excited by the potential of color Doppler imaging. We also hope that each chapter will be the inspiration for the reader to become involved personally in new and different applications of this powerful technology.

Many years ago the late Professor Ian Donald stated that "the day may come that every gravida would have an ultrasound examination." Could he have envisioned that this examination would be in the multiple colors of the rainbow?

Ultimately, we hope that as a result of our effort the pursuit of knowledge has been advanced slightly, that the fetal-uterine environment will be better understood, and that this will lead to an improvement in maternal and child health.

Finally, we would like to thank all the authors for their timely contributions and adherence to production deadline.

BASIC PRINCIPLES OF DOPPLER ULTRASONOGRAPHY

WILLIAM J. MEYER
RICHARD JAFFE

Real-time ultrasonic assessment of the fetus has become an essential component of obstetrical and perinatal practice. Ultrasound has provided a noninvasive method of monitoring and evaluation of the advancing gestation. Ultrasound is a simple, reliable method for pregnancy dating, evaluation of fetal anomalies, and assurance of fetal well-being. The advent of Doppler ultrasound has further enhanced our ability to diagnose specific fetal abnormalities such as structural and functional cardiac anomalies. Doppler velocimetry utilizes advanced technology to assess the hemodynamic status of the uterine-placental-fetal unit. Doppler ultrasound allows a unique opportunity to study the fetal and uterine circulations in normal and abnormal pregnancies, as well as enhancing our understanding of intrauterine physiology. This chapter briefly reviews the basic principles of Doppler ultrasound use in clinical medicine.

PHYSICS OF ULTRASOUND

Transmission of sound waves requires alternate compression and rarefaction of particles in a medium to create a wave.[1] Wavelength is determined by measurement of one cycle of compression and rarefaction. The frequency of this sound is the number of cycles of compression or rarefaction which pass a given point in 1 s. One cycle per second is called *one hertz* (Hz). Ultrasound is defined as a frequency greater than 20 kHz (20,000 Hz). Sound at this frequency is inaudible to the human ear. In diagnostic applications, ultrasound frequencies range between 2 and 10 MHz.[2] The transmitted sound wave has a beam width which varies with the distance from the transducer. This determines the lateral resolution of the ultrasound image. The higher the frequency employed, the better the spatial (axial) resolution[1] but the lower the depth of penetration.

Ultrasound transducers produce high-frequency sound by short bursts of electrical stimulation of piezoelectric crystals located in the transducer. Electric voltages can produce an alteration in the crystal lattice structure of these crystals causing the crystals to vibrate and produce sound waves. This is known as the *piezoelectric phenomenon*[3] and was discovered by the Curies in 1888. The applied electrical stimulus determines the frequency and intensity of the sound wave. The same crystal receives sound, which also causes distortion of the crystal lattice, and produces electrical energy, which can be amplified and recorded. Most diagnostic transducers, which consist of many single piezoelectric elements, spend most of the time in a receiving mode with a transmit-to-receive ratio of approximately 1:1000. Sequential stimulation of the piezoelectric elements produces real-time images by conversion of reflected sound waves to ultrasonic images. In humans, tissue density is variable and therefore transmission speed of the ultrasound beam is variable in the various tissues. The average velocity of sound in soft tissue is approximately 1540 m/s.[4]

When an ultrasound beam travels through medium of variable density and strikes a very dense object, such as bone, most of the incident wave energy is reflected back and the transmitted wave is attenuated. This produces a bright reflected echo. Only incident waves reflected back toward the transducer produce images. The speed with which an echo returns and the intensity of returning echoes are proportional to the depth and reflectivity of objects struck by the incident wave. This is the basis of gray-scale ultrasound imaging.

THE DOPPLER EFFECT

When sound is produced by a stationary source, a wave is propagated with a given wavelength and frequency, as described above. When the source emitting sound moves relative to the receiver, the perceived frequency changes as the distance between the emitter and receiver changes. As the two objects move toward each other, the observed frequency increases, and if they move away from each other, the observed frequency decreases. The change in observed frequency is called the *Doppler shift,* which was first described by the Austrian physicist Johann Christian Doppler in 1842.[5] Doppler realized that the color emitted by a moving star changes relative to its traveling toward or away from earth. The Dutch scientist Buys-Ballot applied Doppler's finding to sound 1 year later,[6] showing that the frequency of a sound wave increases when the source of the sound approaches the receiver and decreases when the source of the sound moves away from the receiver.

This principle is applicable to any form of energy that propagates waves such as sound, light, or radio waves.

The Doppler shift occurs irrespective of whether the source, the object, or both are moving. In terms of diagnostic Doppler ultrasound, the echoes reflected by a moving echogenic object will have Doppler-shifted frequencies that depend on the velocity of the moving object and the angle between the insonating beam and the direction of motion.

The relationship between velocity of blood flow and Doppler shift is expressed by the following equation:

$$F_t - F_r = F_d = \frac{2F_t \times \cos\Theta \times v}{c}$$

where F_d = Doppler shift, F_t = transducer transmission frequency, F_r = received frequency, Θ = incident angle (between ultrasonic beam and long axis of vessel), c = velocity of sound in tissue, and v = velocity of blood flow (Fig. 1-1).

The angle between the ultrasound beam and direction of motion of the red

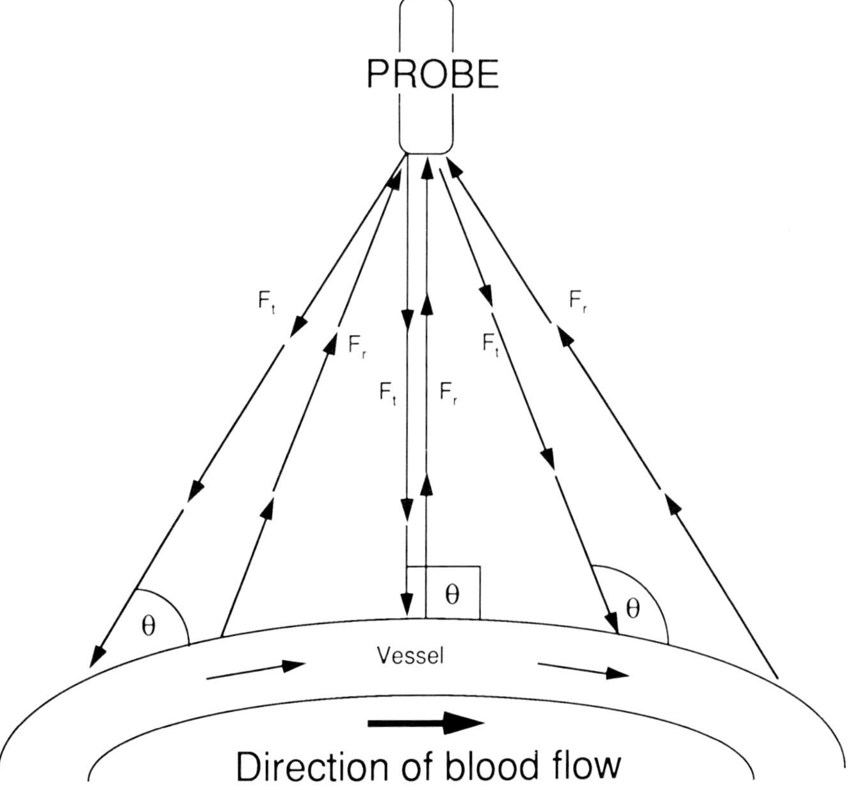

Figure 1-1   Schematic demonstration of the Doppler effect. The difference between the transmitted (F_t) and the received (F_r) frequencies is the Doppler shift (F_d), and it is dependent on the velocity of sound in the tissue (c), the transmitted frequency, the velocity of the blood (v), and the angle of insonation (θ).

blood cells is an important factor in the equation, as the Doppler shift is a consequence of motion along this line and the component of velocity is given by $v \times \cos \Theta$. Figure 1-1 shows that if the motion is perpendicular to the beam, the angle will be 90°, and as $\cos \Theta = 0$, there will be no $v \times \cos \Theta$ component and no Doppler shift. This phenomenon of zero Doppler shift is of considerable importance when evaluating color Doppler images and is discussed further in Chap. 2.

As mentioned above, the Doppler shift produced by a moving object is relative to the velocity of the object moving and the angle of the ultrasonic beam if the transmission frequency and velocity of sound in the tissue are known. When using Doppler ultrasonography to assess blood flow in an artery, the incident ultrasound beam is reflected not by one but by millions of red blood cells. When the ultrasound beam is reflected by moving red blood cells, it undergoes a reflective phenomenon called *backscattering*.[7–9] Backscattering occurs because the size of the reflective surface of the red cell is smaller than the wavelength of the ultrasonic beam. The produced echoes are scattered and reflected in all directions. The frequency shift determined by the transducer is a collection of all the Doppler shifted echoes produced by the red cells and is proportional to the velocity of the moving column of cells in the vessel. The power of the Doppler frequency shift is affected by both the RBC's concentration (hematocrit) and the turbulence of flow within the vessel.[10]

OPERATIONAL PARAMETERS

Volume Estimation

From the above equation the Doppler shift can be precisely calculated only if the angle of incidence and the velocity of blood flow in a given artery are known. Blood flow volume is measured as the product of the mean blood flow velocity and the vessel cross-sectional area (flow = velocity × cross-sectional area). Several methods have been used to estimate volumetric flow, but they all have significant limitations.[11,12] They are as follows:

1. *The uniform insonation technique.* With this technique the ultrasound beam is considered uniform, red blood cells are assumed to reflect sound equally, flow direction is assumed constant, and the sample volume is large enough to include the whole vessel. The mean velocity calculated is then multiplied by the vessel area to give volume of blood flow. Sources of error with this technique are the changes which occur in vascular shapes and diameters during the cardiac cycle, the inability to accurately measure the vessel diameter,[7,13,14] and the turbulence along vessel walls. In smaller vessels it is practically impossible to correctly measure both diameter and angle of insonation, and the error in quantitating the volume of flow can be as high as 25 to 50 percent.[15] Another source of error when employing a large sample volume is the erroneous addition of signals from outside the vessel that will affect the calculations.

2. *The velocity profile technique.* With this technique a multigated pulsed Doppler system that can assess the entire vessel at one time is used, and the individual velocity components throughout the cardiac cycle are measured and integrated. This technique also suffers from severe limitations and is not employed in clinical medicine.[2]
3. *The assumed velocity profile method.* With this method measurements are made at one point in a vessel, and the mean flow velocity assumed equal to the maximal velocity near the center of flow. This flat velocity profile is present only in large vessels such as the aorta, whereas in the smaller fetal vessels the flow profile is parabolic. Several experimental measurements have shown that this assumption is erroneous because velocity profiles were found to change over the cardiac cycle and to differ depending on location within the vessel.[2]

Because of these limitations, methods independent of incident angle and vessel diameter have been developed to estimate blood flow and analyze waveforms. These techniques all involve the calculation of different ratios derived from the shape of the spectrum maximum envelope and are discussed later in this chapter.

Sampling Volume

Sampling volume refers to that region of the Doppler system that can receive Doppler-shifted echoes and can be determined by the operator. Echoes produced within a sample volume are used to calculate the Doppler shift within that sample. In the case of blood-flow estimation, the red cells in the vessel are randomly and independently distributed within the vessel. Red cells within the sample volume generate independent echoes, which are added together to produce the final signal detected and displayed by the monitor. The sample volume is adjusted to approximate the diameter of the blood vessel being studied.[8] When the sample volume equals the vessel diameter, all parts of the vessel cross section contribute equally to the final Doppler signal, and this represents an accurate estimation of blood velocity in the given vessel. It can also be assumed that the maximum Doppler shift is proportional to the maximum velocity and that the mean Doppler shift is proportional to the mean velocity of blood flow.

In estimating flow, the diameter of the vessel may approach the lower limit of spatial resolution of the machine, and therefore vessel diameter cannot be accurately estimated. For this reason the sample volume must be sufficiently large to insolate the entire lumen of the vessel being studied.

Signal Processing

Processing the Doppler echoes involves a complex series of steps. In simple terms, the final Doppler-shifted signal which is displayed on the monitor is a summation of the scattered Doppler shifts produced by the moving column of red cells within the sample volume. This composite signal is composed of a spectrum of Doppler-shifted echoes of variable frequency and amplitude.

The first step in signal processing is separation of Doppler-shifted echoes from the red cells from other echoes returning to the transducer. This process is called *demodulation.* There are many Doppler demodulation schemes. One commonly used demodulation process in diagnostic ultrasound is called *phase quadrant demodulation.*[10] After demodulation, the Doppler signal is analyzed as a function of time. In diagnostic applications the most commonly used method is called *spectral analysis.* Spectral analysis involves quantitating the amplitudes of each frequency of Doppler-shifted signals and also temporal changes in the mean or peak frequency during a cardiac cycle. The frequency information is expressed as a power spectrum in which the amplitude for each frequency component is calculated.[2,16,17] Fast Fourier transform is the most commonly used form of spectral analysis in diagnostic Doppler ultrasound equipment. This is a complex mathematical process which converts the time-dependent Doppler wave signal into a frequency spectrum, useful in study of the hemodynamics of maternal-fetal circulation.[2,18] Newer, nontraditional methods for analysis of Doppler signals have been suggested.[19] These methods have the advantage of being heart-rate-independent and easier to interpret but are still in the developmental stages and not available for clinical use.

Signal Filtering

Any moving object can create a Doppler frequency shift relative to the transducer. Not only does the transducer collect Doppler-shifted echoes produced by the moving objects under study but it also detects echoes from any tissue that moves, thus introducing artificial pulsatility into the tracing. To separate the desired signals from background noise, a collection of filters is employed that can be manipulated by the operator. By employing a low-pass filter, high-frequency signal artifacts can be eliminated. A high-pass filter will eliminate low-frequency signals. In general, most high-frequency artifacts are machine-generated as a result of operator use of too high power or gain. Elimination of these signals by use of a low-pass filter will not generally affect interpretation of results. Venous blood flow will produce low-frequency signals, and use of a high-pass filter (wall thump filter) when studying the fetal circulation can falsely eliminate end-diastolic flow information from these vessels, leading to inaccurate interpretation of the final signal obtained (Fig. 1-2). Filters with low cutoff frequencies of 100 to 150 Hz are generally used.

DOPPLER MODES

Three different types of Doppler ultrasound are used in modern diagnostic equipment. They are *continuous wave* (CW) *Doppler, pulsed wave* (PW) *Doppler,*

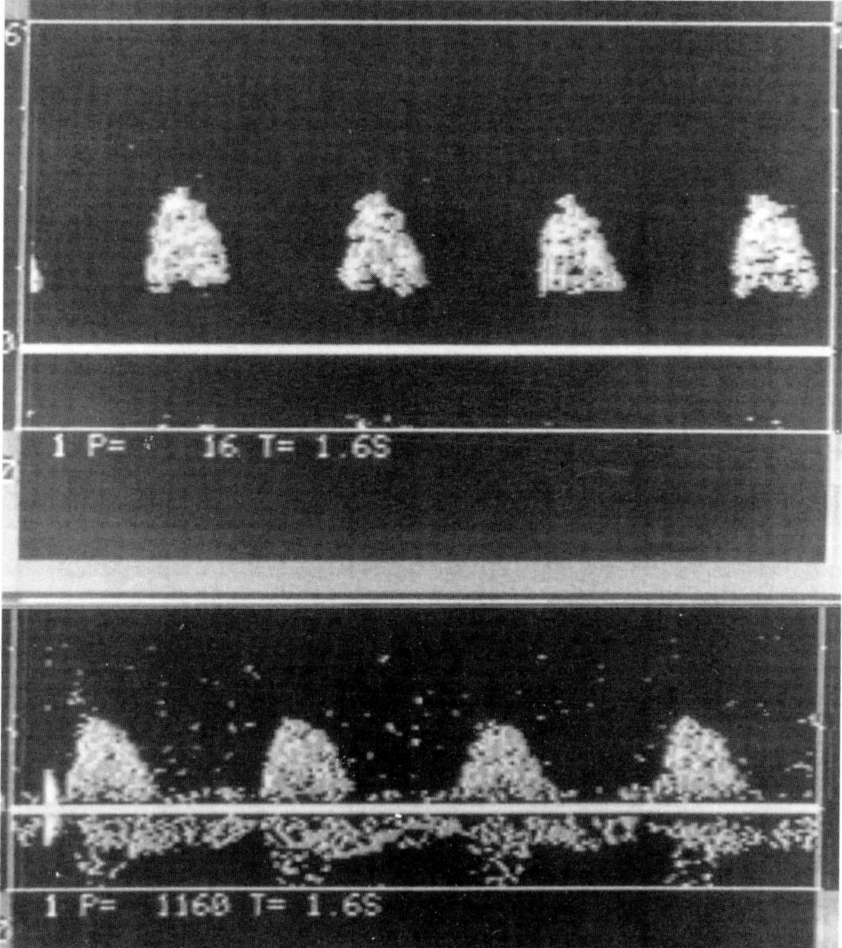

Figure 1-2 Loss of important flow information (*top*) with the use of a high-pass filter (wall-thump filter). With the reduction in the high-pass filter, important low diastolic and venous flow clearly appears (*bottom*).

and *two-dimensional color flow mapping*. Each has advantages and disadvantages that are briefly discussed here.

Continuous Wave Doppler Imaging

In a continuous wave Doppler system a single transducer both transmits and receives the ultrasonic signals. This is accomplished with two piezoelectric elements within the transducer: one continuously transmits while the other continuously receives reflected echoes. The elements are positioned in the transducer in such a way that the transmitted beam and the area of reception of echoes overlap. This allows reception of Doppler-shifted reflected echoes when motion occurs within the sensitive area. A major limitation of continuous wave Doppler is the inability to discriminate the origin of Doppler-shifted echoes. A continuous wave system will receive all Doppler-shifted waves from the reception zone but is unable to differentiate the site of origin of the echo signals. Continuous wave Doppler is widely used for fetal heart rate monitoring. It has also been used in the Doppler assessment of uterine-umbilical blood flow, but the inability to precisely define the origin of echoes has limited the use of continuous wave systems in detailed studies of fetal central circulation.

Pulsed Wave Doppler Systems

The major difference between pulsed and continuous wave systems is that the former uses a single crystal to both transmit and receive. Ultrasound beams are transmitted in a pulsed fashion, and when not transmitting, the same crystal serves as a receiver for returning echoes. The interval time between transmission of the beam and reception of the echoes can be varied, and by doing so the range of the target can be determined. A process called *range gating* allows selection of target depth. Range gating precisely localizes a specific target vessel and allows measurement of flow velocities in a particular vessel such as fetal aorta or middle cerebral artery. Current pulsed Doppler machines are of the duplex type, which allows the same transducer to ultrasonically guide placement of the sample volume over the desired vessel and assess Doppler shift signals indicating flow velocity.[20] Doppler capabilities have been combined with both mechanical and electronic scanners to give the simultaneous display of Doppler and imaging modes. These machines allow axial rotation of the sample volume to obtain optimal incident angles for Doppler samples, usually 30 to 60°. The smaller the incident angle, the better the Doppler signal. If the sample volume is too small for the diameter of the vessel, an inaccurate representation of flow will be obtained. On the other hand, if the sample volume is much larger than the vessel, background noise is intensified, decreasing the signal-to-noise ratio affecting the final signal.

Color Doppler Imaging

Color flow mapping involves the addition of color to the ultrasound image to indicate direction of blood flow. Flow is first determined as being either toward or away from the transducer based on the Doppler shift frequency and then assigned a color code. In most systems, flow toward the transducer is assigned the color red and flow away from the transducer is assigned the color blue. Color flow mapping of the fetal circulation offers a new and exciting method of studying fetal circulation and the hemodynamics of pregnancy in both normal and abnormal pregnancies. Its use in perinatal medicine is addressed in subsequent chapters.

ARTIFACTS AND PITFALLS

Low-Velocity Flow

As already mentioned above, one of the main artifacts of Doppler ultrasonography is the loss of low-flow information owing to the use of a high-pass filter set at a high level. This can be avoided by adjusting the high-pass filter properly or changing the Doppler angle. As previously described, the velocity of the Doppler shift is inversely proportional to the cosine of the Doppler angle. Therefore, the Doppler frequency shifts fall steadily as the angle to flow approaches 90°, and low flows can be amplified artificially by reducing the angle of insonation.

Aliasing

The most well-described Doppler artifact is *aliasing*. Aliasing is a sampling phenomenon that occurs when the sampled frequency is greater than half the pulse repetition frequency (PRF), or sampling rate. This is known as the *Nyquist limit*. When the Doppler shift frequency exceeds the Nyquist limit, the spectral tracing shows the "wraparound" effect (Fig. 1-3). The sampling rate is limited by the depth of the tissue under study because an ultrasound pulse cannot be emitted before the echo produced by the previous pulse is received. The PRF limitation placed on sampling from deep vessels reduces the maximum velocity that can be detected in these vessels. For this reason the more superficial the vessel, the higher the velocities that can be measured and the lower the possibility of aliasing. Different methods can be employed to overcome the occurrence of

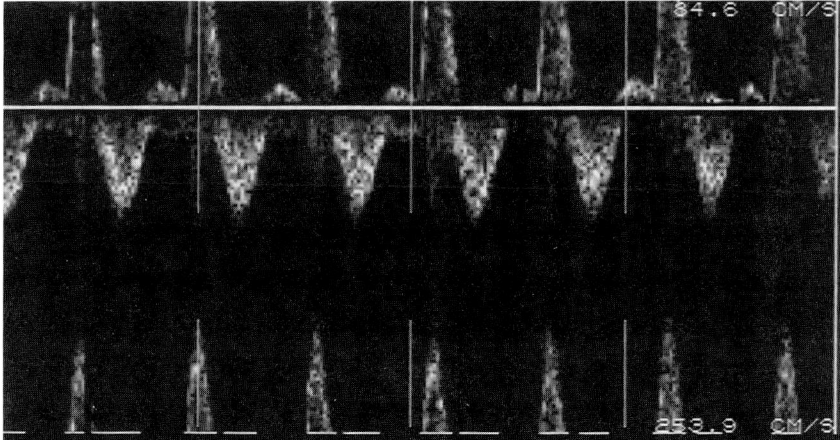

Figure 1-3   Spectral aliasing demonstrated in an iliac artery. The "wraparound" effect of the spectral tracing is due to a sampling frequency that is greater than half the pulse repetition frequency (PRF) and is called the *Nyquist limit.*

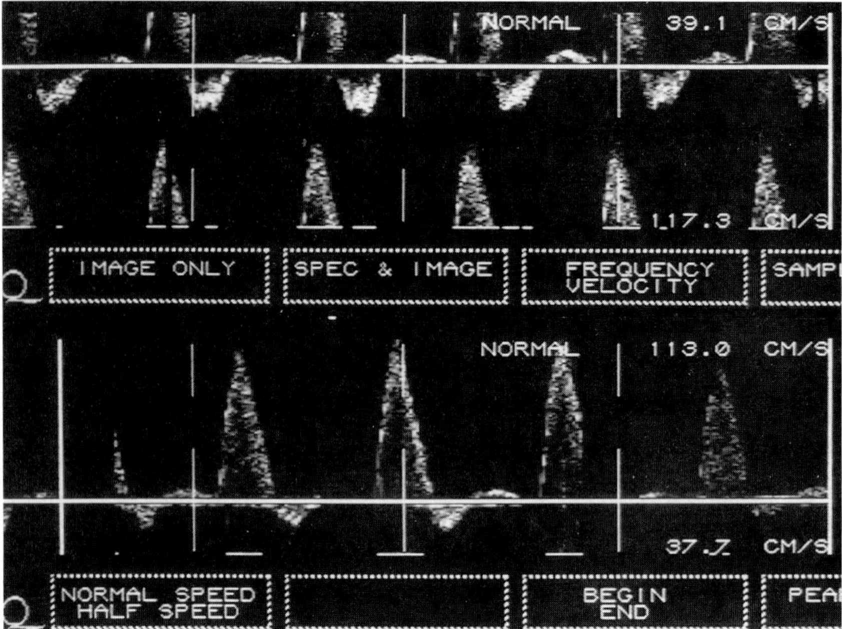

Figure 1-4 An aliased Doppler shift can be corrected either by changing the Doppler scale (increasing the PRF) or by changing the baseline to include a wider frequency range for either positive (above the baseline) or negative signals (below the baseline). Thus, with a high velocity producing an aliased signal, the baseline can be moved down so that most of the available frequency range will be assigned to the positive signal with a high-peak velocity.

an aliased Doppler-shifted frequency. One is to increase the PRF by adjusting the Doppler scale until a normal spectral signal is obtained. The PRF can also be increased by decreasing the field of view or changing the baseline (Fig. 1-4). Other methods are the decrease of the Doppler shift frequency by scanning at an angle closer to 90° or by changing to a transducer with a lower frequency.

Gain Setting

The gain setting is also of great importance when Doppler ultrasonography is performed. With a low gain setting valuable information may be lost, as low flow will not be picked up. Too high a gain setting will degrade the spectral display, as high spikes of noise will project across the tracing (Fig. 1-5).

Mirror Image Artifacts

Another important source of error are the mirror-image artifacts. In the same fashion an optical mirror produces duplication of a visible object, a completely reflected sound wave will produce an acoustic mirror image. This phenomenon

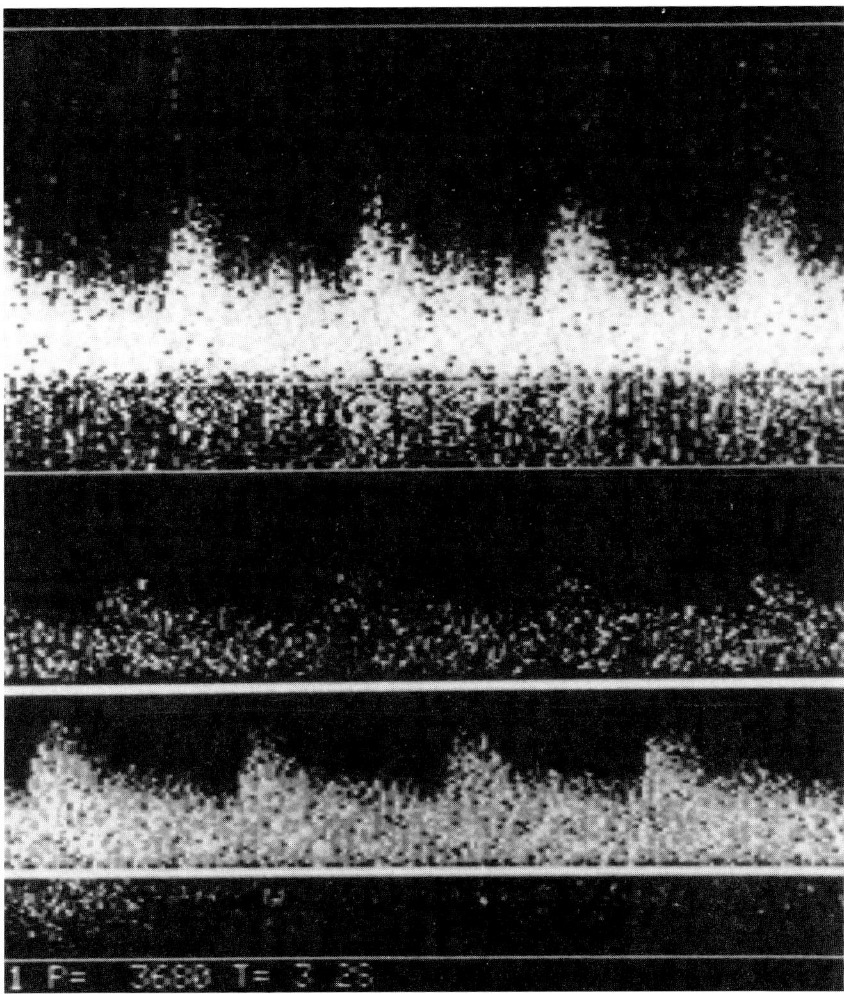

Figure 1-5   Example of a spectral image displayed with too high a gain setting (*top*), low gain setting (*center*), and optimal gain setting for display of whole range of frequencies without noise (*bottom*).

is of utmost importance with the employment of color Doppler imaging and is discussed in Chap. 2.

The Uncertainty Principle

An additional issue to be addressed is the uncertainty principle. It is well known that axial resolution is improved with a shorter ultrasound pulse or a broad-banded pulse. On the other hand, it is also known that the best frequency resolution is obtained with continuous wave sampling, which is a narrow-banded transmission. For practical purposes this implies that if better velocity information is sought, the ability to localize the target is reduced. For this reason, continuous wave systems provide better velocity information but without depth resolution.

ANALYSIS OF DOPPLER WAVEFORMS

The relationship between the variables of the spectral waveform and the velocity of blood flow depends on several factors. The first factor is often referred to as *broadening of the spectrum caused by multiple velocities passing through the beam width*. The effects of these multiple velocities are similar to those of the introduction of additional frequencies above and below the main Doppler shift frequency, or simply a wider spread of frequencies. This causes a conflict between the wish to localize the target by narrowing the beam and causing broadening of the spectrum and the wish to analyze the velocity by narrowing the spectrum.

With a short sample volume employed in duplex Doppler, a large spectral broadening is often found. The spectral waveform will not enable us to determine whether the broadening is a result of an artifact caused by the time broadening phenomena or a result of many scatterers moving at different velocities. This affects the ability of the pulsed Doppler system to measure flow velocity with good axial resolution.

A second factor is the form of the acoustic beam, which has an important influence on the flow-velocity waveform. If the sample volume is smaller than the vessel being studied, the flow-velocity waveform will change according to the velocity of the flow passing the sample volume. As is well established, the beam of the transmitted ultrasound pulse is not uniform, and in most cases flow elements will not contribute equally to the spectral signal.

The final Doppler signal displayed on the monitor is a waveform produced by and representing the Doppler shifts created by circulating red cells during a cardiac cycle. Those Doppler signals producing a shift toward the transducer will be displayed as an upward displacement of the baseline on the monitor, and those signals producing a shift away from the transducer will be displayed as a downward shift from baseline. While it is not possible to accurately measure velocity and volume of blood flow for reasons already discussed, it is possible to analyze these waveforms to determine resistance to blood flow in vessels. This forms the basis of Doppler velocimetry in perinatal medicine and estimation of resistance to flow within a given vessel of the uteroplacental and fetal circulation. The estimation of blood flow and resistance has clinical implications and has been studied extensively.

There are several methods for analysis of waveforms and estimation of resistance to flow, all dependent on a pulsatile blood flow. The most commonly used include the systolic-diastolic ratio (S/D), the resistance index (RI), and the pulsatility index (PI) (Fig. 1-6). They are all based on the ratio of systolic to

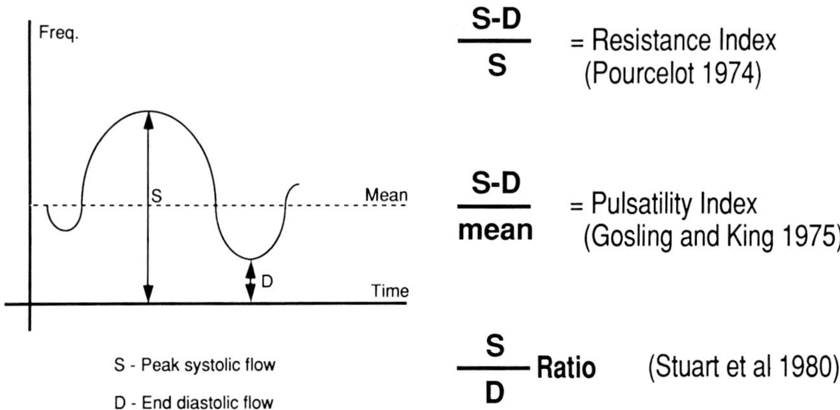

Figure 1-6 Qualitative methods for waveform analysis.

diastolic flow as measured by the amplitude of the Doppler shift. The shape of the curve is relative to the incident angle of the ultrasonic beam with best waveforms being obtained at small incident angles. The waveforms are peaked in shape. As the incident angle approaches 90°, or perpendicular to the study vessel, the waveform is progressively rounded. At 90° no Doppler shift occurs and no waveform is produced.

The S/D ratio is the easiest method of resistance calculation and was described by Stuart et al.[21] The ratio is obtained by measuring the peak systolic and end-diastolic shifts. Normally the ratio is determined over a number of cardiac cycles. Numerous studies have shown that the S/D ratio decreases toward term, indicating decreased downstream resistance to flow with subsequent increased diastolic flow in normal human gestation.

The PI was developed by Gosling and King[22] and describes a method of resistance estimation involving the measure of entire waveforms and relating peak systolic and end-diastolic shift to the mean Doppler shift (Fig. 1-6). The RI was first described by Pourcelot[23] and is another method of resistance estimation that is calculated by taking the systolic minus the diastolic shift divided by the systolic. Both the PI and RI, as well as the S/D ratio, measure the pulsatility of flow and are independent of the incident angle. Campbell et al.[24] reported the technique called the *frequency index profile,* based on normalization of the entire waveform. Other techniques for waveform analysis have been described by Maulik et al.[25] and Thompson et al.,[26] but they do not seem to have any advantages over the simple Doppler ratios that have been extensively employed in the evaluation of maternal and fetal hemodynamics.

In normal pregnancy, as mentioned earlier, resistance to flow decreases in the uteroplacental-umbilical circulation as gestational age increases. The fetal circulation is unique in that forward flow of blood is maintained during the whole cycle, including diastole. Forward diastolic flow increases with gestational age. Estimation of this flow has important diagnostic and prognostic implications in perinatal medicine. The changes in flow are reflected in the decrease of the Doppler indices: S/D, RI, PI.

These ratios can be affected by fetal breathing,[27–29] fetal heart rate abnormalities,[29–31] and fetal movements,[27,32] limiting their usefulness in those situations. In general, the peak systolic shift will be quite variable in periods of fetal breathing activity, and the ratios should not be measured at this time. Diastolic flow when preserved during fetal breathing can be interpreted as a reassuring sign. The S/D ratio, PI, and RI should be measured in periods of fetal apnea.

Fetal arrhythmias cause alteration of the diastolic filling time of the ventricles and therefore will affect the Doppler waveform.[30,31] In fetal bradycardia, the entire cardiac cycle is lengthened, and the diastolic filling time is increased. This reduces the amplitude of the Doppler shift produced during this time. The contractility of the heart is unchanged, and the peak systolic Doppler shift also remains unchanged. The resulting S/D ratio, PI, and RI will be elevated in these cases[30] (Fig. 1-7).

In fetal tachyarrhythmias the opposite occurs with decreased diastolic filling time and, therefore, increased Doppler shift at end-diastole. In these cases, with the systolic shift (contractility) maintained, the Doppler indices will be decreased. There have been some studies which show that these indices vary at different positions along the umbilical cord, which may indicate differential resistance to flow within the cord itself.

Detailed description of the uses and interpretation of Doppler signals, especially color flow signals, are presented in subsequent chapters.

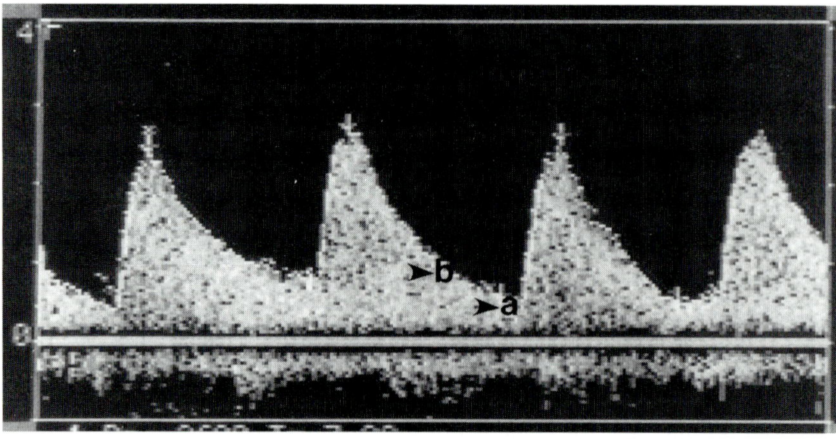

Figure 1-7 A spectral waveform obtained during fetal bradycardia. At point *a* the end-diastolic velocity is low and the calculated indices will be high. At a faster heart rate, the new cycle will start at point *b*, the end-diastolic velocity is higher, and the indices will be lower.

REFERENCES

1. Christensen EE, Curry TS, Dowdey JE: *An Introduction to the Physics of Diagnostic Radiology,* 2d ed. Philadelphia, Lea and Febiger, 1978.

2. Maulik D: Basic principles of Doppler ultrasound as applied in Obstetrics. Clin Obstet Gynecol 32:628–644, 1989.

3. Curie J, Curie P: Development par pression de l'electricite polaire des cristaux hemiedres a faces inclinees. CR Acad Sci Paris 93:1137, 1880.

4. Wells PNT: *The Physical Principles of Ultrasonic Diagnostics.* London, Academic Press, 1969.

5. Doppler CJ: Uber das farbige licht der Doppelsterne und einiger anderer Gestirne des Himmels. Abhandlungen d. Konigl. Bohmischen Gesellshaft der Wissenschaften U. Folge bd. 2, 1842.

6. Buys-Ballot CHD: Akustische versuche auf der Niederlandischen Eisenbahn nebst gelegentlichen Bemerkungen zur Theorie des Hrn. Prof. Doppler. Poggendorf Annalen B. 66:321–351, 1843.

7. Burne PN: The physical principles of Doppler and spectral analysis. J Clin Ultrasound 15:567–590, 1987.

8. Sigelmann RA, Reid JM: Analysis and measurement of ultrasound backscattering from an ensemble of scatters excited by sine-wave bursts. J Acoust Soc Am 53:1351–1355, 1973.

9. Shung KK, Siegelman RA, Reid JM: Scattering of ultrasound by blood. IEEE Trans Biomed Engl 23:460, 1976.

10. Atkinson P, Berry MV: Random noise in ultrasonic echoes diffracted by blood. J Phys A 11:1293–1301, 1974.

11. Gill RW: Measurements of blood flow by ultrasound: accuracy and source of error. Ultrasound Med Biol 11:625–641, 1985.

12. Burns PN: "Doppler flow estimations in the fetal and maternal circulation: principles, techniques and some limitations," in Maulik D, McNellis D (eds), *Doppler Ultrasound Measurements of Maternal-Fetal Hemodynamics.* Ithaca N.Y., Perinatology Press, 1987.

13. Eik-Nes SH, Marsal K, Kristoffersen K: Methodology and basic problems in blood flow studies in human fetus. Ultrasound Med Biol 10:329–337, 1984.

14. Griffin DR, Taegue MJ, Tallet P, Willson K, Bilardo C, Massini L, Campbell S: A combined ultrasonic linear array scanner and pulsed Doppler velocimeter for the estimation of blood flow in the fetus and adult abdomen II: clinical evaluation. Ultrasound Med Biol 11:37–41, 1985.

15. Erskine RLA, Ritchie JWK: Quantitative measurement of fetal blood flow using Doppler ultrasound. Br J Obstet Gynaecol 92:600–605, 1985.

16. Skidmore R, Follet DH: Maximum frequency follower for the processing of ultrasonic Doppler shift signals. Ultrasound Med Biol 4:145–147, 1978.

17. Saini VD, Maulik D, Nanda NC, Rosenzweig MS: Computerized processing of Doppler signals for blood flow measurements. Ultrasound Med Biol 9:657–660, 1983.

18. Cooley JW, Tukey JW: An algorithm for the machine calculation of complex Fourier series. Math Comp 19:297, 1985.

19. Kierney CMP, Zimmerman III GH: "Approaches to Doppler velocity signal analysis," in Maulik D, McNellis D (eds), *Doppler Ultrasound Measurement of Maternal-Fetal Hemodynamics.* Ithaca, N.Y., Perinatology Press, 1987.

20. Taegue MJ, Willson K, Battye CK et al.: A combined ultrasonic linear array scanner and pulsed Doppler velocimeter for the estimation of blood flow in the foetus and adult abdomen I: technical aspects. Ultrasound Med Biol 2:27–36, 1976.

21. Stuart B, Drumm J, Fitzgerald DE, Dugnan VM: Fetal blood velocity waveform in normal pregnancy. Br J Obstet Gynaecol 87:780–785, 1980.

22. Gosling RG, King DH: "Ultrasound angiology," in Macus AW, Adamson J (eds), *Arteries and Veins.* Edinburgh, Churchill-Livingstone, 1975.

23. Pourcelot L: "Applications clinique de l'exame Doppler transcutane," in Pourcelot L (ed), *Velocimetric Ultrasonaire Doppler.* Paris, INSERM, 1974, pp 213–240.

24. Campbell S, Griffin DR, Pearce JM, Diaz-Recasans J, Cohen-Overbeek TE, Willson K, Teague

MJ: New Doppler technique for assessing uteroplacental blood flow. Lancet 1:675–677, 1983.

25. Maulik D, Saini VD, Nanda NC, Rosenzweig MS: Doppler evaluation of fetal hemodynamics. Ultrasound Med Biol 8:705–710, 1982.

26. Thompson RS, Trudinger BJ, Cook CM: Doppler ultrasound waveforms in the fetal umbilical artery: quantitative analysis technique. Ultrasound Med Biol 11:707–718, 1985.

27. Arabin B: *Doppler Blood Flow Measurements in Uteroplacental and Fetal Vessels. Pathophysiological and Clinical Significance.* Berlin, Springer-Verlag, 1990.

28. Eik-Nes SH, Marsal K, Brubaak AM, Ulstein M: Ultrasonic measurements of human fetal blood flow in aorta and umbilical vein: influence of fetal breathing movements. Adv Ultrasound 2:233, 1982.

29. Indik JH, Reed KL: Variation and correlation in human fetal umbilical Doppler velocities with fetal breathing: evidence of the cardiac-placental connection. Am J Obstet Gynecol 163:1792–1796, 1990.

30. Yarlagadda P, Willoughly L, Maulik D: Effect of fetal heart rate on umbilical arterial Doppler indices. J Ultrasound Med 8:215–218, 1989.

31. Reed KL, Sahn DJ, Marx GR, Anderson CF, Shenker L: Cardiac Doppler flows during fetal arrhythmias: physiologic consequences. Obstet Gynecol 70:1–6, 1987.

32. van Eyck J, Wladimiroff JW, Wijngard JAGW, van der Noordam MJ, Prechtl HFR: The blood flow velocity in the fetal descending aorta: its relationship to fetal behavioral states in normal pregnancy at 37–38 weeks gestation. Early Hum Dev 12:137–143, 1985.

COLOR DOPPLER IMAGING— A NEW INTERPRETATION OF THE DOPPLER EFFECT

RICHARD JAFFE

Two-dimensional echocardiography and Doppler techniques have been invaluable in the field of noninvasive clinical cardiology.[1-5] These techniques have made it possible to detect shunts, septal defects, vessel patency, and flow abnormalities in structural heart disease. Although Doppler ultrasonography has been available for over two decades, its clinical use has been restricted almost solely to the study of the heart and major vessels and only recently have other applications emerged. The principal reason for the slow incorporation of Doppler ultrasonography into clinical areas other than cardiology is that there are several limitations to the conventional pulsed Doppler technique. The main limitation is that in conventional Doppler systems flow information is obtained only along the path of the beam with continuous wave Doppler and from a single area, or "gate," if pulsed Doppler is used. In both cases Doppler signals are sampled only from a restricted area, and flow cannot be evaluated over the whole ultrasonic image. The second limitation is that with conventional two-dimensional ultrasonography and Doppler techniques, it is often impossible to establish direction of flow and angle between beam and sampled vessel, both important parameters in the calculation of flow (Chap. 1). These two limitations make the process of obtaining maximum information a time-consuming task, and the sonographer must be highly skilled and motivated to search multiple sample volume positions within each plane to detect disturbances of flow. Another problem with conventional Doppler techniques is that we do not get instantaneous "right-wrong" feedback. If during scanning any unwanted effect disturbs the picture, the plane of scanning or machine setting has to be changed to receive an improved image.

Growing interest in the use of Doppler ultrasonography for abdominal, obstetrical, gynecological, and neonatal applications has enhanced the development of a new technique that overcomes the limitations of conventional Doppler ultrasonography. This technique allows evaluation of flow characteristics over selected areas of the image with simultaneous real-time two-dimensional ultrasonography of the vessels and surrounding tissue. The technique that has been developed is based on converting detected frequency shifts to color based on direction of flow, turbulence, and flow velocity.

This new technique has been primarily used in clinical cardiology and is described by a variety of terms such as *color Doppler imaging* (CDI), *Doppler color flow mapping* (DCFM), *Doppler angiography, color-coded Doppler,* and *angiodynography.*[6,7] With conventional Doppler, information received from a vessel may be displayed as an audible signal or as a graph of blood velocity versus time. With CDI we get diagnostic information from spatial representation of flow within the selected area of the image itself.

COLOR GENERATION

The process of generating color Doppler images occurs in two phases. In phase one we acquire echo-amplitude signals from the ultrasound beam and process them to conventional B-mode two-dimensional gray scale images. In the second, color Doppler phase, multiple ultrasound beams are processed to estimate blood flow velocity in each sample volume.[8] The echoes that return from red blood cells during this phase are analyzed for frequency, phase, and amplitude, and simultaneously fed into the memory and a color convertor. Analysis of a large number of sample volumes gives estimates of direction of flow, mean velocity, and variance (turbulence), which will be coded into appropriate colors for display in a color image.[9]

The signals obtained from nonmoving perivascular tissue are very large and can inhibit the detection of the weaker Doppler signals from the moving red blood cells. As the transmitted signal in most systems is broad-banded (multiple frequencies), the backscattered signal from the nonmoving tissue is frequency shifted from the original signal. This interference is avoided by the autocorrelation detector or moving target indicator.[10] As the name implies, the process is the subtraction of all nonmoving components from the received signal and calculation of the frequency shift by comparing the phase difference between successive measurements of the Doppler-shifted spectrum. The final signal displayed will consist only of shifts generated by moving red cells, whereas in case there are no moving structures giving rise to echoes, the autocorrelator output will be 0.

The estimation of frequency in CDI improves with increasing number of samples, although this increases sampling time, and adversely affects the frame rate and resolution. As frequency sampling in CDI has to be minimized to maintain an acceptable frame rate for real-time imaging, adjustments have to be made in the imaging process. One possibility is to decrease the field of color Doppler sampling. By reducing the field, the sampling time decreases and the frame rate is increased.

COLOR VELOCITY IMAGING

As already outlined in this chapter, the basis for color generation is the acquisition of frequency shifts from the moving red blood cells. The Doppler equation is used to calculate the velocity (Chap. 1), which is assigned a color displayed at the appropriate point on the ultrasound image. The main source of inaccuracy with this technique is occurrence of fluctuations in both transmitted and received frequencies, whereas the Doppler equation assumes a single, constant frequency. With CDI there is a compromise between the color accuracy and the gray-scale resolution, known as the uncertainty principle and explained in Chap. 1.

To try to overcome these limitations, a new technique, called *color velocity imaging* (CVI), was proposed.[11] This technique measures velocities directly, employing the time-domain process, and is independent of the frequency shift. Color velocity imaging is based on the recording of the distance red blood cells move in a given time and the calculation of the velocity from the equation: $v = d/t$, where v = velocity, d = the distance the red blood cell has traveled, and t = time between two ultrasound pulses in microseconds. With CVI the uncertainty principle does not exist. Color velocity imaging uses the same obtained information for gray-scale and color imaging, fewer samples per line are needed, and the gray-scale resolution is not adversely affected. Color velocity imaging may therefore improve the color profile and give more information on the velocity spectrum across the investigated vessel.

The clinical potentials of CVI have to be evaluated, bearing in mind the fact that this technique provides a more accurate velocity profile without compromising the gray-scale resolution.

COLOR ASSIGNMENT

In color Doppler imaging, the choice of color is determined by the direction of flow relative to the transducer. In most commercially available systems, flow toward the transducer is coded red and flow away from the transducer is coded blue. This coding is arbitrary and can be changed on most equipment to the operator's preference (Fig. 2-1). The degree of turbulence is estimated and coded as the amount of green mixed with red and blue.[9] Color shading is another important factor in the interpretation of the color image. Color shading is determined by the frequency shift with higher shifts coded in lighter shades and lower shifts coded in darker shades (Fig. 2-2).

Even though the mean frequency shift can be determined from different

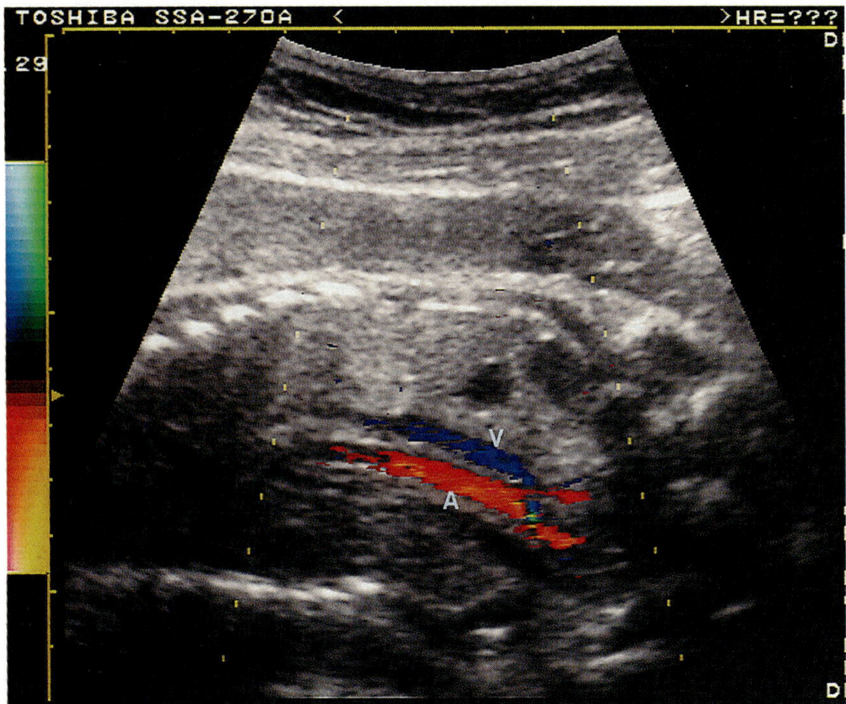

Figure 2-1 Change of color assignment. Flow in the aorta (A) is directed away from the transducer and will appear red, whereas flow in the vena cava (V) is toward the transducer and will appear blue.

portions of the vessel, the maximum Doppler shift can be calculated only by analysis of the flow-velocity waveform. The color shading is also related to the angle of the transmitted beam. As already described in Chap. 1, the frequency shift decreases as the angle of insonation increases. Therefore the color shading will be darker as the angle of insonation approaches 90° and lighter as it approaches 0°.

The angle to flow is crucial in interpreting color Doppler images with sector transducers. Positioning the transducer just above the vessel makes the color displayed go from red to blue, as the direction of flow relative to the transducer changes, with a small black area at the point where the beam insonates the vessel at a 90° angle (Fig. 2-3). This phenomenon is caused by the fact that at the center the calculated flow is zero as cos 90° = 0, making the equation $F_d = (2F_t \times \cos \Theta \times v)/c = 0$ (Fig. 1-1). When a sector transducer is used, we must be aware of the angle of flow at all times not to wrongly interpret the information displayed.[12]

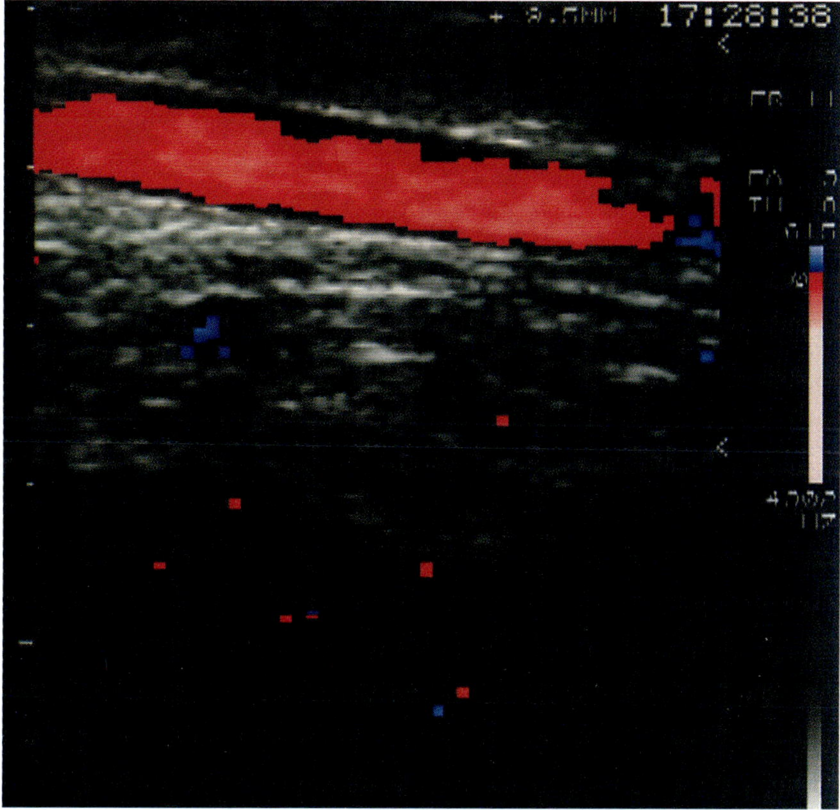

Figure 2-2   Color Doppler image of the carotid artery showing lighter shades in the central part of the vessel. The lighter shades represent higher peak velocities in the middle of the stream.

OPERATIONAL CONSIDERATIONS

Before beginning color Doppler imaging studies, several operational parameters have to be adjusted.[9,11]

Transducer Frequency

The first operational parameter to be considered is the *choice of the transducer frequency*. The Doppler equation clearly shows that the Doppler shift is directly proportional to the transmitted frequency. As higher frequencies have less depth penetration, there has to be a compromise between Doppler shift frequency and depth resolution. The choice of transducer frequency has to be made according to the opacification obtained of the vessel being studied.

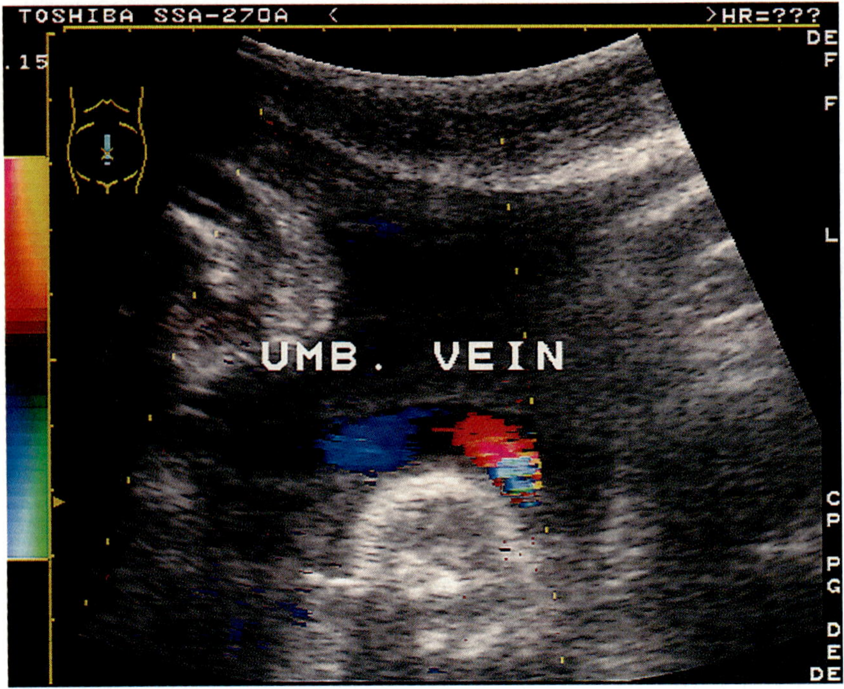

Figure 2-3 Color Doppler imaging of the umbilical vein employing a sector transducer. The change in direction of flow relative to the transducer is clearly demonstrated by the change of color in the same vessel. At the point where the ultrasound beam is insonating at an angle of 90°, there is no Doppler shift and there will be no display of color.

Gain Setting

Flow sensitivity is adjusted by appropriate *gain setting*. Low color gain setting will result in decreased detection of slow flow. The maximum sensitivity is obtained when the color occupies the total anteroposterior diameter of the vessel and there is no color noise from perivascular tissues. Gain settings that are too high will result in images clustered with a snowstorm pattern of color (Fig. 2-4).

Pulse Repetition Frequency

Pulse repetition frequency (PRF) plays an important role in the sensitivity of the color Doppler system. Decreasing the PRF, by decreasing the Doppler scale, will improve sensitivity and better detect slow flow. Changes in PRF will also affect the shading of the colors in the vessel examined. With a decrease in the Doppler scale, higher velocities will be shaded lighter as their frequency will be positioned in the higher part of the scale.

As previously described, the decrease of the field of view will result in a

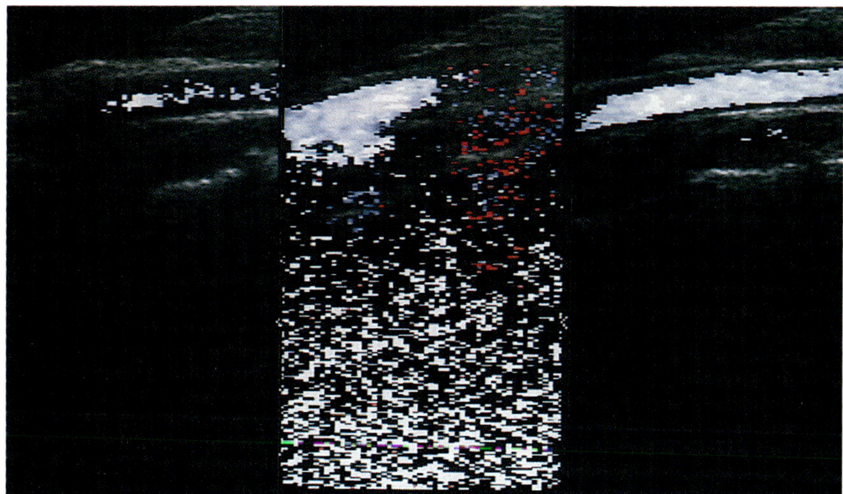

Figure 2-4   Color gain setting is important to enable correct evaluation of signals obtained from a vessel. If the gain setting is too low, important information will be lost (*left*); too high a gain setting will produce an image clustered with a snowstorm pattern (*center*); and maximum sensitivity will be obtained when the color fills the anteroposterior diameter of the vessel (*right*).

decreased time spent on sampling, and consequently the PRF will increase. This will cause an increase in the Doppler scale and darker shades of the displayed colors.

Motion Discrimination

Motion discrimination capability is an important factor in the sensitivity of a color Doppler system. Transmitted respiratory and cardiac motions exist in most parts of the body as well as soft-tissue vibration caused by speech and movements related to bowel peristalsis. These aberrant tissue motions generate frequency shifts that are usually displayed as flashes of color[12] (Fig. 2-5A and *B*), and they have to be differentiated from blood flow. The color artifacts produced by these motions are usually not centered around the vessel, and they are not related to the cardiac cycle.

Velocity filters (wall-motion or thump filters) that minimize flash artifacts also filter out low blood flow velocities, thus reducing the sensitivity of the system. To overcome this problem it is necessary to discriminate moving red blood cells from moving tissue so that valuable information is not lost in the process of filtering out artifacts. This can be achieved by a color/gray-scale priority function that determines the gray-scale echo that will override the color pixel, thus suppressing all color information.

ARTIFACTS AND PITFALLS

As spectral Doppler and CDI are based on the same principles, we can expect the same artifacts described with the use of duplex Doppler to occur with CDI. Even so, there are understandable differences in the appearance of some artifacts with CDI, and they are discussed here.[8,9,12,13]

Angle of Insonation

The importance of the angle of insonation in Doppler ultrasonography has already been explained. In CDI the angle is very important in the determination of direction of flow. The artifact most commonly encountered is the mixture of red and blue within the vessel. This is caused by an insonation angle of close to 90°, where flow will be displayed above and below the baseline in duplex Doppler and as a mixture of colors in CDI. With this display we will have a directional ambiguity, and the transducer has to be angulated to avoid an insonation angle of 90° (Fig. 2-6).[9]

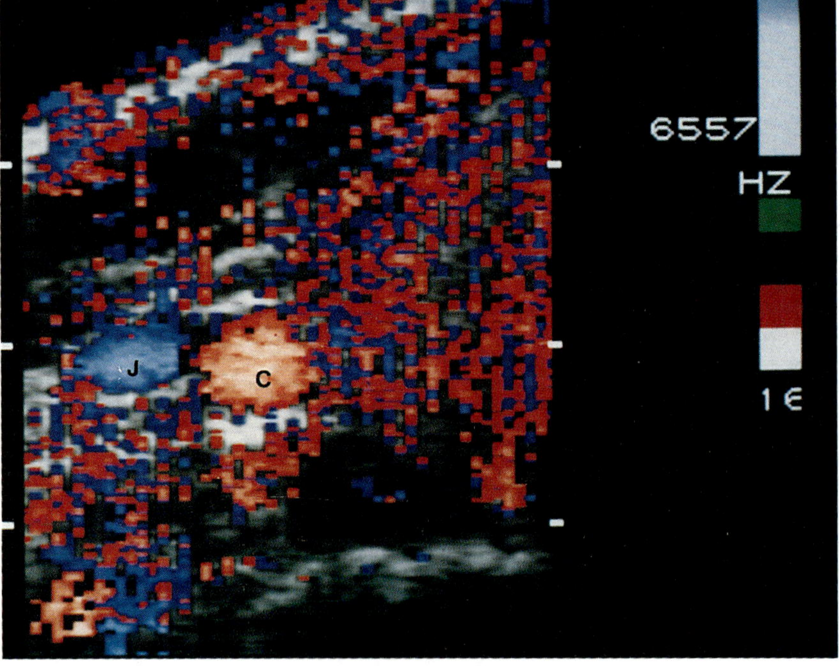

A

Figure 2-5 *A*. Laryngeal vibration transmitted to soft tissue of the neck. During phonation, tissue vibrations result in extravascular assignment of mixed red and blue that is not perivascular in location and does not vary with the cardiac cycle. C = carotid artery; J = jugular vein. *(Printed with permission from Middleton WD, Erickson S, Melson GL: Perivascular color artifact: pathologic significance and appearance on color Doppler US images. Radiology 171:647–652, 1989.)*

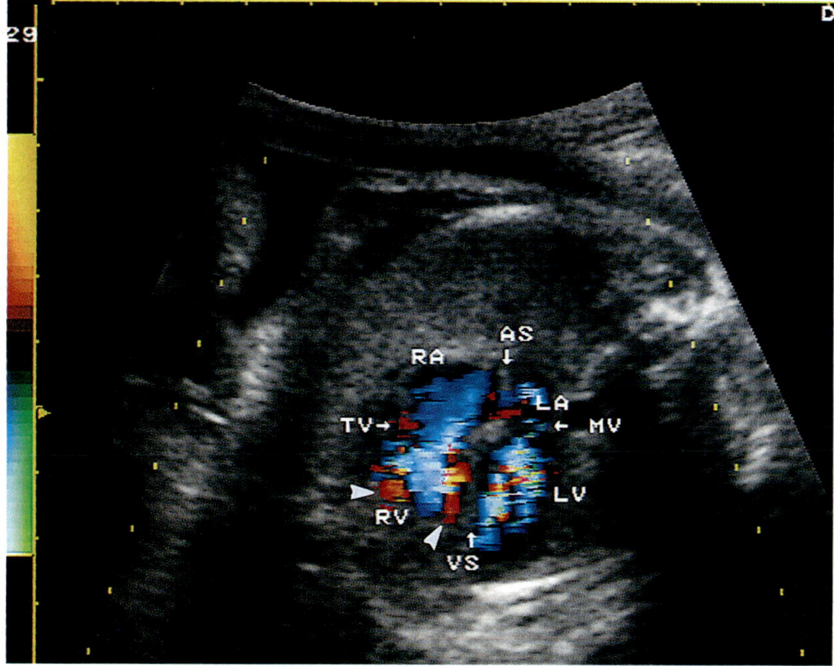

B

Figure 2-5 (*Continued*) *B*. A four-chamber view of the heart with superimposed color imaging. Image taken during diastole with flow going from atria to ventricles. Motion of ventricular walls is clearly identified (*arrowheads*) and assigned a mixture of red and blue. RA = right atrium; LA = left atrium; AS = atrial septum; TV = tricuspid valve; MV = mitral valve; RV = right ventricle; LV = left ventricle; VS = ventricular septum.

Aliasing

Aliasing was described in detail in Chap. 1. With CDI the shading of the assigned color becomes lighter as the frequency shift increases. When the Nyquist limit is exceeded, the color assignment is folded over into the opposite color and we get a light blue color in the center of a vessel displayed in red. As with spectral Doppler, this can be avoided by increasing the PRF by adjusting the Doppler scale (Fig. 2-7) and by decreasing the baseline (Figs. 2-7 and 2-8) or field of view. Other methods are repositioning of the transducer so the angle of insonation approaches 90° or choosing a transducer with a lower frequency. It is important to notice that in the presence of color aliasing there is no black stripe between the opposite colors, the stripe seen when direction of motion changes in relation to the transducer (Fig. 2-3).[9]

Wall Motions

When flow turbulence is present in a vessel, the vessel walls often vibrate. These movements of the vessel wall and surrounding tissue produce frequency shifts,

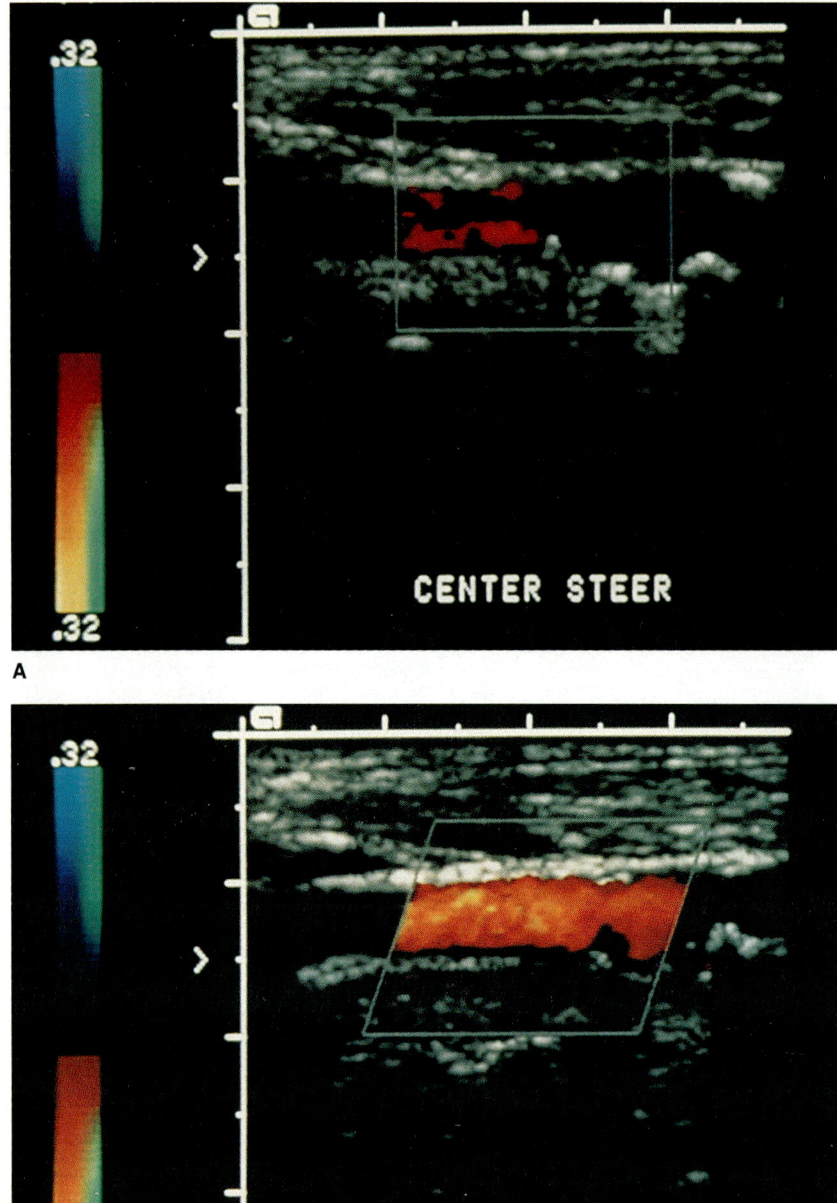

Figure 2-6 With the angle of insonation being close to 90°, the frequency shifts obtained are very low (*A*) and the direction of flow is difficult to determine. When the transducer is angled, the frequency shifts increase, color signals are stronger, and direction of flow can be determined (*B*). (*Courtesy of Acuson Ltd., Mountain View, California.*)

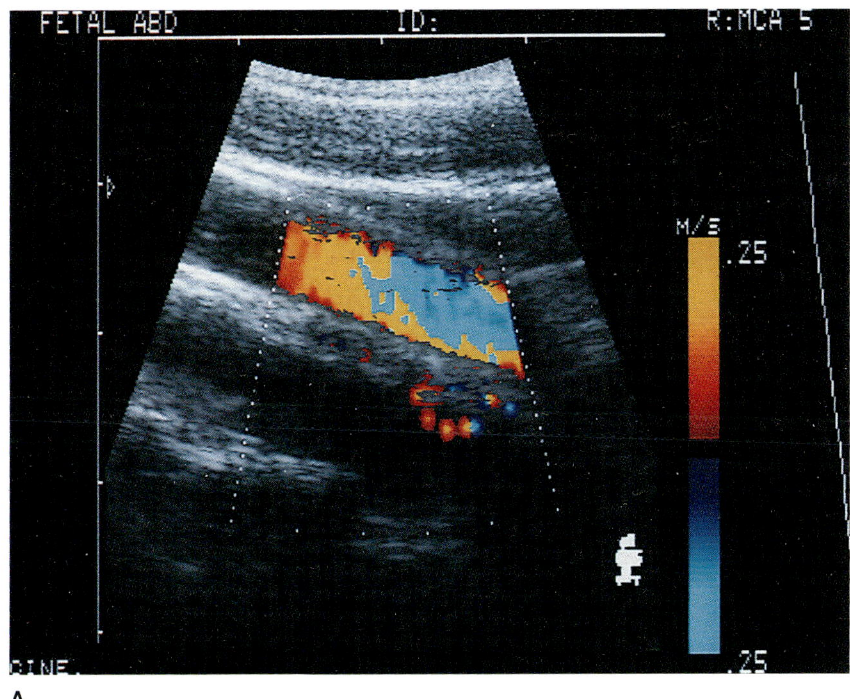

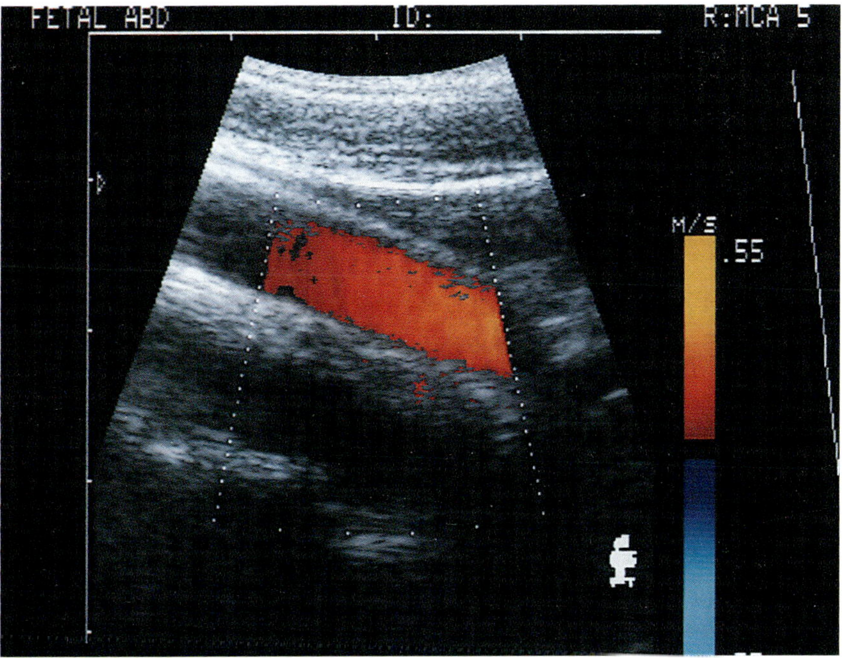

Figure 2-7   Color aliasing displayed as light shades of blue appearing in the center of a vessel with flow displayed in red (*A*). The aliasing is corrected by changing the Doppler scale (increasing the PRF) (*B*) or by moving the baseline (*C*). *(Courtesy of General Electric, Milwaukee, Wisconsin.)*

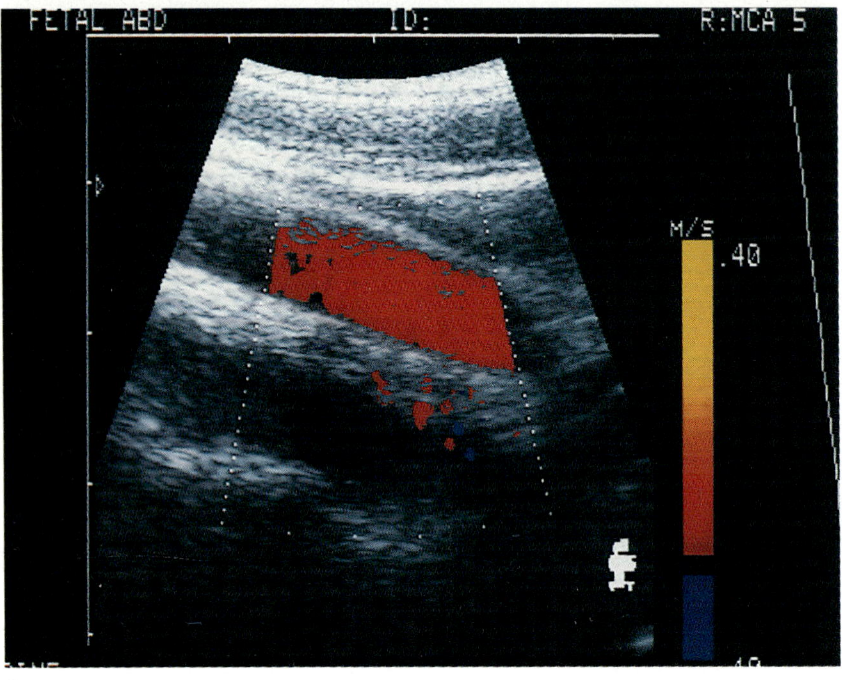

C

Figure 2-7 (*Continued*)

and they will be assigned a color[12] (Fig. 2-9). These vibrations are directed both toward and away from the transducer, and we will get a mixture of red and blue with CDI and artificial pulsatility in the spectral Doppler waveform. In contrast to color artifacts produced by moving tissue, this artifact varies with the cardiac cycle and rate of flow. This artifact can be ignored if it is properly recognized or avoided if sensitivity gain or angle are changed.

Mirror Artifacts

Mirror artifacts were mentioned in Chap. 1 but are potentially more likely to be recognized with CDI. As this phenomenon occurs with complete reflection of sound, it is usually detected in regions close to the lungs, as gas reflects close to 100 percent of sound. This phenomenon will thus occur mostly in the sub-diaphragmatic and subclavicular regions[13] (Fig. 2-10).

Color Flashes

While performing CDI, flashes of color are often observed. It has to be remembered that the frequency shift derived from the Doppler equation is not limited

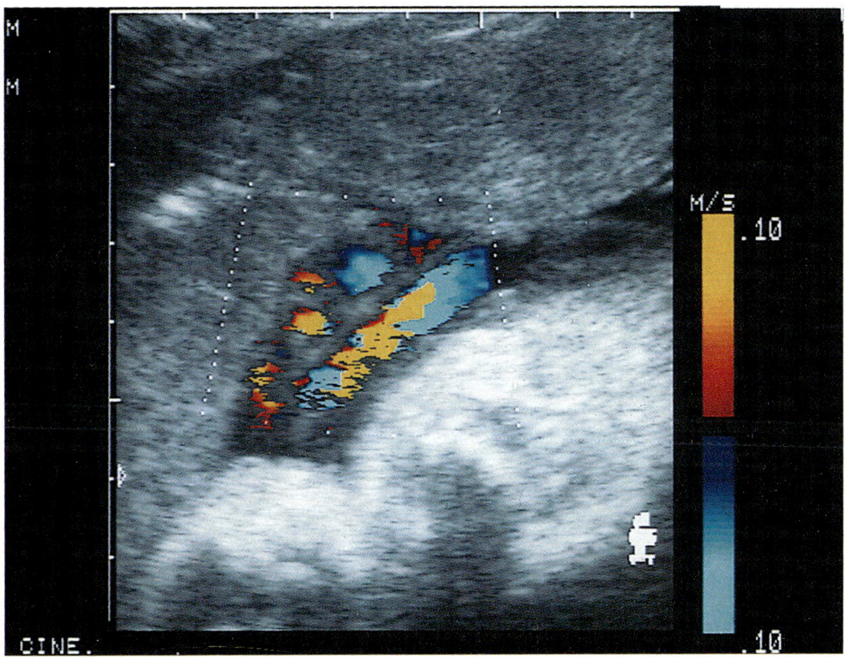

A

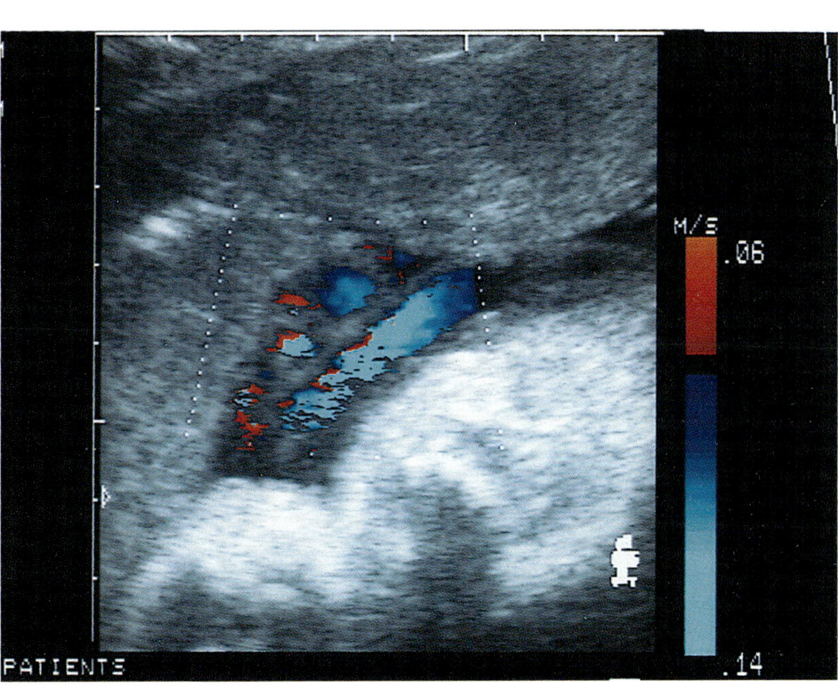

B

Figure 2-8 An umbilical vessel demonstrating aliasing (*A*) that is corrected by change of baseline (*B*).

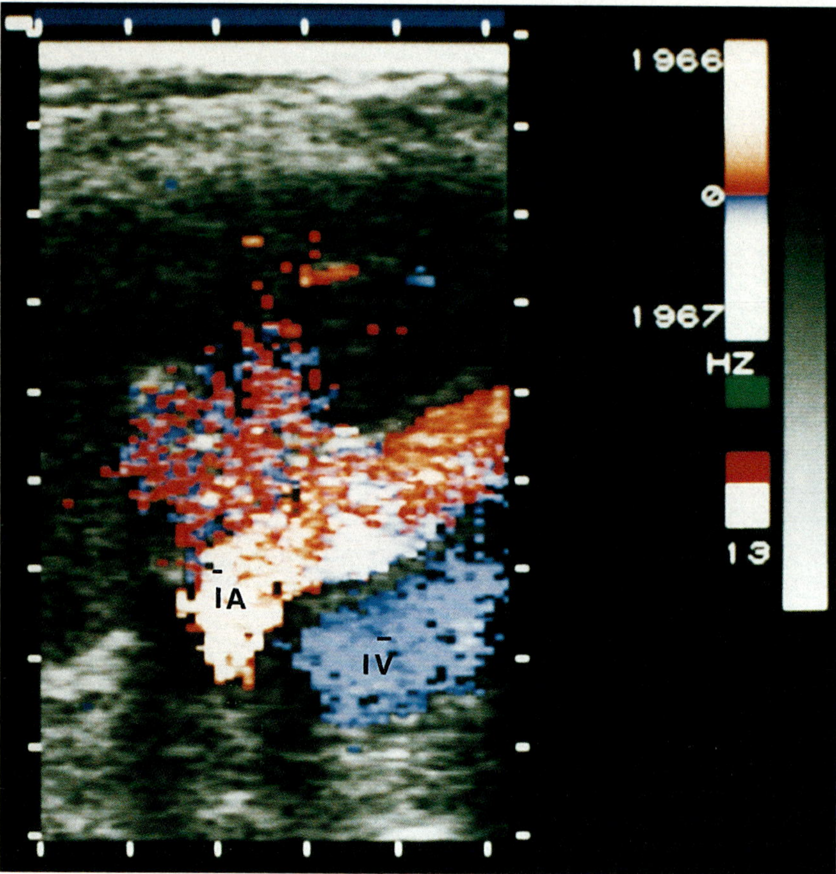

Figure 2-9 Stenosis of main renal artery after renal transplantation. Longitudinal color Doppler image shows perivascular color artifact in the region of the origin of the donor renal artery. Iliac artery (IA) and iliac vein (IV) are deep to the renal transplant. *(Printed with permission from Middleton WD, Erickson S, Melson GL: Perivascular color artifact: pathologic significance and appearance on color Doppler US images. Radiology 171:647–652, 1989.)*

to moving red blood cells but can be generated by any movement of other fluids or soft tissue. With the movement of the transducer, any fluid can be set into motion and subsequently produce color flashes on the screen. This phenomenon can clearly be seen in the bladder at the outflow from the ureters (Fig. 2-11), in the fetal nose or mouth as amniotic fluid is swallowed or expelled (Fig. 2-12), or in any cystic structure containing moving fluid.

COLOR IMAGING

Color Doppler sensitivity is based on the ability of the system to obtain maximum blood flow information from ultrasound echoes and display it with correct an-

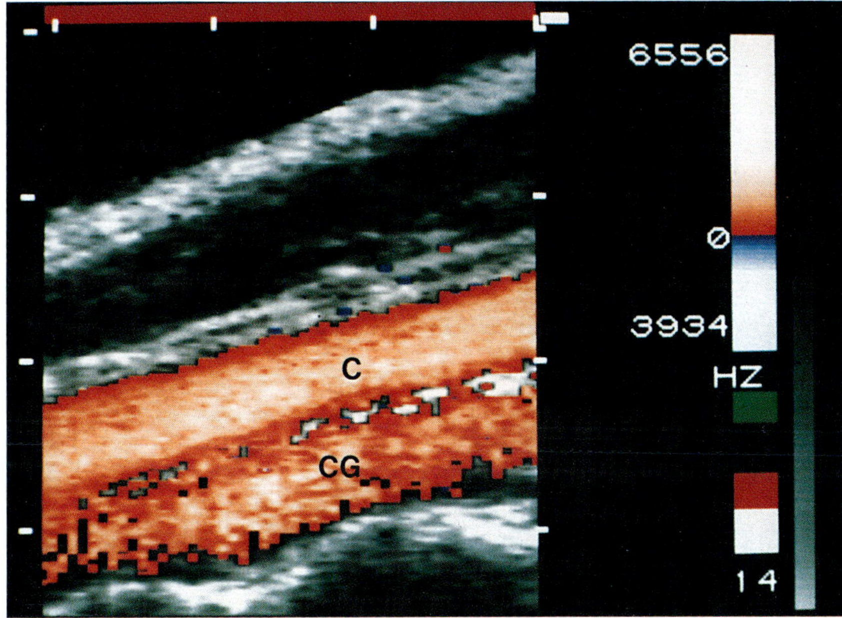

A

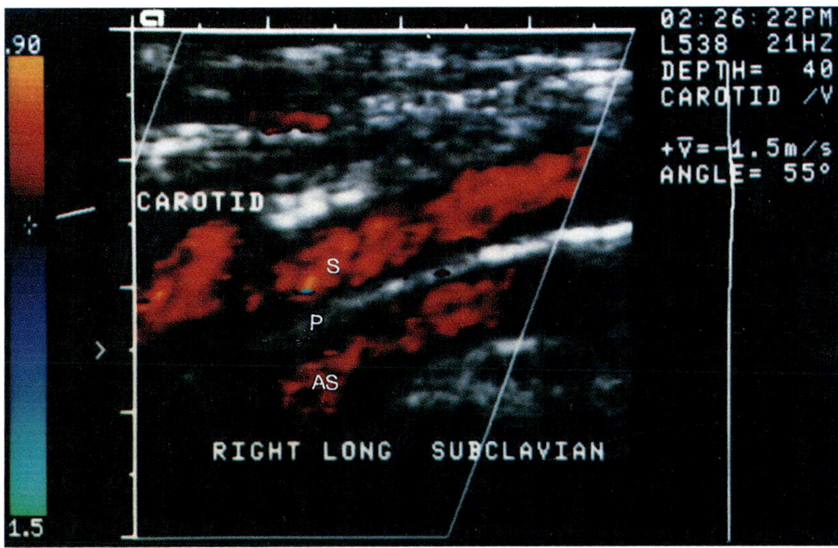

B

Figure 2-10 *A*. Longitudinal color Doppler image showing the carotid artery (C) and the carotid mirror-image artifact (CG = carotid ghost) *(Printed with permission from Middleton WD, Melson G: The carotid ghost: a color Doppler ultrasound duplication artifact. J Ultrasound Med 9:487–493, 1990.) B*. Longitudinal color Doppler sonogram of the subclavian artery demonstrates the real artery (S) and mirror-image artifact (AS) on opposite sides of the lung apex-pleura interface (P). *(Printed with permission from Reading CC, Charboneau JW, Allison JW, Cooperberg PL: Color and spectral Doppler mirror-image artifact of the subclavian artery. Radiology 174:41–42, 1990.)*

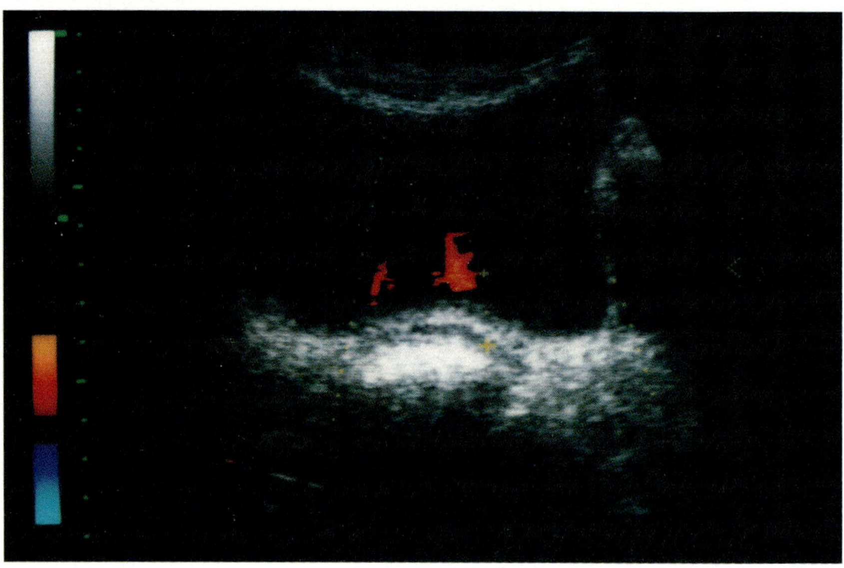

Figure 2-11 Color flashes produced by the rapid flow of urine at the outflow of the ureters in a distended bladder.

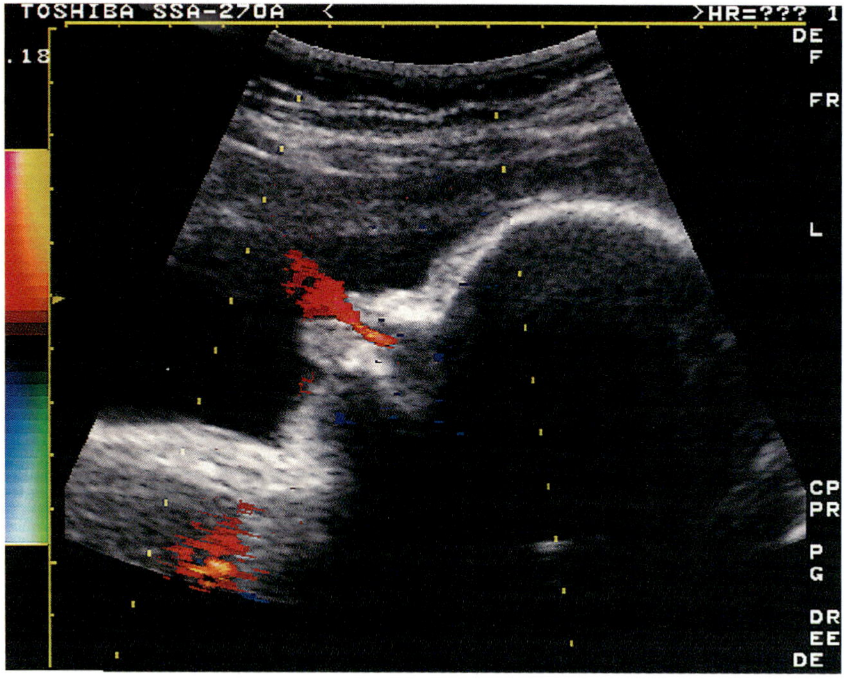

Figure 2-12 Color flashes produced by the flow of amniotic fluid expelled by the fetus through the nose.

atomic relationships. Sensitivity of the color Doppler system is therefore directly related to the amount of new physiologic information added to the gray scale. The information presented with color superimposed on the two-dimensional real-time gray scale images is still limited and confined primarily to the presence of flow in a specific region. Therefore, in order to perform spectral analysis and hemodynamic evaluations, present systems have combined color Doppler imaging with conventional two-dimensional duplex scanners.

An optimized color Doppler imaging system requires the simultaneous adjustment of all parameters used for gray scale, spectral Doppler, and color Doppler. Without high-level computer control, the system would be too complicated for routine use and clinical sensitivity would be severely compromised.

The value of color Doppler imaging is already recognized in fetal heart studies.[1–5,14–18] This technique also enables the study of blood flow in fetal peripheral vessels.[19–22] The observation of flow characteristics in fetal peripheral vessels provides a new dimension to the understanding of fetal circulatory physiology and pathophysiology.

The major problem with conventional pulsed Doppler systems is the low reproducibility due to difficulties in vessel localization and identification of flow direction. Use of CDI makes it possible to define the point of measurement, to visualize the direction of flow, and to accurately calculate the size of vessels so that a more reliable volumetric estimation of flow can be performed.[19] The improved reproducibility and reduction in examination time will expand the scope of research applications of the Doppler technique in the field of obstetrics, some of which are discussed in the following chapters.

REFERENCES

1. Winsberg F: Echocardiography of the fetal and newborn heart. Invest Radiol 7:152–158, 1972.
2. Kleinman CS, Hobbins JC, Jaffe CC, Lynch DC, Talner NS: Echocardiographic studies of human fetus: prenatal diagnosis of congenital heart disease and cardiac dysrhythmias. Pediatrics 65:1059–1067, 1980.
3. Wladimiroff JW, Voster R, McGhie JI: Normal cardiac ventricular geometry and function during the last trimester of pregnancy and early neonatal period. Br J Obstet Gynaecol 89:839–844, 1982.
4. DeVore, GR: The prenatal diagnosis of congenital heart disease: a practical approach for the fetal sonographer. J Clin Ultrasound 13:229–245, 1985.
5. DeVore GR, Siassi B, Platt LD: Fetal echocardiography IV. M-mode assessment of ventricular size and contractility during the second and third trimester of pregnancy in the normal fetus. Am J Obstet Gynecol 150:981–988, 1984.
6. Switzer DF, Nanda NC: Doppler color flow mapping. Ultrasound Med Biol 11:403–416, 1985.
7. Merrit, CRB: Doppler color flow imaging. J Clin Ultrasound 15:591–597, 1987.
8. Taylor KJW, Holland S: Doppler US. Part I- Basic principles, instrumentation and pitfalls. Radiology 174:297–307, 1990.
9. Mitchell DG: Color Doppler imaging; principles, limitations and artifacts. Radiology 177:1–10, 1990.

10. Namekawa K, Kasai C, Tsukamoto M, Koyano A: Imaging of blood flow using autocorrelation. Ultrasound Med Biol 8:138–143, 1982.
11. Bonnefous O, Pesqué P: Time domain formulation of pulsed Doppler ultrasound and blood velocity estimation by cross correlation. Ultrasonic Imaging 8:73–85, 1986.
12. Middleton WD, Erickson S, Melson GL: Perivascular color artifact: pathologic significance and appearance on color Doppler US images. Radiology 171:647–652, 1989.
13. Reading CC, Charboneau JW, Allison JW, Cooperberg PL: Color and spectral Doppler mirror-image artifact of the subclavian artery. Radiology 174:41–42, 1990.
14. Ortiz E, Robinson PJ, Deanfielad JE: Localization of ventricular septal defects by simultaneous display of superimposed colour Doppler and cross-sectional echocardiographic images. Br Heart J 54:53–60, 1985.
15. Dagli SV, Nanda NC, Roitman D: Evaluation of aortic dissection by Doppler color flow mapping. Am J Cardiol 56:497–498, 1985.
16. DeVore GR, Horenstein J, Siassi B, Platt LD: Fetal echocardiography VII. Doppler color flow mapping: a new technique for the diagnosis of congenital heart disease. Am J Obstet Gynecol 156:1054–1064, 1987.
17. Chiba Y, Kanzaki T, Kobayashi H, Murakami M, Yutani C: Evaluation of fetal structural heart disease using color flow mapping. Ultrasound Med Biol 16:221–229, 1990.
18. Maulik D, Nanda NC, Hsiung MC, Youngblood J: Doppler color flow mapping of the fetal heart. Angiology 37:628–632, 1986.
19. Arduini D, Rizzo G, Boccolini MR, Romanini C, Mancuso S: Functional assessment of uteroplacental and fetal circulation by means of color Doppler ultrasonography. J Ultrasound Med 9:249–253, 1990.
20. Arduini A, Rizzo G: Normal values of pulsatility index from fetal vessels: a cross-sectional study on 1556 healthy fetuses. J Perinat Med 18:165–172, 1990.
21. Stewart PA, Wladimiroff JW, Stijnen T: Blood flow velocity waveforms from the fetal external iliac artery as a measure of lower extremity vascular resistance. Br J Obstet Gynaecol 97:425–430, 1990.
22. Kurjak A, Alfirevic Z, Miljan M: Conventional and color Doppler in the assessment of fetal and maternal circulation. Ultrasound Med Biol 14:337–354, 1988.

THREE

FROM OVULATION TO IMPLANTATION

ROGER A. PIERSON

The events which begin at the moment of ovulation and end with implantation lay the foundation for the continuum of gynecology and obstetrics. Ultrasonographic studies of the female reproductive organs to elucidate the normal processes which occur from the moment of follicular rupture to implantation of the early conceptus have just begun. These studies have been greatly facilitated by the advent of transvaginal ultrasonography, which allows almost microscopic examination of the female reproductive tract. High-resolution ultrasonography may be used to perform serial examinations assessing minute detail in the same patient over time. This new technology has therefore overcome many of the difficulties associated with detailed evaluation of normal reproductive processes in living subjects. Transvaginal color flow Doppler ultrasonography has opened a new window in these endeavors. Vascular changes in vessels as small as the arteries supplying the preovulatory follicle, corpus luteum, oviduct, and endometrium may be evaluated, and much physiologic information revealed. In addition, the minute vascular changes associated with early relationship of the embryonic vesicle and the endometrium may be investigated.

The goal of this chapter is to provide a brief synopsis of the very early events in the reproductive cascade leading to the development of an embryo and to explore the potential for high-resolution color flow imaging in the events from ovulation to implantation. It is noteworthy that all the events involved in ovulation, luteogenesis, fertilization, and embryogenesis occur within the field of view of a high-resolution transvaginal ultrasonographic imaging instrument (Fig. 3-1).

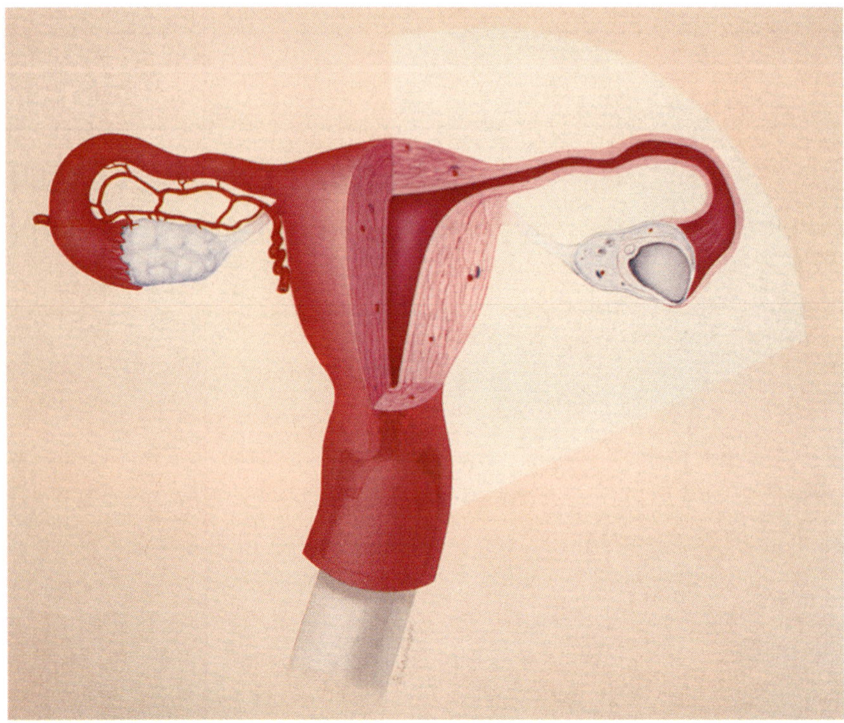

Figure 3-1 Schematic diagram showing the relationships among the reproductive organs and a transvaginal probe oriented in an oblique plane. A preovulatory follicle and the ovarian and oviductal arteries are seen on the right and left sides of the illustration, respectively.

OVARIES

The role of the ovary as the master gland of the female reproductive tract necessitates a dynamic morphology. In this role, the ovarian follicle has both endocrine (production of estrogens and nonsteroid hormones) and exocrine (nurture and release of the oocyte) functions. The primary functions of a preovulatory follicle may be considered to be the nurture and release of an oocyte capable of being fertilized and subsequent structural and functional transformation into a luteal gland capable of adequate progesterone production. It must be considered that follicular development is a concomitant, concerted development of all the components of the follicle. The follicular portion of the ovarian cycle has been divided into functional divisions describing the events that occur during folliculogenesis. They are the *recruitment phase*, during which many receptive follicles are recruited and develop; the *selection* and *dominance phases*, during which one follicle undergoes favored growth and development while other follicles in the recruited cohort are committed to atresia; and the *ovulation phase*, during which the dominant follicle ruptures and expels the oocyte-cumulus complex.

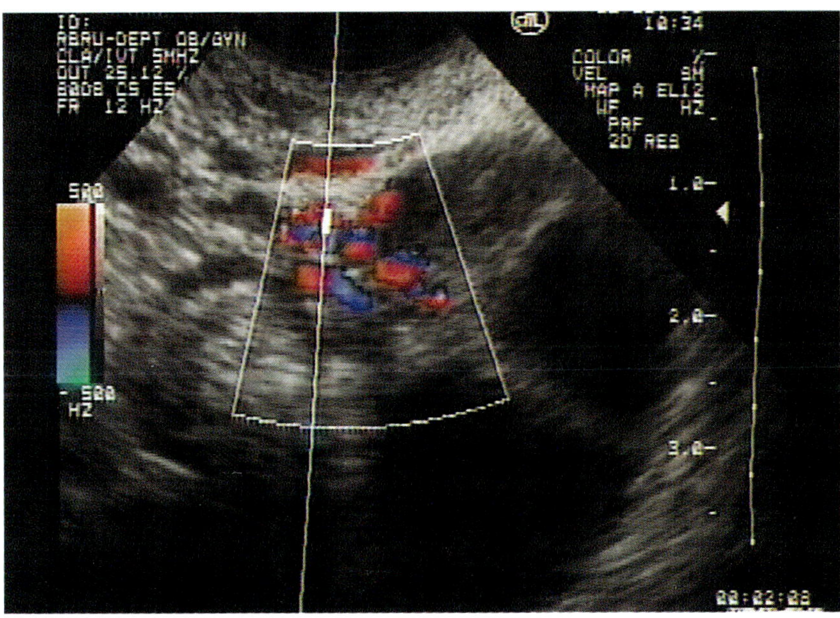

A

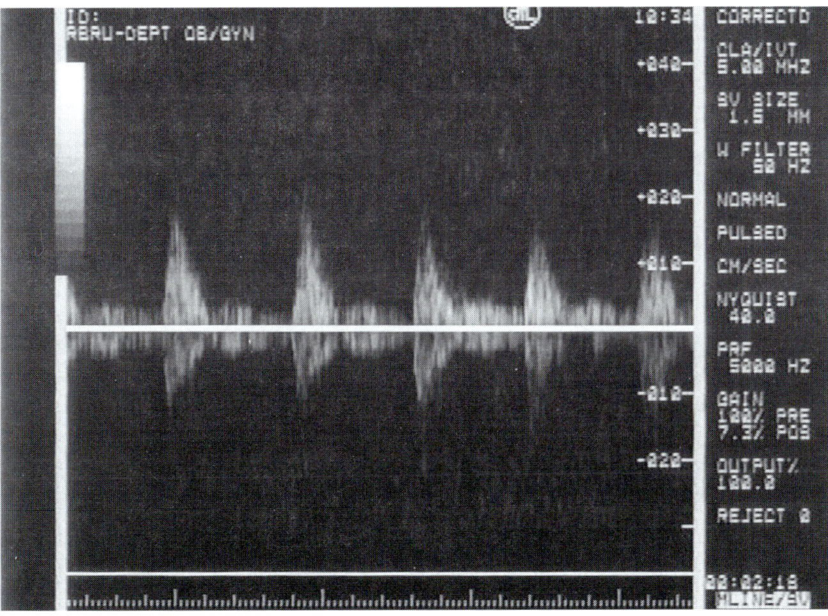

B

Figure 3-2   *A*. Image of an ovary on the day before ovulation. The plane of section is through the ovarian hilus. The ovarian artery is clearly seen as it enters the ovary. The dominant preovulatory follicle (inferior) and a subordinate follicle (superior) are seen to the lower right of the image of the ovary. *B*. Flow velocity waveform taken from image *A*.

Transvaginal ultrasonography has afforded a unique opportunity to evaluate changes in the ovaries during the ovarian cycle. Transvaginal color flow Doppler imaging has been used to identify the ovarian arteries, and the blood flow impedance has been studied at various times during the ovarian cycle. Color flow mapping greatly enhances the ability to identify accurately the ovarian vessels. In most cases, the ovarian vessels may be identified as they enter the ovarian hilus, removing all doubt as to the identity of the ovarian vasculature (Fig. 3-2). The lowest impedance to blood flow during the ovarian cycle reportedly occurs on the day of the luteinizing hormone (LH) peak, while highest resistance to blood flow was observed on day 1 of menses.[1] The temporal relationships of blood flow and ovarian status in regard to development of the preovulatory follicle, ovulation and development and regression of the corpus luteum apparently have not been fully investigated.

Preovulatory Follicle

The follicle destined to ovulate is physiologically selected for preferential development and eventual ovulation. The processes by which the selection mechanism occurs have not been determined and remain among the great mysteries in reproductive biology. Current concepts regarding physiologic selection of the dominant follicle in women and nonhuman primates have been critically evaluated. It has been determined, in primates, that the selection process is completed only during the ovarian cycle in which the individual ovulation occurs.[2–5] In this regard, it has been postulated that selection, final growth, and maturation of the ovulatory follicle may be due simply to chance development of a follicle within the recruited cohort coincident with luteal regression and increased preovulatory follicle stimulating hormone (FSH) levels.

Preovulatory follicles have a more extensive and permeable capillary network than other follicles.[6–8] The considerable vascularity which exists around the dominant follicle may allow it to accumulate more of the circulating gonadotropins and thus survive while the other members of its cohort undergo atresia. However, enhanced vascularity may be either a cause or reflection of selection. Increased blood flow to and hyperemia of the preovulatory follicle are apparently mediated by increased prostaglandin E_2, although histamine and bradykinins also have been implicated.[8,9] Edema of the theca interna is induced by dramatically increased fenestration of capillaries. In addition, there is a noticeable increase in mast cell infiltration of the tissues surrounding the follicle prior to ovulation.[10]

Studies using transvaginal color flow mapping to assess the intraovarian blood flow to the follicle and the vascular perfusion of the follicular wall during the dominance phase are ongoing.[1,11] Although data have not yet been critically evaluated, it appears that there is a very gradual decrease in impedance to blood flow in the vessels immediately surrounding the follicle as the interval to ovulation decreases. Immediately prior to ovulation, the perifollicular vessels are easily identified, and flow velocity waveforms may be generated (Fig. 3-3A and B). It

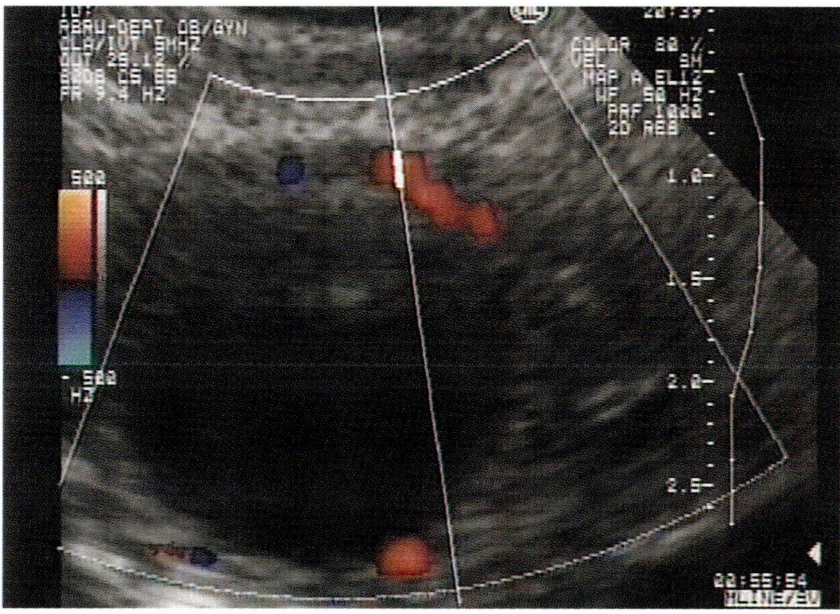

A

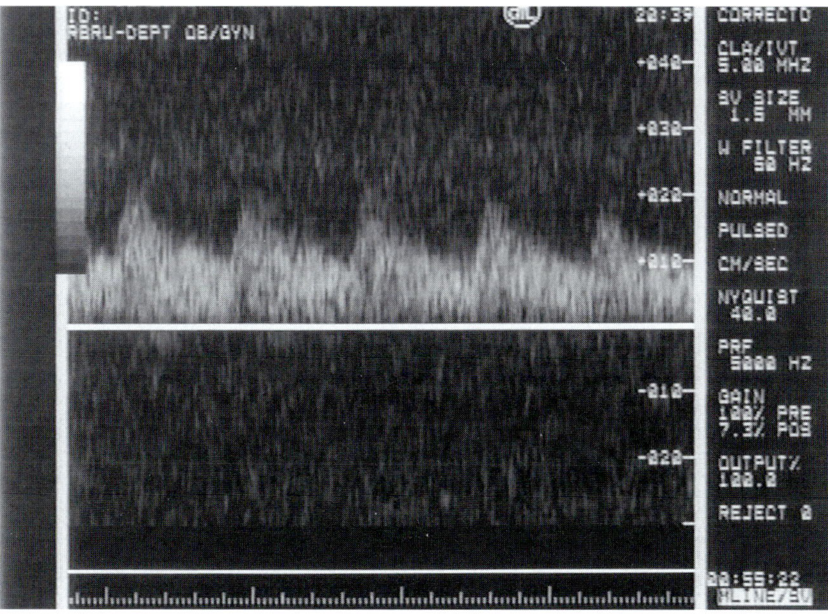

B

Figure 3-3   Series of images taken from a single patient during a study designed to visualize ovulation. *A*. Preovulatory follicle 60 s before the onset of follicular rupture. *B*. Flow velocity waveform associated with image *A*.

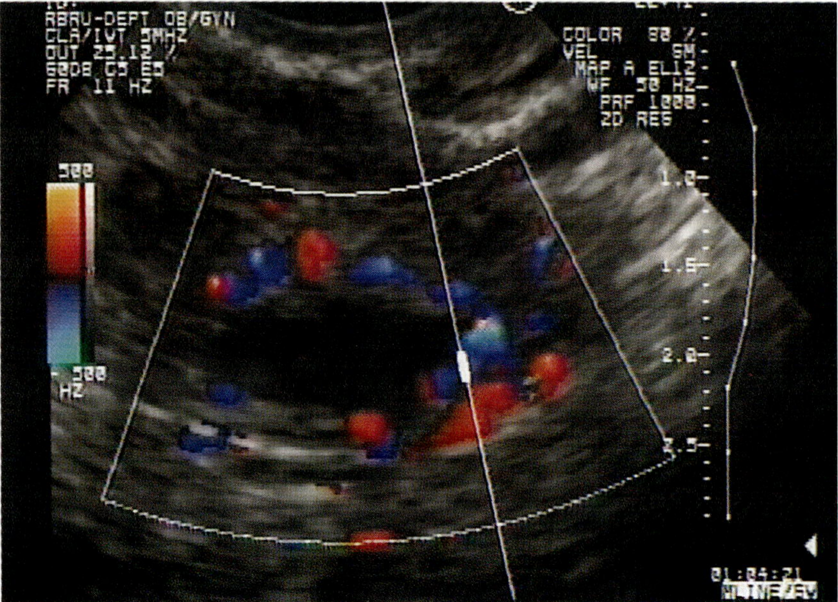

C

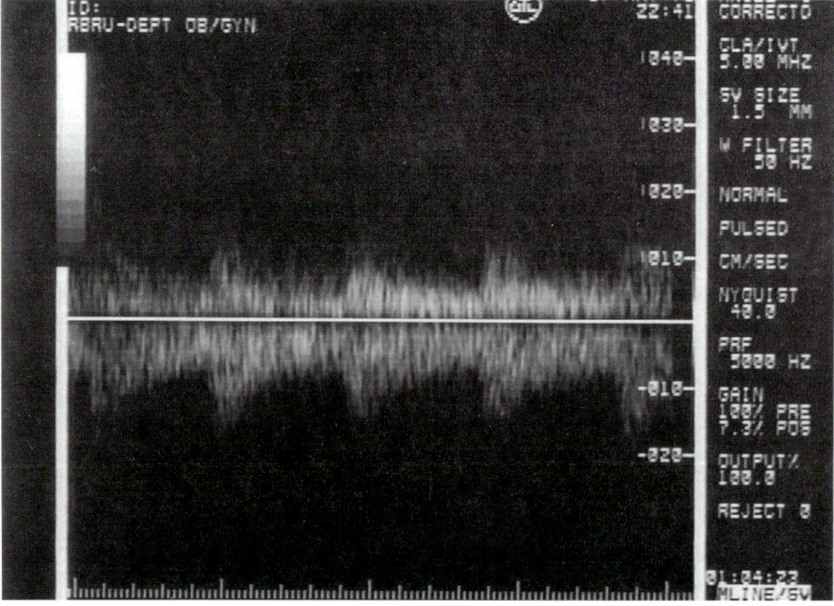

D

Figure 3-3 (*Continued*) *C*. Follicle 60 s following follicular rupture. The follicle lost 85 percent of the follicular fluid volume in the first 60 s. *D*. Flow velocity waveform associated with image *C*.

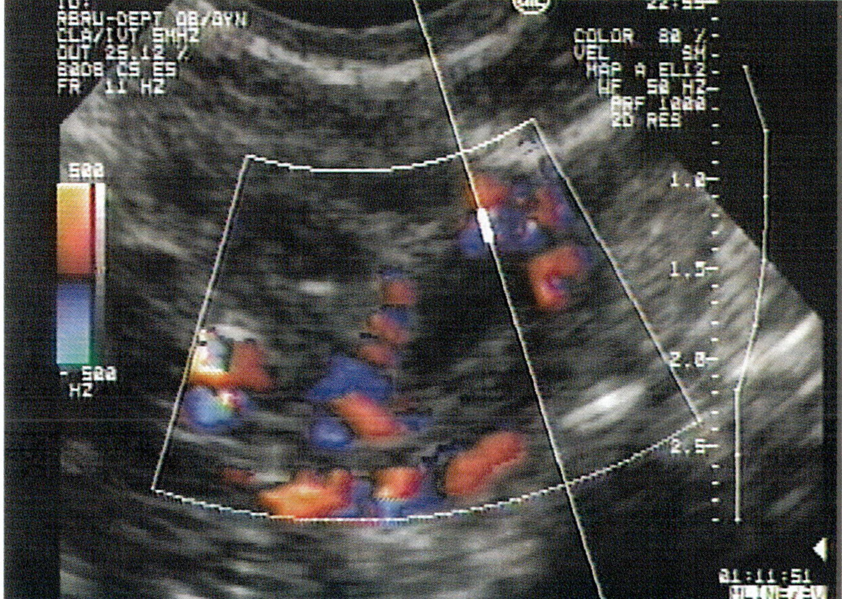

E

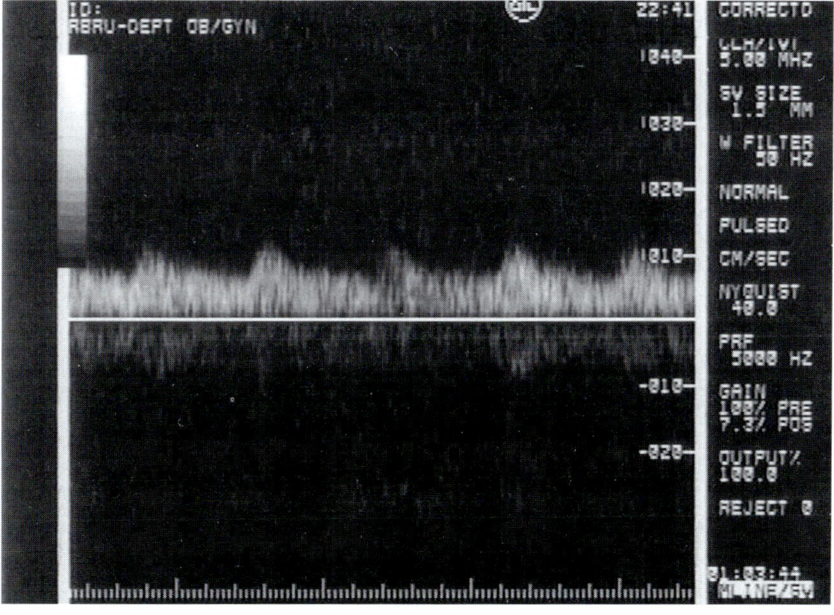

F

Figure 3-3 (*Continued*) *E*. The ovulatory follicle 15 min after the onset of follicular rupture. The follicular fluid volume was reduced to 5 percent of the original volume. Complete follicular evacuation and apposition of the follicular walls did not occur in this patient. A 5 to 2 percent residual fluid volume was observed at 30-min, 60-min, 120-min, and 12-h follow-up examinations. Corpus hemorrhagicum formation was observed at a 24-h postovulation examination. *F*. Flow velocity waveform associated with image *E*. Images were taken from a videotape of continuous scanning of the ovulatory process. The transverse plane of section is the same for all images.

is rare, however, to visualize the perifollicular vessels in one image plane due to their tortuous path around the periphery of the follicle.

Ovulation

Ovulation is the culmination of a complex series of events which is set into motion with elevated circulating LH concentrations and results in the evacuation of the follicular fluid, collapse of the preovulatory follicle, and expulsion of the oocyte from the follicle.[9,12,13] The primary stimulus for ovulation in women is a sudden, very brief rise in peripheral LH concentrations.[9] Disintegration of the apex of the follicle, final maturation of the oocyte, and evacuation of the follicular fluid must be closely coordinated for successful ovulation. Subsequent functional and morphologic changes in the cells which formerly made up the follicular epithelium and theca interna also must be completed to form the luteal gland. While the direct observation of ovulation by laparoscopy or ultrasonography may be quite dramatic, it must be remembered that the event of ovulation is the result of a long series of biochemical, physiologic, and morphologic changes in the tissues of the follicle.[13]

The LH trigger is followed by increased prorenin concentration in the pre-ovulatory follicle; thus, the prorenin-renin-angiotensin system has been implicated in the final microvascular aspects of ovulation.[9,14] Vasoconstriction and reduced blood flow which occur at the apex of the follicle as rupture of the follicle approaches may be mediated by prostaglandin $F_{2\alpha}$.[9] Ovulation has been compared to an inflammatory response in an interesting hypothesis.[10] Many of the similarities between ovulation and inflammation, especially regarding microvascular aspects, are profound; however, further exploration of these ideas is beyond the scope of this brief synopsis.

The first noticeable micromorphologic alteration following the LH surge is that the capillaries which surround the preovulatory follicle become increasingly fenestrated and the theca interna becomes edematous due to plasma effusion from the newly fenestrated vasculature.[7,8] The collagen networks making up the theca externa and tunica albuginea dissociate because of increased plasmin released by granulosa cells and increased collagenase activity originating from the fibroblasts of the albuginea. Weakening of the follicle wall occurs over the entire wall; however, rupture is localized to the apex. The cells making up the wall of the follicle are not destroyed but reorganized, facilitating transformation to the corpus luteum.[6,7,12,15]

Ovulation occurs on approximately day 14 postmenstruation in a classic "textbook" 28-day menstrual cycle.[16-20] Transabdominal ultrasound scanning has been used for many years to detect ovulation in women.[16] However, rupture of the follicle and evacuation of the follicular fluid and cumulus-oocyte complex has only recently been demonstrated by ultrasonography.[21] On average, ovulation appeared to take approximately 10 min from the first detected release of follicular fluid to complete follicular evacuation. However, the time required for ovulation varied from less than 1 min to more than 20 min. The site of the former follicle was immediately identifiable. The point of follicular rupture from the surface of the ovary could be recognized for up to a week. The luteal gland formed following ovulation typically remained ultrasonographically detectable until the subsequent ovulatory cycle.[14,20]

Color flow mapping studies of the follicular vasculature have begun only recently. There is a single report of a single ovulation in the literature.[22] Studies regarding vasculature changes during ovulation are ongoing.[11,21,22] In our series of color flow studies, volumetric estimations of the follicular fluid are made from follicular measurements at defined times before and during ovulation. Color flow maps and waveforms also are generated at defined times during follicular evacuation. Two sets of images from this series are shown (Fig. 3-3A to F). The patterns of blood flow during collapse of the follicle have not yet been critically evaluated. However, variation in resistance to blood flow appears to be quite dramatically decreased between preovulatory measurements and those taken following initiation of follicular rupture. Variations in flow characteristics appear very slight once follicular evacuation has begun.

Corpus Luteum

The walls of the follicle are in close apposition immediately following evacuation of the follicular fluid. The cells of the former follicular wall begin structural and functional transformation to the cells which will make up the corpus luteum. It appears that following approximately 60 percent of ovulations in women, there is a slight hemorrhage into the evacuated follicle. The degree of hemorrhage is extremely variable; however, there does not appear to be any effect of luteal morphology on progesterone production during the luteal phase of the menstrual cycle.[11]

Over the 48 to 72 h following ovulation, the walls of the evacuated follicle become profoundly vascularized. Blood and lymphatic vessels follow angiogenic factors and colonize the developing corpus luteum (Fig. 3-4A and B). The cells of the former follicular wall become luteinized and greatly increase in size. Progesterone secretion increases during this time. Four days following ovulation, the cells of the corpus luteum have attained maximal size and have completed the transformation to luteal cells.[23] A discernible layer of connective tissue typically lines the cavity of the corpus luteum if a central cavity is present. In the absence of a central cavity, a thin, highly echoic line is usually seen in the center of the corpus luteum. There is typically a pronounced ring of vascularity which appears to follow the path of the vascular supply surrounding the former preovulatory follicle and which becomes even more apparent as the corpus luteum matures (Fig. 3-5A and B).

Transvaginal color flow ultrasonography has been used to evaluate luteal blood flow in pregnant and nonpregnant women. Low rates of luteal flow were observed in nonpregnant women, while highest rates of blood flow were observed

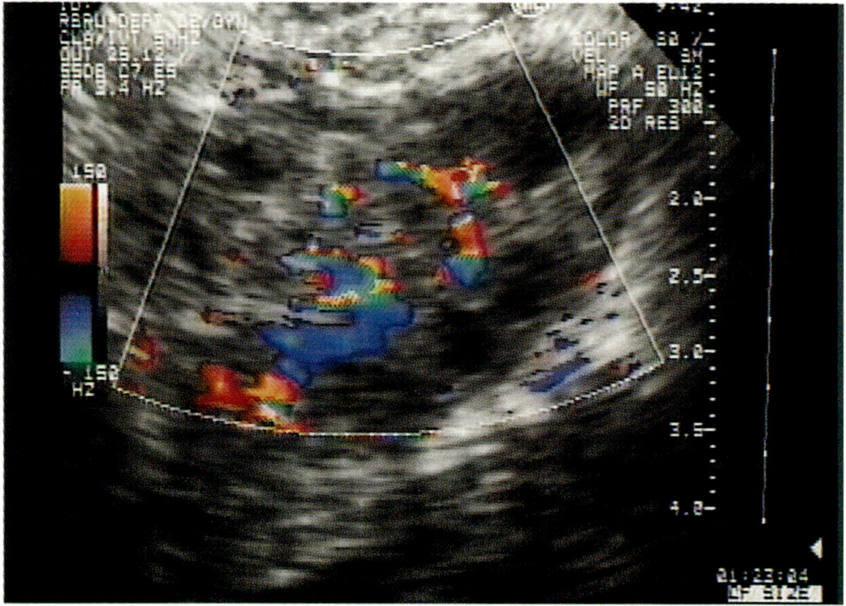

Figure 3-4 *A*. Image of a developing corpus luteum taken 24 h following ovulation. The color flow map shows the development of a ring of vascularity apparently around the walls of the former follicle. The intraovarian vessel supplying the corpus luteum is seen entering the lower left side of the color flow box. This individual corpus luteum did not form a central blood clot associated with corpus hemorrhagicum. *B*. Flow velocity waveform associated with image *A*.

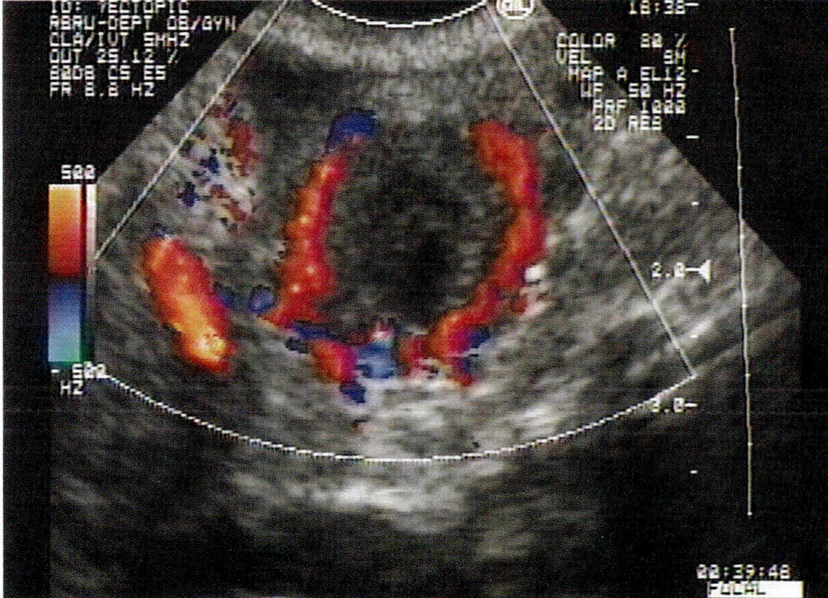

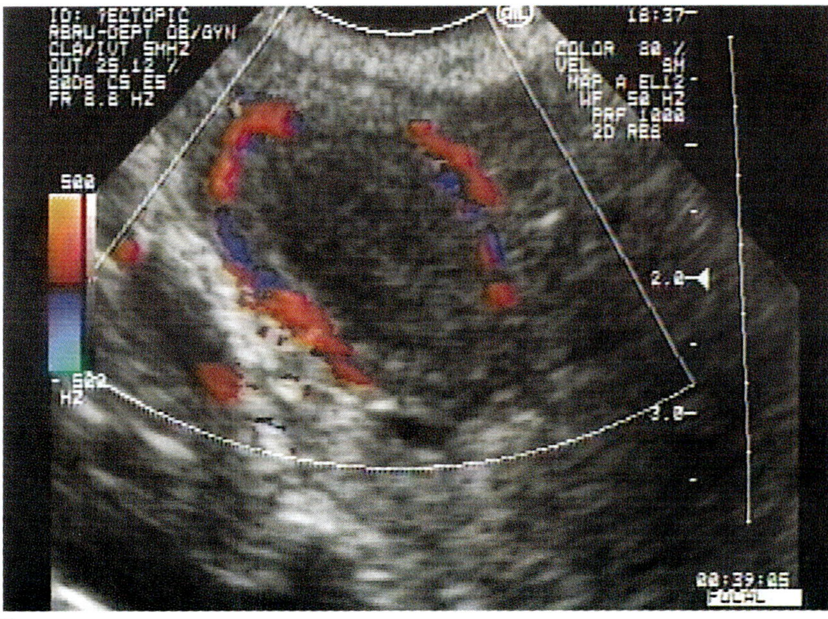

Figure 3-5 Images of a corpus luteum of pregnancy 3 weeks and 4 days following ovulation in the transverse (*A*) and sagittal (*B*) planes. The ring of vascularity typical of color flow maps of corpora lutea is clearly seen in both images. The luteal gland has a centrally located hypoechoic area characteristic of luteal glands in pregnancy.

in the luteal glands of women with intrauterine pregnancies.[24] A precise role for color flow Doppler assessment of luteal vascularity has yet to be defined; it seems probable that there is a profound role for this imaging modality in the study of luteal angiogenesis.

To maintain a level of progesterone sufficient to support a developing pregnancy, it is necessary for the conceptus to prevent the luteal regression usually associated with impending menstruation. Maternal recognition of pregnancy is the mechanism by which the conceptus signals the maternal host to maintain luteal secretion of progesterone. In women, the mechanism for maternal recognition of pregnancy is the production of a chorionic gonadotropin (hCG). The embryo initiates production of hCG at approximately the time of implantation. Increased circulating levels of β-hCG are observed as early as 8 to 12 days following conception, that is, approximately 4 to 8 days before the gestational sac may be visualized with high-resolution ultrasonography.[23–28] The syncytiotrophoblastic cells of the developing embryonic vesicle are responsible for the production of hCG and thus the enhanced secretion of progesterone. Peak levels of hCG are reached at approximately the 14th week of gestation, and the levels then begin to decline. Although the human placenta begins to elaborate progesterone by the sixth week following conception, quantities sufficient to maintain the pregnancy are not available until approximately the tenth week. Morphologic regression of the corpus luteum is observed beyond approximately the 20th week of gestation.[29]

The corpus luteum of pregnancy increases in size until approximately the 12th week of gestation. A large, anechoic (fluid-filled) central cavity typically develops in concert with the increased size of the luteal gland. Active progesterone secretion is observed from the earliest detection of pregnancy until the end of the 16th week of gestation. By the end of the 16th week of pregnancy, the central cyst of the corpus luteum begins to regress. There is usually no luteal cavity observed at term; however, the corpus luteum may be still recognizable.[23,29]

OVIDUCTS

The oviducts are the site of fertilization and very early embryonic development. In this regard, the oviducts are important to consider in imaging of the female reproductive tract, although the oviducts are difficult to visualize under routine circumstances.[30] Improvements in the resolving power of ultrasound instruments and transvaginal imaging are making the routine identification of the oviduct easier. It is possible for a skilled ultrasonographer to identify the oviduct from the uterine cornu through the mesosalpinx to the infundibulum in most patients. Patients with profoundly retroverted uteri present the most difficulty in imaging of the oviduct.

The oviduct is a tortuous structure approximately 10 mm in diameter at the proximal end. The diameter of the tube gradually increases toward the ampulla.

Occasionally the fimbria may be visualized waving freely in surrounding free pelvic fluid (Fig. 3-6*A*). The tortuous, almost serpentine nature of the oviduct usually yields a series of cross-sectional images rather than a linear image of the tube. Imaging of the oviduct is dramatically improved if there is free fluid in the cul-de-sac. Normally there is insufficient peritoneal fluid to outline the oviducts. However, following ovulation there is substantially more free fluid surrounding the reproductive tract as a result of evacuation of the ovulated follicle, and the oviducts may usually be thoroughly evaluated. When the oviducts are isolated from surrounding tissues, the vascular patterns may be followed along the entire length of the oviduct using color flow mapping (Fig. 3-6*B* to *D*). The vascular supply for most of the oviduct arises from tubal branches of the ovarian vessels. The portion of the oviduct proximal to the uterus is supplied by branches of the uterine vessels. Although critical studies have apparently not been performed, resistance to blood flow in the oviductal vessels does not appear to change during the normal menstrual cycle.

Imaging pathologic conditions of the oviduct is easier than imaging normal oviducts. Fluid accumulation in the oviduct appears as anechoic areas within the defined contours of the oviduct. Hydrosalpinx is easily diagnosed.[30,31] Typically the dilated infundibulum and ampulla, apparently contiguous with the ovary, are seen. Small, nonpathologic aggregates of fluid may also be identified in the oviduct immediately following ovulation, intrauterine insemination, or saline-enhanced ultrasound examination. The ability to image the entire oviduct from the uterus to the fimbria adjacent to the ovary also is important as high-resolution transvaginal ultrasonography has become widely used to search for and evaluate very early ectopic pregnancies. Vascular changes associated with early ectopic pregnancies have not been reported.

UTERUS

The uterus is the site of embryonic implantation and continued fetal development. In this regard it is of utmost importance for detailed ultrasonographic examination. The vascular supply to the uterus is primarily through the uterine artery which approaches the uterus at the level of the cervix and lower uterine segment in the plane where the ureter passes the uterus. Superior branches of the uterine artery supply the uterus, and inferior branches supply the cervix and vagina. Doppler flow studies have been used to demonstrate increased uterine perfusion via the uterine artery correlated with increased circulating levels of estrogen and pro-gesterone.[32,33] Decreasing perfusion was associated with low levels of estrogen following ovulation.[32] Further critical studies are needed which precisely equate particular waveforms and flow characteristics with circulating levels of repro-ductively active hormones (Fig. 3-7*A* and *B*).

The uterine artery may be identified as it enters the uterus and followed through the vascular cascade of the arcuate arteries, between the outer and middle

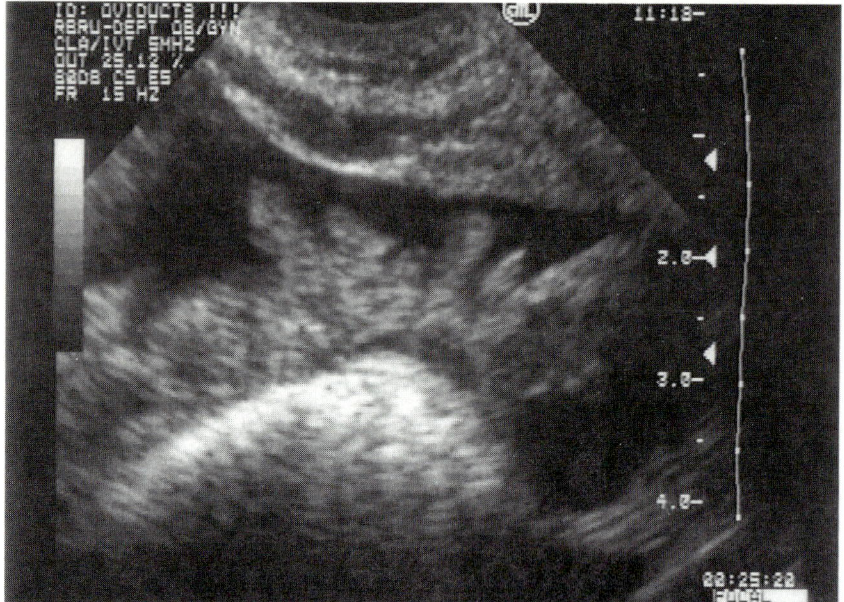

A

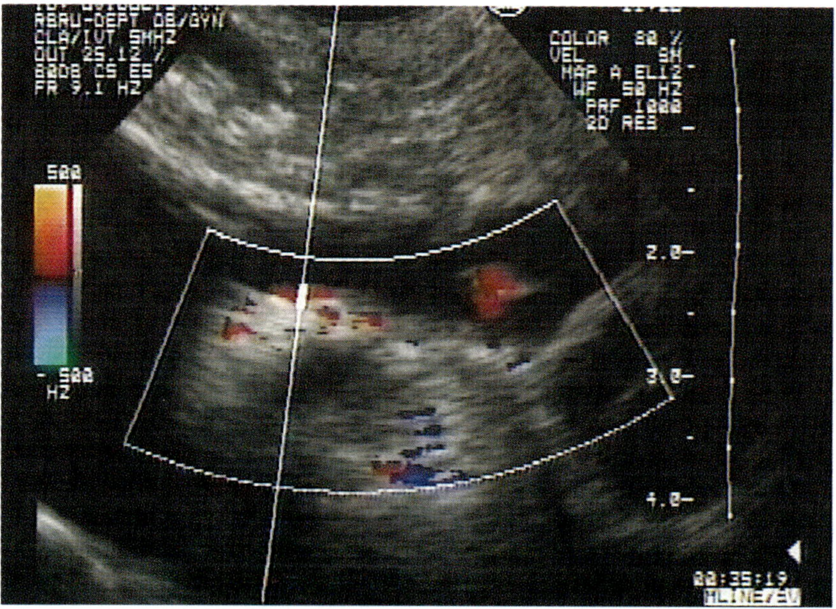

B

Figure 3-6 Series of oblique images of oviducts. *A.* The fimbriae are seen clearly because of surrounding fluid. In real time, the fimbriae could be seen to be waving in the fluid. The image was recorded approximately 10 h following a multiple ovulation. *B* and *C*. Two images of color flow maps of oviductal arteries. In both cases surrounding fluid outlined the oviducts allowing easy identification. The color maps follow the courses of small arteries apparently originating from tubal branches of the ovarian vessels.

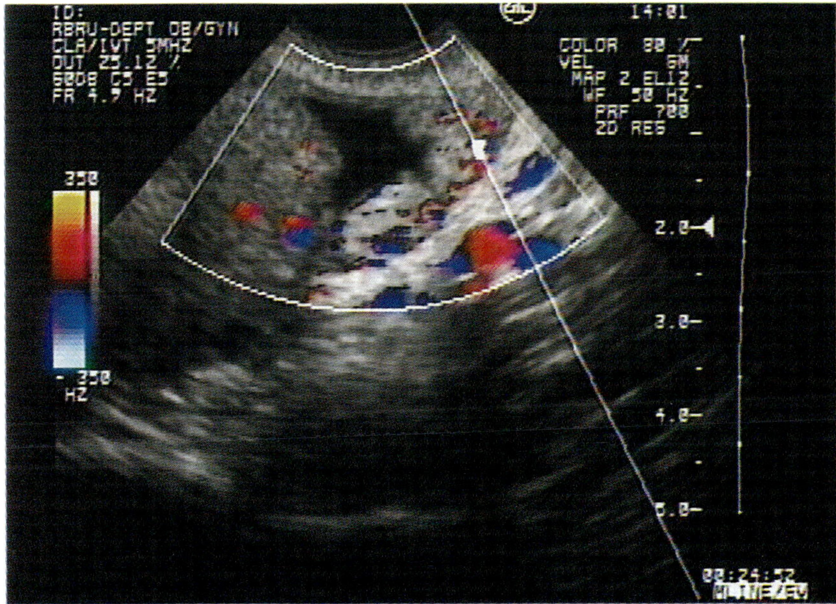

C

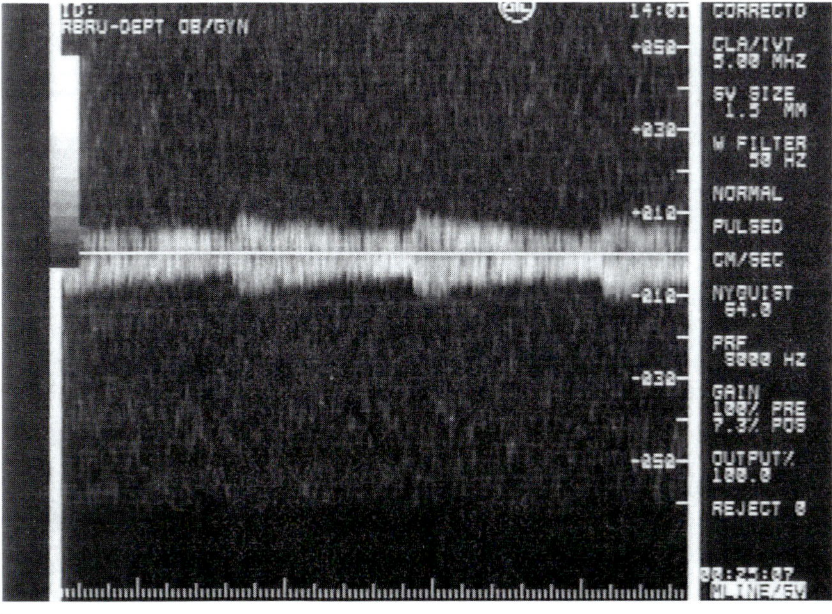

D

Figure 3-6 (*Continued*) *D*. Flow velocity waveform taken from image *C* showing waveform typical of oviductal vessels.

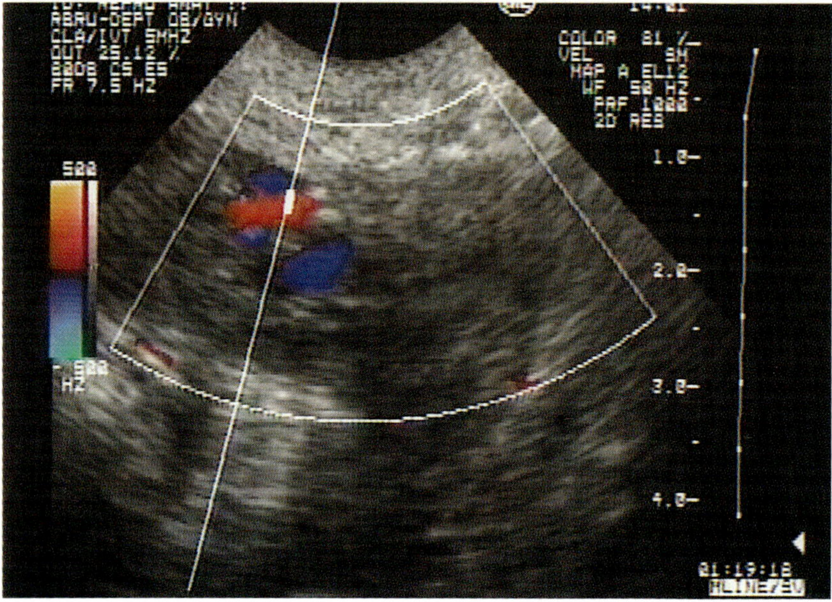

A

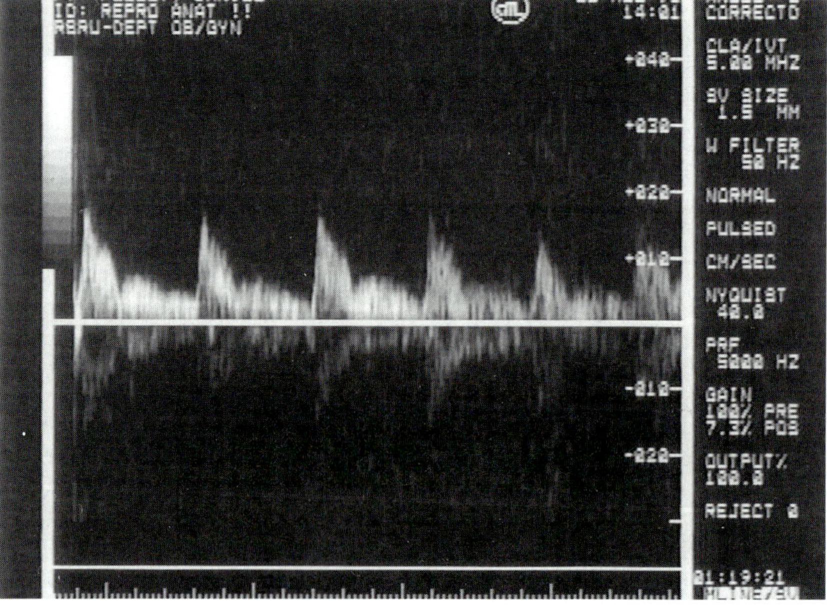

B

Figure 3-7 *A*. Transverse image showing the left uterine vessels 10 days following ovulation. The corpus luteum was ipsilateral to the image. *B*. Uterine arterial waveform taken from image *A*. Note the pronounced diastolic notch in the waveform.

thirds of the myometrium and their radial branches which branch inward to supply the endometrium (Fig. 3-8*A*). Occasionally, color flow interrogation yields glimpses of the spiral arteries as they pass through the basal layer of the endometrium and into the functional zone (Fig. 3-8*B*).

The myometrium does not appear to exhibit quantifiable changes during the menstrual cycle. The echotexture appears homogenous throughout the body of the uterus except when disrupted by various pathologic changes (e.g., leiomyomata). The vasculature of the uterus is distinct, especially at the interface with the broad ligament. Uterine blood vessels in women who have previously been pregnant are demonstrably larger than those of nulligravida women. Doppler waveforms may vary quite dramatically with both age and parity.

From an ultrasonographic perspective, the endometrium is the most important aspect of the uterus for routine evaluation in both early pregnant and nonpregnant women. The endometrium undergoes dramatic morphologic changes during a normal menstrual cycle which may be rapidly assessed with ultrasonographic imaging technology. Endometrial changes throughout the menstrual cycle are well described in the literature.[34–37] The endometrial detail which may be appreciated with high-resolution transvaginal ultrasound is striking. It is possible to discern the inner and outer strata of the endometrium and to assess changes in echotexture of the stratum spongiosum during the follicular and luteal phases of the menstrual cycle.[37]

The morphologic changes in the endometrium are directly related to the circulating concentrations of estrogen and progesterone and provide a conceptual bioassay for the reproductively active hormones. The degree of synchronicity between the ovaries and uterus may be serially evaluated and may be indicative of subtle defects in reproductive hormone production or action. There have been several studies on the correlation of the probability of implantation with the thickness of the endometrium when fertilized ova are transferred into the uterus following in vitro fertilization; however, definitive results remain inconclusive.[38]

Endometrial echoes associated with the time of conception and implantation are those typical of an estrogen-primed progestational phase uterus. During the late follicular phase of the menstrual cycle, images of the endometrium are displayed as a halo of light grays with a central echoic line representing the uterine lumen. The halo surrounds the deep grays of the edematous, central endometrial tissue. This ultrasonographic morphology is indicative of exposure to estrogen. Following ovulation and subsequent exposure of the endometrium to circulating progesterone, the central deep gray echoes lighten and the echotexture appears homogenous. The lumen is usually detectable, although it may be masked by the surrounding tissues. Vascular perfusion may be evaluated by color flow mapping and an impression of the degree of perfusion made. A technique for routine evaluation of endometrial perfusion has not yet been developed; however, such a strategy would represent a tremendous step forward in the evaluation of endometrial response to endogenous and exogenous hormones. In this regard, decreased uterine perfusion has been implicated as a cause of infertility.[39]

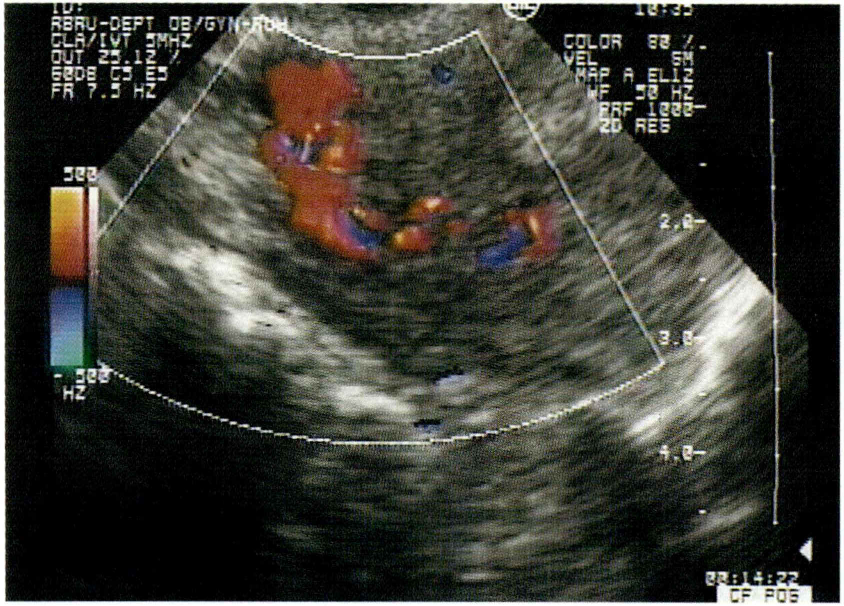

A

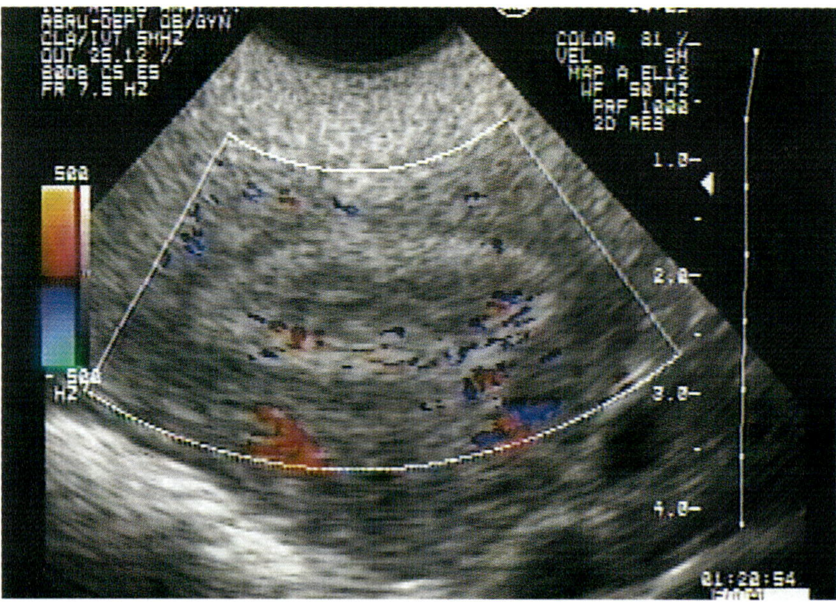

B

Figure 3-8 *A.* Image of the cascade of right uterine vessels entering the myometrium and continuing to the stratum basalis layer of the endometrium as the circumferentially oriented arcuate arteries. Flow velocities decrease with the continued branching of the vessels as they approach the endometrium. *B.* Color flow map of a transverse section of the uterus 6 days following ovulation. The endometrium shows ultrasonographically detectable characteristics of progesterone exposure. Vascularity is seen scattered in a roughly circular fashion around the stratum spongiosum.

CONCEPTION AND EARLY PREGNANCY

Fertilization

Fertilization describes the process in which the male and female gametes fuse to form a zygote. Fertilization normally occurs at the junction of the oviductal isthmus and ampulla. Spermatozoa pass rapidly through the vagina, uterus, and oviduct following ejaculation, although there is great attrition in the numbers of spermatozoa as they transverse the female tract. Of the 200 to 400 million spermatozoa typically present in the ejaculate, only 200 to 500 are usually found in the distal oviduct. In the female reproductive tract the spermatozoa must undergo the final maturation processes of capacitation and the acrosome reaction before they are able to fertilize an ovum. Capacitation describes the loss of surface proteins and the glycoprotein coat covering the acrosomal region of the spermatozoa. The acrosome reaction involves loss of the acrosomal membrane and release of hyaluronidase, trypsinlike substances, and zona lysin.[40–42]

The corona radiata is the first layer of the oocyte-cumulus complex through which the spermatozoa must pass before reaching the female gamete. The spermatozoa must penetrate the coronal cells and burrow down to the zona pellucida. Penetration of the second barrier, the zona pellucida, is achieved by enzymatic digestion of the proteins that make up the extracellular matrix of the zona pellucida. The permeability of the zona pellucida changes with the attachment of a spermatozoon, resulting in the zona reaction. The zona reaction describes a series of structural alterations which make it virtually impassable to other spermatozoa. Following penetration of the zona, the cell membranes of the spermatozoon and oocyte fuse, and the oocyte releases cortical granules, which serve as an immediate block to polyspermy.[40–42]

The oocyte resumes the second meiotic division immediately after spermatozoon entry, and the metabolic activity of the oocyte increases. These two phenomena are responsible for initiation of the cellular and molecular events of embryogenesis. Fertilization results in establishment of the full complement of chromosomes in the zygote, establishment of the gender of the zygote, and initiation of cleavage.[40–42]

Embryogenesis

Development of the zygote progresses from the two-cell stage, which is reached approximately 30 h following fertilization, to the four-cell stage at approximately 40 h postfertilization. The 16-cell stage is attained approximately 3 days following fertilization and the late morula stage 1 day later, just as the embryo is about to enter the uterus. The blastomeres, the individual cells that make up the early embryo, are surrounded by the zona pellucida until the morula stage. Morulae derived their name from visually having the appearance of a mulberry upon light microscopy. The late morula hatches from the zona pellucida and enters the uterine lumen at approximately 4.5 to 5 days following fertilization and consists of the inner cell mass and surrounding outer cells. The inner cell mass becomes the embryo proper, and the surrounding cells give rise to the trophoblast. Concurrently, that is, 4.5 to 5 days following fertilization, fluid begins to penetrate the zona pellucida into the interstitial spaces around the inner cell mass. The fluid pockets coalesce to form a single cavity called the blastocoele. Acquisition of the blastocoele marks the transformation of the morula to a blastocyst.[40–43]

Implantation

Six days following fertilization, the trophoblastic cells over the inner cell mass come into intimate contact with epithelial cells lining the endometrium. The cells of the trophoblast secrete proteolytic enzymes and subsequently begin to erode the uterine mucosa. The lining of the uterus promotes the invasion of the trophoblast; thus implantation is the result of interaction of embryonal and maternal tissues.[40–42,44]

Twelve days following fertilization, the blastocyst has become completely embedded in the uterine stoma. The inner cell mass, which will become the embryo proper, has formed a bilaminar germinal disk which consists of an ectodermal and endodermal layer. The area of the uterine endometrium surrounding the site of implantation is highly edematous. There is also a profound increase in the vascularity of the localized region surrounding the conceptus.[40–42,44] However, differences in the edema, thickening, and vascularity of endometria of pregnant and nonpregnant women may not yet be differentiated by ultrasonography.[26,44] Lacunae are present in the syncytiotrophoblast, and greatly enlarged blood vessels are seen in the surrounding uterine stroma. Syncytiotrophoblastic cells invade the stroma and contact and erode the maternal capillaries. The resulting maternal sinusoids become continuous with the trophoblastic lacunae, and maternal blood enters the lacunae. As the trophoblast erodes more sinusoids, the uteroplacental circulation is established. Thirteen to fourteen days following fertilization the definitive yolk sac has formed from a group of cells that originated as an evagination of the endodermal germ layer.[40–42,45]

Early Pregnancy

The embryonic period is usually described as ending at the eighth week of development. The period of the embryo is that in which the three germ layers give rise to the organs and tissues and the major features of the body are established.[40–42] The resolving powers of the current generation of ultrasound instruments enable the detection of a gestational sac as early as 15 to 18 days postovulation.[46] The gestational sac is first visualized as a small anechoic sphere within the thickened, progestational phase endometrium. The average diameter of the very early gestational sac is approximately 2 mm, and the average serum

B-hCG level at 15 to 18 days following conception is 400 to 800 mIU/mL.[26,27,46] A very thin halo of echoes of a slightly lighter gray than those of the surrounding endometrium may frequently be observed circumscribing the gestational sac (Fig. 3-9).

By 5 weeks after the last menstrual period (LMP) the gestational sac measures approximately 5 to 6 mm in diameter and the definitive yolk sac may be visualized within the gestational sac (Fig. 3-10*A*).[26,27,46,47] Application of color flow mapping yields the impression of profound microvascular development immediately surrounding the gestational sac. Additionally, the vessels supplying the endometrium may be clearly visualized as they approach the gestational sac and embryonic vesicle (Fig. 3-10*B*). Occasionally, anechoic areas in the decidua may be visualized and represent lacunae in the developing placenta.[26] At approximately 5.5 weeks following the LMP the embryonal pole may be differentiated from the adjacent yolk sac and will have a crown-rump length of 4 to 5.5 mm.[26,48] The "flicker" of the embryonic heartbeat may be visualized within the embryonal pole.[48] The embryo may be clearly differentiated from the yolk sac and surrounding amnion at approximately 7.5 weeks after the LMP. The amnion and definitive yolk sac join the embryo at the site of the future umbilical cord. The embryonic heart has established pronounced pulsatile activity. The allantois has not yet begun to evaginate and is not detectable. The chorion is represented at

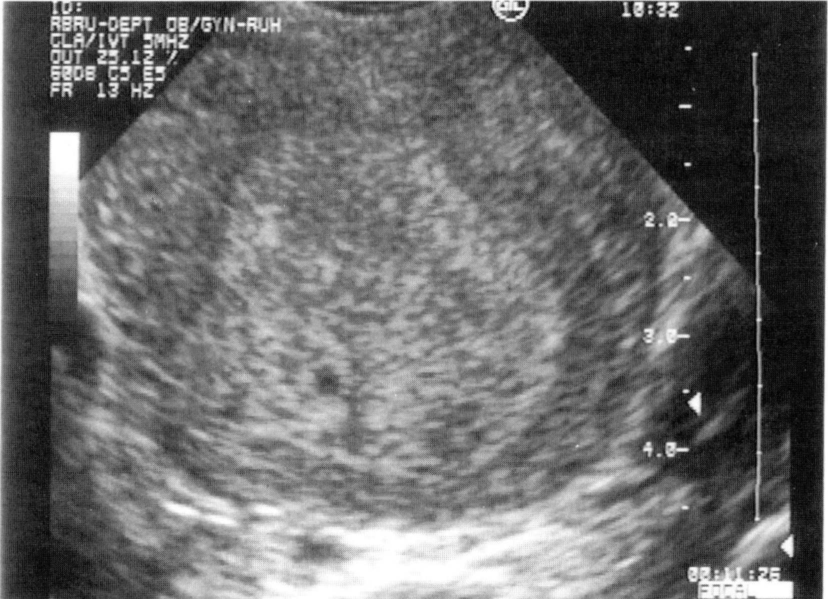

Figure 3-9 Transverse image of the uterus showing a 4-week and 2-day (from LMP) gestational sac. The conceptus has undergone nidation, and the endometrium shows a strong decidual reaction. The gestational sac is 3.4 mm in diameter and the β-hCG level was 425 mIU/mL.

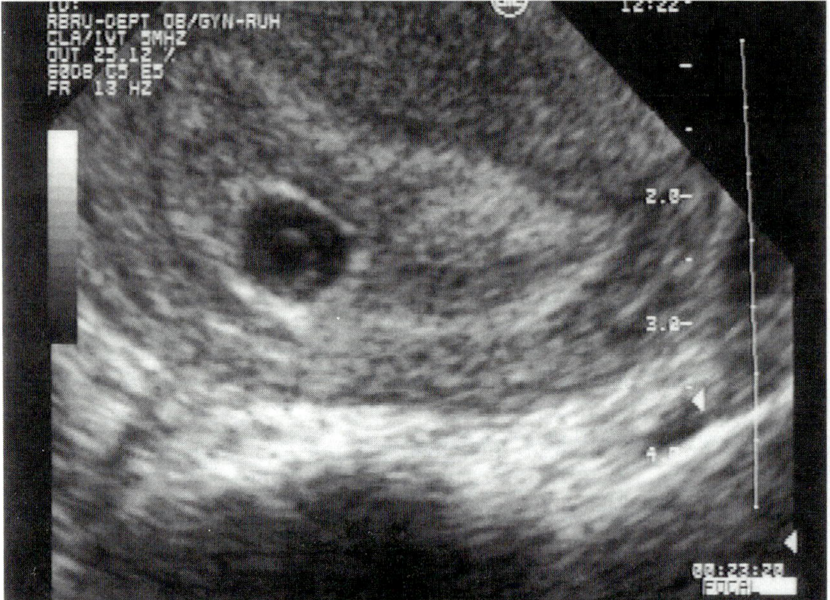

A

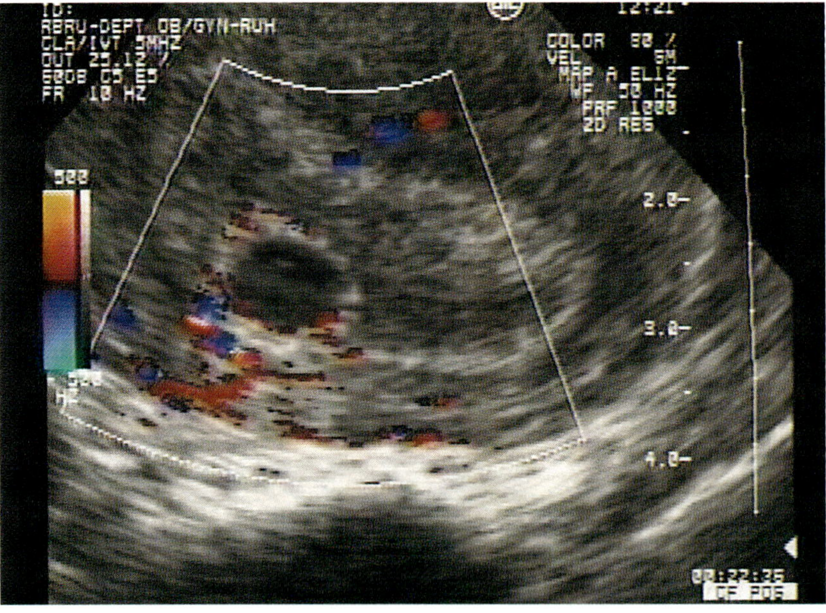

B

Figure 3-10 *A* and *B*. Image of a 5-week and 3-day (from LMP) pregnancy. The yolk sac is clearly visualized within the gestational sac, and the endometrium shows a very strong decidual reaction. *B*. Color flow map shows the vascular pattern surrounding the gestational sac. The primary vessels supplying the gestational sac are seen entering the color flow box at the lower left aspect of the image. A vessel approaching the stratum basalis of the endometrium is also seen at the upper right aspect of the color flow box.

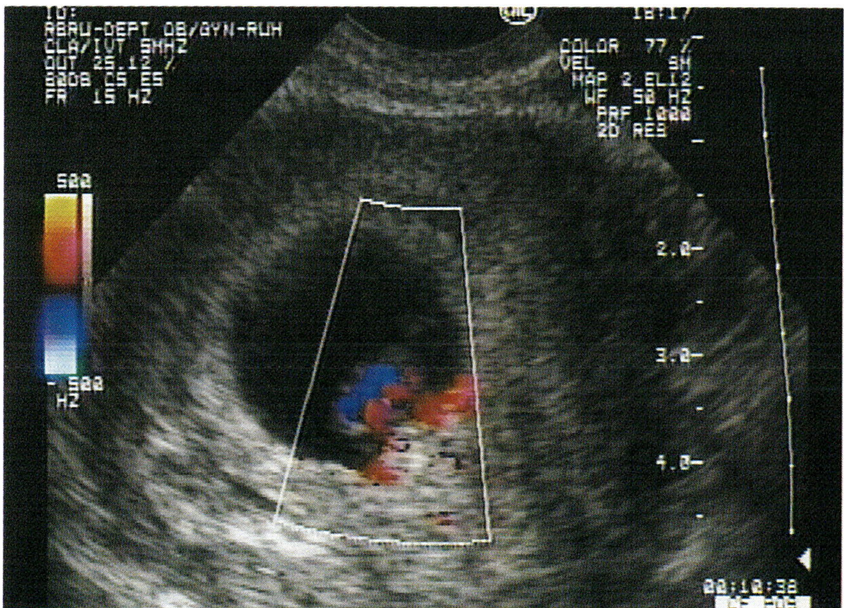

Figure 3-11   Transverse image of a 7-week and 5-day (from LMP) intrauterine pregnancy. A strong decidual reaction is seen in the surrounding endometrium. The color flow map shows the strong vascular flow pattern in the embryonic circulation. Vascular flow from the interface of the embryonic and maternal circulation is seen at the superior and inferior aspects of the embryo distal to the umbilical surface.

the fluid-endometrial interface. Color flow mapping reveals the intimate vascular association between the placenta and the embryo. The viability of the embryo may also be incontrovertibly established by visualization of vascular flow through the embryonic circulation (Fig. 3-11).

CONCLUDING REMARKS

The events from ovulation to implantation are among the most interesting aspects of human reproduction. These early phenomena remain among the crucial aspects of reproduction about which there are the fewest data. Transvaginal color flow Doppler ultrasonography is a remarkable tool for the elucidation of both normative and pathologic processes in reproductive biology. The technique provides rapid, noninvasive, visual access to the morphologic, physiologic, and vascular status of the structures involved in early human reproduction. The potential is great for new discoveries in both clinical and basic science aspects of human reproduction as the time courses of reproductive events are integrated with the already standardized methods of assessing reproductive function.

ACKNOWLEDGMENTS

The author is supported by the Medical Research Council of Canada and the Saskatchewan Health Research Board. Appreciation is expressed to D. R. Chizen, M. D. Hanna, and K. A. Pierson for review and discussion of the manuscript.

REFERENCES

1. Collins W, Jurkovic D, Bourne T, et al.: Ovarian morphology, endocrine function and intra-follicular blood flow during the peri-ovulatory period. Hum Reprod 6:319–324, 1991.
2. Hodgen GD: The dominant ovarian follicle. Fert Steril 38:281–300, 1982.
3. Gougeon A: Dynamics of follicular growth in the human: a model from preliminary results. Human Reprod 1:81–87, 1986.
4. Baird DT: A model for follicular selection and ovulation: lessons from superovulation. J Steroid Biochem 27:15–23, 1987.
5. Greenwald GS, Terranova PF: "Follicular selection and its control," in Knobil E, Neill J (eds), *The Physiology of Reproduction*. New York, Raven Press, 1988, pp 387–446.
6. Moor RM, Seamark RF: Cell signalling, permeability, and microvascular changes during follicle development in mammals. *J Dairy Sci* 69:927–943, 1986.
7. Guraya SS: *Biology of Ovarian Follicles in Mammals*. New York, Springer-Verlag, 1985, p 320.
8. Carson R, Findlay J, Mattner P, Brown B: Relative levels of thecal blood flow in atretic and non-atretic ovarian follicles of the conscious sheep. Aust J Exp Biol Med Sci 64:381–387, 1986.
9. Lipner H: "Mechanism of mammalian ovulation," in Knobil E, Neill J (eds), *The Physiology of Reproduction*. New York, Raven Press, 1988, pp 447–488.
10. Espey LL: Ovulation as an inflammatory reaction—A hypothesis. Biol Reprod 22:73–106, 1980.
11. Pierson RA: unpublished.
12. Balboni GC: "Structural changes: ovulation and luteal phase," in Serra GB (ed), *The Ovary: Comprehensive Endocrinology*. New York, Raven Press, 1983, pp 123–142.
13. Morioka N et al.: "Mechanisms of mammalian ovulation," in *Development of Preimplantation Embryos and Their Environment*. New York, Alan R. Liss, 1989, pp 65–85.
14. Richards JS: Maturation of ovarian follicles: actions and interactions of pituitary and ovarian hormones on follicular cell differentiation. Physiol Rev 60:51–89, 1980.
15. Woessner JF et al.: Connective tissue breakdown in ovulation. Steroids 54: 491–499, 1989.
16. Bomsel-Helmreich O: Ultrasound and the preovulatory human follicle. Ox Rev Reprod Biol 7:1–72, 1985.
17. Hackelöer BJ, Fleming R, Robinson HP, et al.: Correlation of ultrasonic and endocrinologic assessment of human follicular development. Am J Obstet Gynecol 135:122–128, 1979.
18. Hall DA, Hann LE, Ferrucci Jr. JT, et al.: Sonographic morphology of the normal menstrual cycle. Radiology 133:185–188, 1979.
19. Nitschke-Dabelstein S, Hackelöer BJ, Sturm G: Ovulation and corpus luteum formation observed by ultrasonography. Ultrasound Med Biol 1:33–39, 1980.
20. Lenz S: Ultrasonic study of follicular maturation, ovulation and development of corpus luteum during normal menstrual cycles. Acta Obstet Gynecol Scand 64:15–19, 1985.
21. Pierson RA, Martinuk SD, Chizen DR, Simpson CW: "Ultrasonographic visualization of human ovulation," in Evers JHL, Heineman MJ (eds), *From Ovulation to Implantation*. Amsterdam, Excerpta Medica, 1990, pp 73–79.
22. Bourne TH, Jurkovic J, Waterstone J, et al.: Intrafollicular blood flow during human ovulation. Ultrasound Obstet Gynecol 1:53–59, 1991.

23. Niswender GD, Nett TM: "The corpus luteum and its control," in Knobil E, Neil J (eds), *The Physiology of Reproduction*. New York, Raven Press, 1988, pp 489–525.

24. Zalud I, Kurjak A: The assessment of luteal blood flow in pregnant and nonpregnant women by transvaginal color doppler. J Perinat Med 18:215–221, 1990.

25. Kosasa TS, Levesque LA, Taymor ML, Goldstein DP: Measurements of early chorionic activity with a radioimmunoassay specific for human chorionic gonadotropin following spontaneous and induced ovulation. Fertil Steril 25:211–216, 1974.

26. Timor-Tritsch IE, Peisner DB, Raju S: Sonoembryology: an organ-oriented approach using a high-frequency vaginal probe. J Clin Ultrasound 18:286–298, 1990.

27. Peisner DB, Timor-Tritsch IE: The discriminatory zone of B-hCG for vaginal probes. J Clin Ultrasound 18:280–285, 1990.

28. Solomon S: "The placenta as an endocrine organ: steroids," in Knobil E, Neil J (eds), *The Physiology of Reproduction*. New York, Raven Press, 1988, pp 2085–2092.

29. Hodgen GD, Itskovitz J: "Recognition and maintenance of pregnancy," in Knobil E, Neil J (eds), *The Physiology of Reproduction*. New York, Raven Press, 1988, pp 1995–2021.

30. Timor-Tritsch IE, Rottem S, Lewit N: "The fallopian tubes," in Timor-Tritsch IE, Rottem S (eds), *Transvaginal Sonography*. New York, Elsevier, 1991, pp 131–144.

31. Tessler FN, Perrella RR, Fleischer AC, Grant EG: Endovaginal sonographic diagnosis of dilated fallopian tubes. Am J Roent 153:523–525, 1989.

32. Taylor KJ, Burns PN, et al.: Ultrasound doppler flow studies of the ovarian and uterine arteries. Br J Obstet Gynecol 92:240–246, 1985.

33. Goswamy RK, Steptoe PC: Doppler ultrasound studies of the uterine artery in spontaneous ovarian cycles. Hum Reprod 3:721–726, 1988.

34. Brandt TD, Levy EB, Grant TH, et al.: Endometrial echo and its significance in female infertility. Radiology 157:225–228, 1985.

35. Fleischer AC, Kalemeris GC, Entman SS: Sonographic depiction of the endometrium during normal cycles. Ultrasound Med Biol 12:271–277, 1986.

36. Fleischer AC, Kalemeris GC, Machin JE, et al.: Sonographic depiction of normal and abnormal endometrium with histopathologic correlation. J Ultrasound Med 5:445–452, 1986.

37. Lenz S, Lindenberg S: Ultrasonic evaluation of endometrial growth in women with normal cycles during spontaneous and stimulated cycles. Hum Reprod 5:377–381, 1990.

38. Casper RF, Gonen Y: Prediction of implantation by the sonographic appearance of the endometrium during controlled ovarian stimulation for in vitro fertilization (IVF). J In Vitro Fert Embryo Transf 7:146–151, 1990.

39. Goswamy RK, Williams G, Steptoe PC: Decreased uterine perfusion—a cause of infertility. Hum Reprod 3:955–959, 1988.

40. Langman J: *Medical Embryology*, 4th ed. Baltimore, Williams and Wilkins, 1981, p 384.

41. Hamilton WJ, Boyd JD, Mossman HW: *Human Embryology*, 4th ed. Baltimore, Williams & Wilkins, 1972, p 646.

42. Yanagimachi R: "Mammalian fertilization," in Knobil E, Neil J (eds), *The Physiology of Reproduction*. New York, Raven Press, 1988, pp 135–186.

43. Pedersen R.A.: "Early mammalian embryogenesis," in Knobil E, Neil J (eds), *The Physiology of Reproduction*. New York, Raven Press, 1988, pp 187–230.

44. Timor-Tritsch IE, Peisner DB, Raju S: Sonoembryology: an organ-oriented approach using a high-frequency vaginal probe. J Clin Ultrasound 18:286–298, 1990.

45. Weitlauf HM: "Biology of implantation," in Knobil E, Neil J (eds), *The Physiology of Reproduction*. New York, Raven Press, 1988, pp 231–264.

46. Goldstein SR, Snyder JR, Watson C, Danon M: Very early pregnancy detection with endovaginal ultrasound. Obstet Gynecol 72:200–204, 1988.

47. Fossum GT, Davajan V, Kletzky OA: Early detection of pregnancy with transvaginal ultrasound. Fertil Steril 49:788–791, 1988.

48. Rempen A: Diagnosis of viability in early pregnancy with vaginal sonography. J Ultrasound Med 9:711–715, 1990.

FOUR

ASSESSMENT OF THE UTEROPLACENTAL CIRCULATION IN THE NORMAL FIRST TRIMESTER PREGNANCY

RICHARD JAFFE

The introduction of diagnostic ultrasonography into clinical medicine has had an unprecedented impact on the practice of obstetrics. Ultrasonography has become one of the most important tools for the obstetrician and is used for evaluation of the gestation from the very first weeks until delivery. The information obtained from the employment of the different ultrasonographic techniques is so valuable to the obstetrician that it is almost impossible to imagine the clinical practice of obstetrics without it.

In recent years dynamic studies of fetal and maternal blood flow by the different Doppler ultrasound techniques have added valuable information to the understanding of the pathophysiology of several conditions affecting pregnancy. The information gained from these studies has modified both follow-up and treatment of several conditions such as intrauterine growth retardation (IUGR),[1–5] hypertensive disorders of pregnancy,[6,7] fetal malformations,[8,9] and chronically stressed fetuses.[10–14] The placenta plays a major role in the normal development of the pregnancy. Placental dysfunction caused by the interference with normal growth of uteroplacental and fetoplacental circulations leads to deficient nutritional and respiratory supplies to the fetus.[15,16]

Several methods have been developed for the measurement of uteroplacental blood flow in animals. These methods include the Fick principle, the diffusion-equilibrium technique, the steady-state diffusion method, the microsphere method, and the flow probe technique. Most of these techniques have not been applied to the measurement of human maternal placental blood flow owing to their invasiveness or the use of radioactive materials.[17] In human pregnancies the rate and extent of metabolism of estrogen precursor substances have been measured. The methods used are the metabolic clearance rate of maternal plasma dehydroisoandrosterone sulfate (DS) and placental clearance rate of DS and androstenedione through estradiol.[18]

With the introduction of Doppler ultrasound we can now perform noninvasive dynamic studies of blood flow in both uteroplacental and fetal circulations. Most Doppler studies of human gestations have been performed by the conventional transabdominal approach employing low-frequency probes with relative poor axial resolution. These low-frequency probes have been used to enable the imaging of maternal blood vessels deep in the pelvis and fetal vessels far from the ultrasound probe. Even so, only larger vessels could be visualized clearly, and most studies were undertaken during the second half of gestation.[3,4,19–26]

Development of the transvaginal probe has greatly improved the accuracy of ultrasound diagnosis of early gestation[27,28] and of nonpregnant pelvic structures.[29–31] With the transvaginal approach, the closer proximity of the probe to the region scanned allows the use of a high-frequency probe with an improved axial resolution.[32] Using a 5- to 7.5-mHz transvaginal probe it is now possible

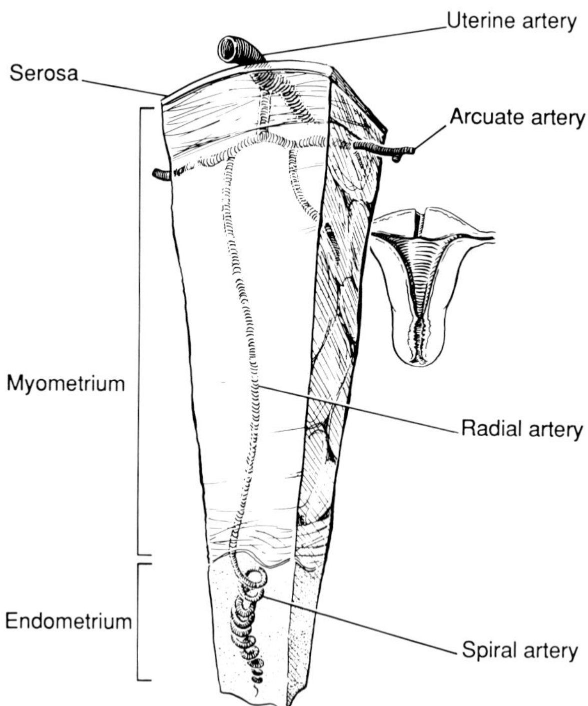

Figure 4-1 Schematic drawing of the blood supply to the uterus.

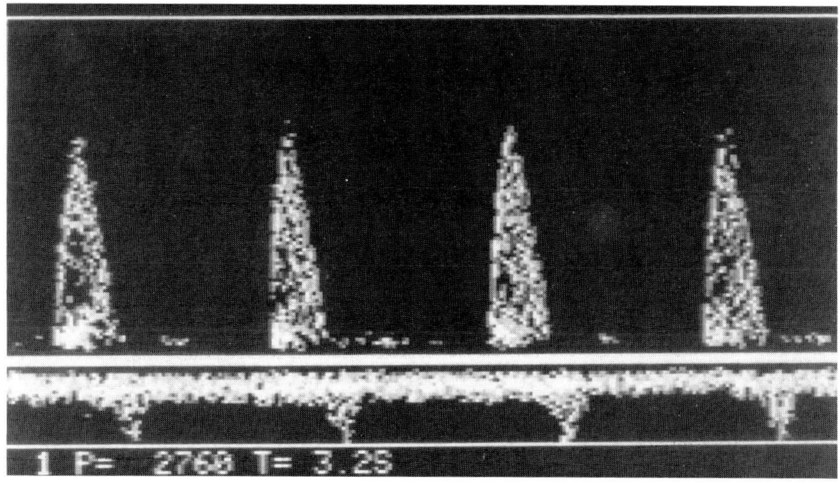

Figure 4-2   A spectral waveform obtained from an iliac artery demonstrating the high peak systolic flow and the reverse flow in diastole.

to detect fetal heart activity and embryonic structures at an earlier stage than with the conventional transabdominal approach.[33]

The uterus is supplied by blood from the uterine arteries which originates from the anterior division of the internal iliac arteries. Branches of the uterine artery, the arcuate arteries, extend inward for a third of the thickness of the myometrium and encircle the uterus. The radial arteries arise from the arcuate arteries and are directed toward the uterine cavity. As these vessels enter the endometrium, they become the spiral arteries which undergo cyclic changes during the menstrual cycle[34] (Fig. 4-1).

The flow velocity waveforms (FVW) of the nonpregnant pelvic circulation have been described.[35,36] Knowledge of the shape of the waveforms of the different vessels is a prerequisite for attempting to analyze signals obtained by color Doppler imaging (CDI) and the pulsed Doppler technique. The FVW of the external iliac artery shows a pattern of high resistance with reverse flow in late systole and during diastole (Fig. 4-2).

The FVW of the internal iliac artery shows a continuous forward flow during diastole with a deep notch related to aortic valve closure.[35] The same pattern of flow is seen in the uterine artery of the nonpregnant uterus[7] (Fig. 4-3).

Flow velocity waveforms of the uterine circulation in pregnancy were initially described by Campbell et al. in 1983[37] using the pulsed Doppler technique for qualitative measurement of blood flow in the uteroplacental circulation. Measurements in that study were performed on FVW received from the arcuate arteries.

There have been numerous studies of uteroplacental and fetal arterial FVWs

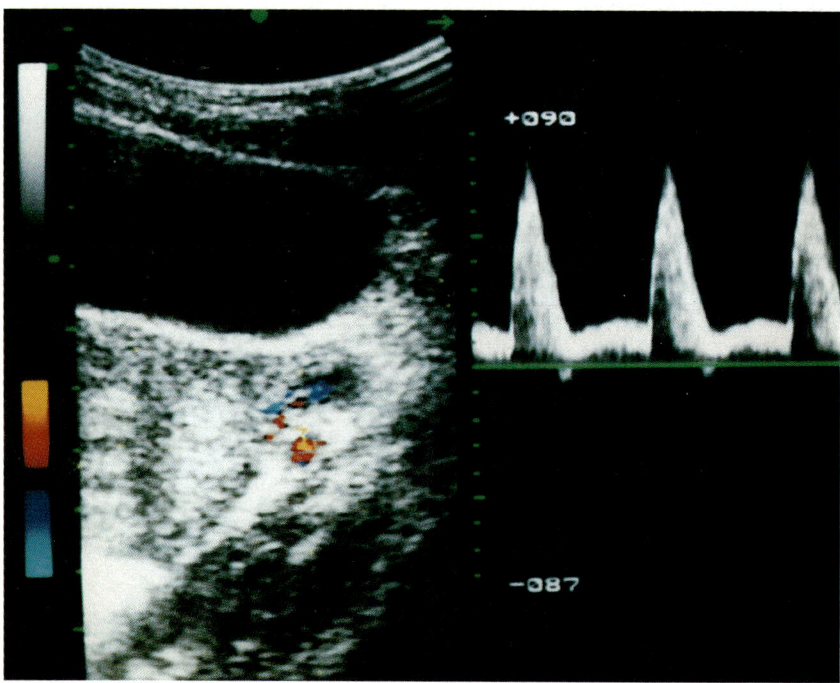

Figure 4-3 A waveform obtained from an uterine artery of a nonpregnant uterus showing the low forward flow with a notch at the beginning of the diastole.

as indicators of fetal well-being and placental function during the second half of gestation.[4,7,25,38,39] These studies evaluated FVWs obtained from the uterine artery or its largest branches and have shown a decrease in resistance to flow as the pregnancy progresses.[1,3,7,19,21] Results from the initial studies showed minimal diastolic blood flow in the first trimester of gestation and revealed the fact that as pregnancy approaches the second trimester the uterus is converted into a low-resistance organ with an increasing diastolic blood flow component[16,21,39] (Fig. 4-4). This is demonstrated by the decrease in the different ratios calculated from FVWs.[1,19,21,26,40] The most common explanation for the physiology behind this phenomenon was given by Brosens et al.[41,42] and DeWolf et al.,[43] who suggested that the trophoblast invades the myometrial segments of the spiral arteries, destroys the elastic lamina, and replaces the smooth muscle elements. This transformation causes defective contractility of these vessels. The decreased ability to contract leads to the formation of a low-resistance vascular system with the characteristic continuous forward flow demonstrated by the high diastolic component (Fig. 4-4).

Several authors have addressed the problem of low reproducibility of Doppler ultrasound waveform analysis of the uteroplacental circulation that is due to different sites of measurements.[25,44–47] Arabin[16] in a recent study clearly dem-

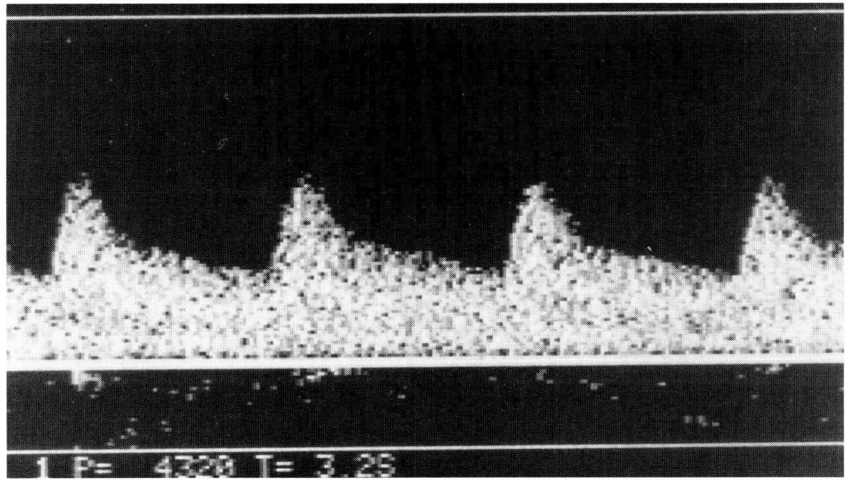

Figure 4-4   A waveform of the uterine artery in pregnancy demonstrating high diastolic flow.

onstrated that the location of the vessel measured by Doppler ultrasound relative to the placental site is of great importance. Her study showed that measurements performed on waveforms obtained from vessels close to the placenta have lower indices than those calculated from vessels far away from the placenta. Similarly, several authors have reported that resistance indices derived from arcuate artery signals obtained from the placental side of the uterus were significantly lower than those derived from signals obtained from the nonplacental side.[48–50] These lower indices reflect lower resistance to flow in vessels close to the placenta, and it is therefore important to exactly define the measurement site to avoid false-positive or false-negative results when using existing nomograms for flow in the uteroplacental circulation.

With the introduction of the transvaginal probe with both CDI and pulsed Doppler, it is now feasible to more accurately study both nonpregnant pelvic vessels and structures and the uteroplacental circulation at the early stages of gestation.[31,35,49,51,52] As already emphasized in Chap. 2, the great advantage of CDI is its area analysis of flow providing quick and easy detection of flow in vessels too small to be detected by the conventional two-dimensional real-time ultrasound.[53,54]

The combined employment of transvaginal CDI and pulsed Doppler has given us the added opportunity to analyze FVWs obtained from blood vessels beneath the trophoblast and better understand the early development of utero-placental circulation. Placental growth disturbance has been associated with elevated indices of waveforms obtained from the uteroplacental vessels.[55] This increase in calculated indices is due to the higher resistance to blood flow in these vessels. Other pathologic conditions of the placenta such as partial abruption and infarction are caused by disturbed uteroplacental circulation.[56]

Doppler ultrasound waveform analysis may detect pathologic changes in the uteroplacental circulation before any clinical manifestation and so alert the physician earlier to the possibility of acute placental insult.

Whether continuous wave (CW) or pulsed Doppler was employed, it is evident from recent studies[50–52,57] that the FVWs obtained from first trimester uterine arteries do not show any significant decrease in calculated ratios compared to nonpregnant ratios of the same vessel.[1,21,40] The systolic-diastolic ratios and resistance indices calculated from the uterine artery FVWs remain high during the first trimester, and a decrease is evident only in the second trimester when the trophoblastic invasion is complete.

The combined use of CDI and pulsed Doppler in the assessment of the pelvic circulation has recently been reported.[40,48,58,59] The guidance of the pulsed Doppler beam by CDI has improved the visualization of the main arteries and the demonstration of vessels that cannot be easily detected with conventional methods.[48,58,60] (Fig. 4-5).

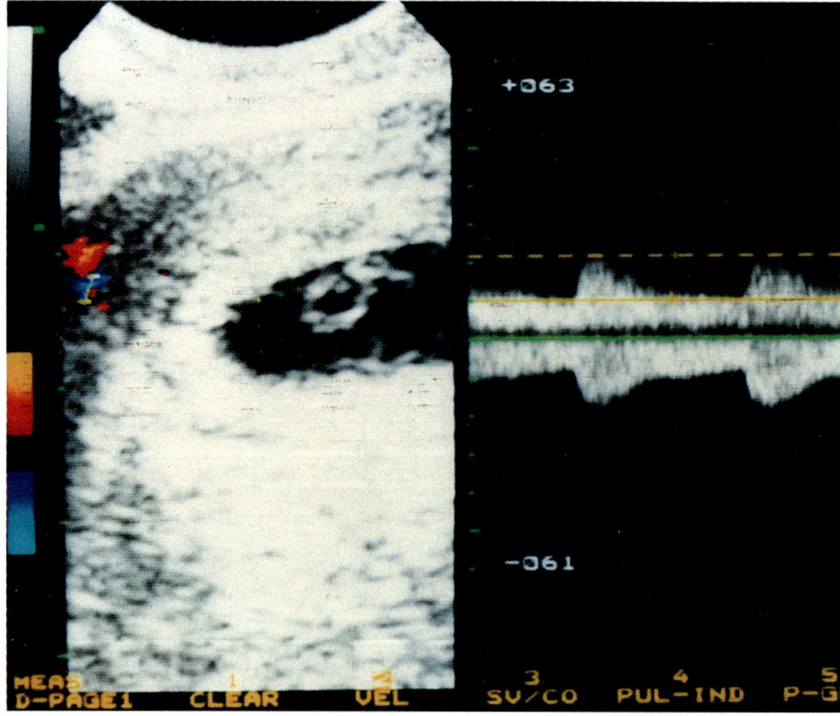

Figure 4-5 Detection of subtrophoblastic flow in early pregnancy by color Doppler imaging. The flow velocity waveforms demonstrate a high diastolic component and continuous forward flow. *(Printed with permission from Jaffe R, Warsof SL: Transvaginal color Doppler imaging in the assessment of uteroplacental blood flow in the normal first-trimester pregnancy. Am J Obstet Gynecol 164:781–785, 1991.)*

Just as Arabin[16] in her study of 20- to 40-week gestations demonstrated an increase in resistance to flow with an increasing distance from the placenta, Jaffe and Warsof's[60] first trimester analysis of FVW from vessels at the level of the trophoblast revealed a different flow pattern compared to that of the larger vessels. These FVWs of trophoblastic vessels show characteristics of low resistance to flow and demonstrate continued forward flow with a prominent diastolic component (Fig. 4-5).

Blood flow can be detected in pregnancy by transvaginal color Doppler imaging at the level of the trophoblast at 5 to 6 weeks amenorrhea in most cases and in all cases at or beyond 7 weeks gestation[60] (Fig. 4-6).

The calculated ratios of FVW obtained from the trophoblast are significantly lower than those reported for the uterine or arcuate arteries at the same gestational age (Fig. 4.7A and B).[1,7,21,51,57,60]

Simultaneous Doppler analysis of FVW from the uterine artery and trophoblast at the early stages of the gestation may help us to understand the development of the low resistance of uterine flow. There are studies which suggest that vessels with larger diameters, such as the uterine and arcuate arteries, retain their ability to contract during diastole in the early stages of gestation. Only as placental volume and trophoblastic invasion increase are changes in blood flow reflected in the FVWs obtained from these vessels. The smaller vessels at the site of the trophoblast, however, are probably affected very early by trophoblastic invasion as shown by their characteristic low impedance waveforms.

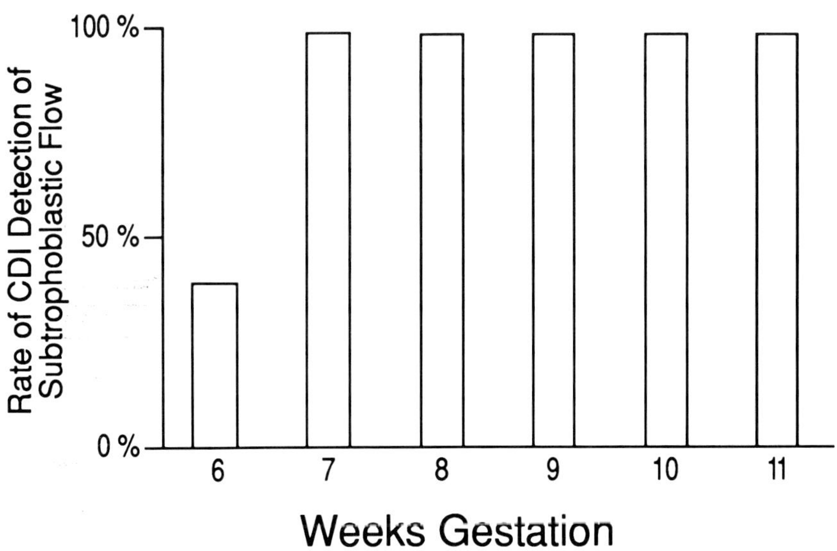

Figure 4-6   Rate of detection of subtrophoblastic flow in early pregnancy by color Doppler imaging.

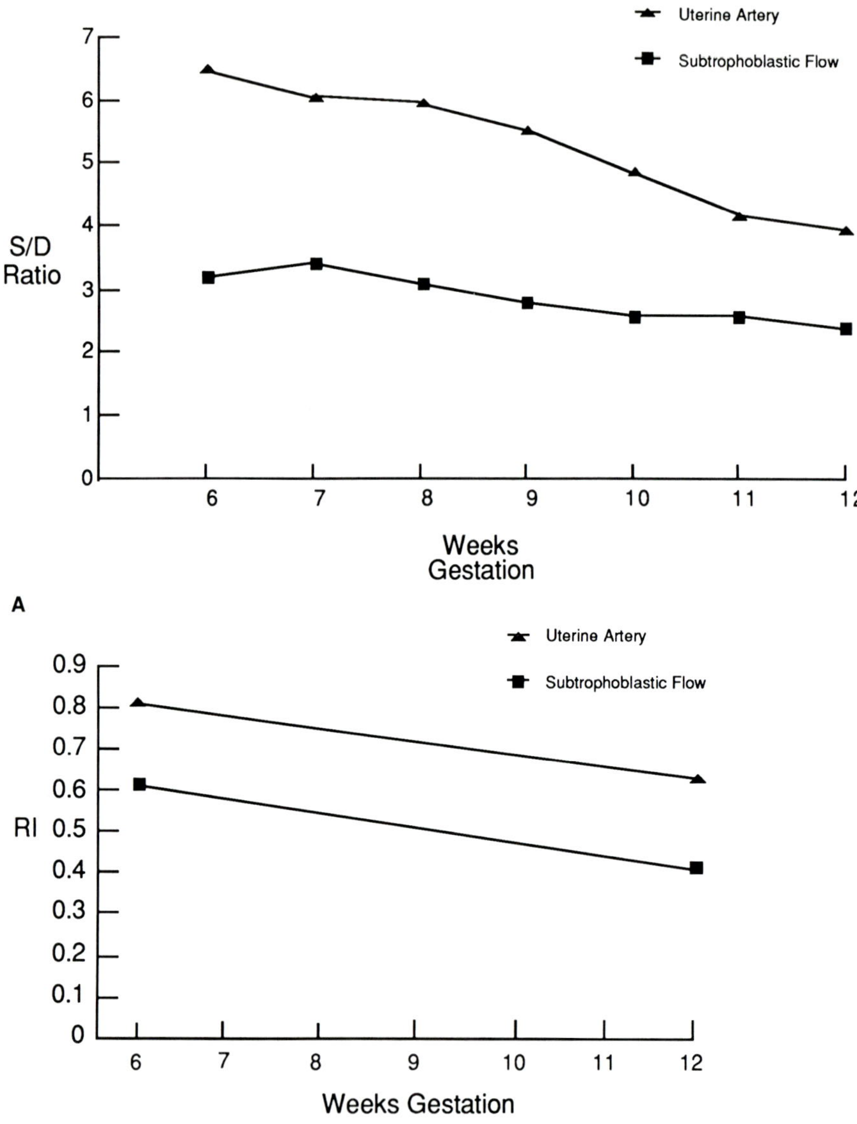

Figure 4-7 The systolic-to-diastolic (S/D) ratios and resistance index (RI) calculated from uterine vessels in early pregnancy. Both figures clearly demonstrate that resistance to flow is much higher in the uterine artery as compared to the trophoblastic vessels.

SUMMARY

Transvaginal ultrasonography combined with pulsed and color Doppler provides an improved method for evaluation of the uteroplacental circulation. Subtrophoblastic vessels show low resistance to flow in the early first trimester, and it was demonstrated that the resistance in the uteroplacental circulation increases as the distance from the placenta increases.

With this new technique we can provide a more accurate assessment of the developing circulation of the normal early pregnancy and better understand the pathophysiology behind some conditions specifically affecting early pregnancies.

Chapter 5 addresses the use of CDI in the assessment of complications of early intrauterine pregnancies.

REFERENCES

1. Griffin D, Cohen-Overbeek T, Campbell S: Fetal and uteroplacental blood flow. Clin Obstet Gynaecol 10:565–603, 1983.
2. Fleischer A, Schulman H, Farmakaides D, Bracero L, Blattner P, Randolph G: Umbilical artery velocity waveforms and intrauterine growth retardation. Am J Obstet Gynecol 151:502–505, 1985.
3. Trudinger BJ, Giles WB, Cook CM: Flow velocity waveforms in the maternal uteroplacental and fetal umbilical circulations. Am J Obstet Gynecol 152:155–163, 1985.
4. Trudinger BJ, Giles WB, Cook CM: Uteroplacental blood flow velocity-time waveforms in normal and complicated pregnancy. Br J Obstet Gynaecol 92:39–45, 1985.
5. Giles WB, Lingman G, Marsal K, Trudinger BJ: Fetal volume blood flow and umbilical artery flow velocity waveform analysis: a comparison. Br J Obstet Gynaecol 93:461–465, 1986.
6. Fleischer A, Schulman H, Farmakaides G, Bracero L, Grunfeld L, Rochelson B, Koenigsberg M: Uterine artery Doppler velocimetry in pregnant women with hypertension. Am J Obstet Gynecol 154:806–813, 1986.
7. Schulman H: The clinical implication of Doppler ultrasound analysis of the uterine and umbilical arteries. Am J Obstet Gynecol 156:889–893, 1987.
8. Trudinger BJ, Cook CM: Umbilical and uterine artery flow velocity waveforms in pregnancy associated with major fetal anomalies. Br J Obstet Gynaecol 92:666–670, 1985.
9. Chan FY, Woo SK, Ghosh A, Tang M, Lam C: Prenatal diagnosis of congenital fetal arrhythmias by simultaneous pulsed Doppler velocimetry of the fetal abdominal aorta and inferior vena cava. Obstet Gynecol 76:200–204, 1990.
10. Trudinger BJ, Cook CM, Jones L, Giles WB: A comparison of fetal heart rate monitoring and umbilical artery waveforms in the recognition of fetal compromise. Br J Obstet Gynecol 93:171–175, 1986.
11. Hackett GA, Campbell S, Gamsu H, Cohen-Overbeek T, Pearce JMF: Doppler studies in the growth retarded fetus and prediction of neonatal necrotizing enterocolitis, haemorrhage and neonatal morbidity. Br Med J 294:13–16, 1987.
12. Soothill PW, Nicolaides KH, Rodeck CH, Campbell S: Uteroplacental velocity resistance index and umbilical venous P_{O_2}, P_{CO_2}, pH, lactate and erythroblast count in growth retarded fetuses. Fetal Ther 41:1–4, 1987.
13. Nicolaides KH, Bilardo CM, Campbell S: Prediction of fetal anemia by measurement of the mean blood velocity in the fetal aorta. Am J Obstet Gynecol 162:209–212, 1990.
14. Vyas S, Nicolaides KH, Campbell: Doppler examination of the middle cerebral artery in anemic fetuses. Am J Obstet Gynecol 162:1066–1068, 1990.
15. Vogel M: "Morphology of placental dysfunction: contribution to the recognition of pathogenetic factors in intrauterine hypoxia and fetal growth retardation," in Braueen DL, Rappourt I, Wauer RR (eds), *Research in Perinatal Medicine.* Leipzig, Thieme, 1987, pp 292–299.
16. Arabin B: *Doppler Blood Flow Measurement in Uteroplacental and Fetal Vessels. Pathophysiology and Clinical Significance.* Berlin, Springer-Verlag, 1990.

17. Meschia G: "Techniques for the study of the uteroplacental circulation," in Rosenfeld CR (ed), *The Uterine Circulation*. Ithaca, New York, Perinatology Press, 1989, pp 35–51.

18. Gant NF, Worley RJ: "Measurement of uteroplacental blood flow in the human," in Rosenfeld CR (ed), *The Uterine Circulation*. Ithaca, New York, Perinatology Press, 1989, pp 53–73.

19. Stuart B, Drum J, Fitzgerald DE, Durigan NM: Fetal blood flow velocity waveform in normal pregnancy. Br J Obstet Gynaecol 87:780–785, 1980.

20. Schulman H, Fleischer A, Stern W, Farmakaides G, Jogani N, Blattner P: Umbilical velocity wave ratios in human pregnancy. Am J Obstet Gynecol 148:985–990, 1984.

21. Schulman H, Fleischer A, Farmakaides G, Bracero L, Rochelson B, Grunefeld L: Development of uterine artery compliance in pregnancy as detected by Doppler ultrasound. Am J Obstet Gynecol 155:1031–1036, 1986.

22. McCowan LM, Erskine LA, Ritchie K: Umbilical artery Doppler blood flow studies in the preterm small for gestational age fetus. Am J Obstet Gynecol 156:655–659, 1987.

23. Arduini D, Rizzo G: Normal values of pulsatility index from fetal vessels: a cross-sectional study on 1556 healthy fetuses. J Perinat Med 18:165–172, 1990.

24. Gudmundsson S, Fairlie F, Lingman G, Marsal K: Recording of blood flow velocity waveforms in the uteroplacental umbilical circulation: reproducibility study and comparison of pulsed and continuous wave Doppler ultrasonography. J Clin Ultrasound 18:97–101, 1990.

25. Campbell S, Pearce JMF, Hackett G, Cohen-Overbeek T, Hernandez C: Qualitative assessment of uteroplacental blood flow: early screening test for high risk pregnancies. Obstet Gynecol 68:649–653, 1986.

26. Fogarty P, Beattie B, Harper A, Dornan J: Continuous wave Doppler blood flow velocity waveforms from the umbilical artery in normal pregnancy. J Perinat Med 18:51–57, 1990.

27. Goldstein SR: Early detection of pathologic pregnancy by transvaginal sonography. J Clin Ultrasound 18:262–273, 1990.

28. Rempen A: Diagnosis of viability in early pregnancy with vaginal sonography. J Ultrasound Med 9:711–716, 1990.

29. Fleischer AC: Transvaginal sonography helps find ovarian cancer. Diagn Imaging 10:124–128, 1988.

30. Kurjak A, Zalud I, Alfirevic Z, Jurkovic D: The assessment of abnormal pelvic blood flow by transvaginal color and pulsed Doppler. Ultrasound Med Biol 16:437–442, 1990.

31. Bourne T, Campbell S, Steer C, Whitehead MI, Collins WP: Transvaginal color flow imaging: a possible new screening technique for ovarian cancer. Br Med J 299:1367–1370, 1989.

32. Thaler I, Manor D: Transvaginal imaging: applied physical principles and terms. J Clin Ultrasound 18:235–238, 1990.

33. Timor-Tritch IE, Farine D, Rosen MG: A close look at early embryonic development with the high frequency transvaginal transducer. Am J Obstet Gynecol 159:676–681, 1988.

34. King BF: "The functional anatomy of the placental vasculature," in Rosenfeld CR (ed), *The Uterine Circulation*. Ithaca, New York, Perinatology Press, 1989, pp 17–33.

35. Taylor KJW, Burns PN, Wells PNT, Conway D, Hull MGR: Ultrasound Doppler flow studies of the ovarian and uterine arteries. Br J Obstet Gynaecol 92:240–246, 1985.

36. Thaler I, Manor D, Rottem S, Timor-Tritch IE, Brandes IM, Itskovitz J: Hemodynamic evaluation of the female pelvic vessels using a high-frequency transvaginal image-directed Doppler system. J Clin Ultrasound 18:364–369, 1990.

37. Campbell S, Griffin DR, Pearce JM, Diaz-Recasans J, Cohen-Overbeek TE, Willson K, Teague MJ: New Doppler technique for assessing uteroplacental blood flow. Lancet 1:675–677, 1983.

38. Trudinger BJ, Giles WB, Cook CM, Bombardieri J, Collins L: Fetal umbilical artery flow velocity waveforms and placental resistance: clinical significance. Br J Obstet Gynecol 92:23–30, 1985.

39. Jacobson SL, Imhof R, Manning N, Mannion V, Little D, Rey E, Redman C: The value of Doppler assessment of the uteroplacental circulation in predicting preeclampsia or intrauterine growth retardation. Am J Obstet Gynecol 162:110–114, 1990.

40. Erskine RLA, Ritchie JWK: Umbilical artery blood flow characteristics in normal and growth retarded fetuses. Br J Obstet Gynecol 92:605–610, 1985.
41. Brosens I.: Morphological changes in the utero-placental bed in pregnancy hypertension. Clin Obstet Gynecol 4:573–593, 1977.
42. Brosens I, Robertson WB, Dixon HG: The physiological response of the vessels of the placental bed to normal pregnancy. J Pathol Bacteriol 93:569–579, 1967.
43. DeWolf F, DeWolf-Peeters C, Brosens I: Ultrastructure of the spiral arteries in the human placental bed at the end of normal pregnancy. Am J Obstet Gynecol 117:833–848, 1973.
44. Pearce JM: "Uteroplacental and fetal blood flow," in Whittle MJ (ed), *Clinical Obstetrics and Gynaecology, Fetal Monitoring.* Eastbourne, Bailliere's, 1987, p 175.
45. Gudmundsson S, Marsal K: Umbilical and uteroplacental blood flow velocity waveforms in pregnancies with fetal growth retardation. Eur J Obstet Gynecol Reprod Biol 27:187–196, 1988.
46. Ruissen CJ, van Vugt JMG, De Haan J: Variability of P.I. calculations. Eur J Obstet Gynecol Reprod Biol 27:213–220, 1988.
47. Arduini D, Rizzo G, Boccolini MR, Romanini C, Mancuso S: Functional assessment of utero-placental and fetal circulations by means of color Doppler ultrasonography. J Ultrasound Med 9:249–253, 1990.
48. Chambers SE, Johnstone FD, Muir BB, Hoskins P, Hadda NG, McDicken WN: The effects of placental site on the arcuate artery flow velocity waveform. J Ultrasound Med 7:671–673, 1988.
49. Deutinger J, Rudelsdorfer R, Bernaschek G: Vaginosonographic velocimetry of both main uterine arteries by visual vessel recognition and pulsed Doppler method during pregnancy. Am J Obstet Gynecol 159:1072–1076, 1988.
50. Stabile I, Campbell S, Grudzinskas J: Doppler assessed uteroplacental blood flow impedance in the first trimester: physiologic variation with site of measurement. J Obstet Gynaecol 9:177–180, 1989.
51. Den Ouden M, Cohen-Overbeek TE, Wladimiroff JW: Uterine and fetal umbilical artery flow velocity waveforms in normal first trimester pregnancies. Br J Obstet Gynaecol 97:716–719, 1990.
52. Alfirevic Z, Kurjak A: Transvaginal colour Doppler ultrasound in normal and abnormal early pregnancy. J Perinat Med 18:173–180, 1990.
53. Kurjak A, Alfirevic Z, Miljan M: Conventional and color Doppler in the assessment of fetal and maternal circulation. Ultrasound Med Biol 14:337–354, 1988.
54. Zalud I, Kurjak A: The assessment of luteal blood flow in pregnant and non-pregnant women by transvaginal color Doppler. J Perinat Med 18:215–221, 1990.
55. Itskovitz J: "Maternal-fetal hemodynamics," in Maulik D, McNellis D (eds), *Doppler Ultrasound Measurement of Maternal-Fetal Hemodynamics.* Ithaca, New York, Perinatology Press, 1987, pp 13–42.
56. Oosterhof H, Aarnoudse JG: Placental abruption preceded by abnormal flow velocity waveforms in the uterine arteries. Br J Obstet Gynecol 98:225–226, 1991.
57. Stabile I, Bilardo C, Panella M, Campbell S, Grudzinkas C: Doppler assessed uterine blood flow in the first trimester of pregnancy. Trophoblast Res 3:301–308, 1988.
58. Kurjak A, Jurkovic D, Alfirevic Z, Zalud I: Transvaginal color Doppler imaging. J Clin Ultrasound 18:227–234, 1990.
59. Kurjak A, Breyer B, Jurkovic D, Alfirevic Z, Miljan M: Color flow mapping in obstetrics. J Perinat Med 15:271–280, 1987.
60. Jaffe R, Warsof SL: Transvaginal color Doppler imaging in the assessment of utero-placental blood flow in the normal first trimester pregnancy. Am J Obstet Gynecol 164:781–785, 1991.

UTEROPLACENTAL BLOOD FLOW ASSESSMENT IN EARLY PREGNANCY FAILURE

RICHARD JAFFE

The introduction of high-frequency transvaginal transducers has greatly improved the accuracy of sonographic diagnosis of early gestations and its complications.[1]

Over the past several years transabdominal real-time ultrasonography and Doppler velocimetry have been extensively used to assess the uteroplacental circulation in normal and abnormal second trimester gestations (Chap. 3). However, before the introduction of transvaginal sonography Doppler flow studies of early gestation were rare because of technical difficulties and low reproducibility. Among the problems were inability to discretely visualize pelvic vessels and the distance between the abdominal wall and the region being evaluated. With the incorporation of color Doppler capabilities into the transvaginal transducer, our assessment of early uteroplacental circulation has entered a new phase in which the physiologic development of the early uteroplacental circulation can be studied. The ability to assess the functional integrity of this circulation is an important step toward better understanding of the normal first trimester gestational development and the role of the circulation in the pathophysiology of early pregnancy failure.

In the normal first trimester pregnancy color Doppler flow studies have demonstrated that flow velocity waveforms of trophoblastic vessels show common characteristics of low resistance to flow with a prominent diastolic component (Fig. 5-1).[2–4] This appears to allow considerable flow to the trophoblast during the entire cardiac cycle assuring large supply of oxygen and nutrients to the developing embryo. Major deviations from this pattern will probably lead to obstetrical complications.

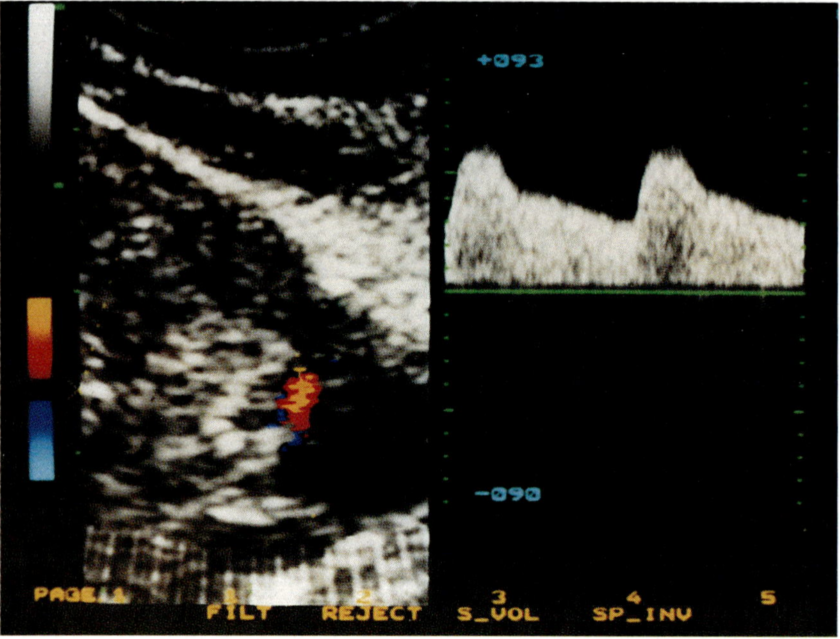

Figure 5-1   The detection of subtrophoblastic flow by color Doppler imaging in a 5-week gestation. *(Printed with permission from Jaffe R, Warsof SL: Transvaginal color Doppler imaging in the assessment of uteroplacental blood flow in the normal first-trimester pregnancy. Am J Obstet Gynecol 164:781–785, 1991.)*

Chapter 4 deals with the evaluation of the uteroplacental circulation in early normal pregnancies. In this chapter we address the subject of Doppler flow studies in early intrauterine pregnancy failure.

MISSED ABORTION AND BLIGHTED OVUM

The transabdominal and transvaginal ultrasonographic criteria for an abnormal intrauterine gestational sac were described by Nyberg et al.[5] These criteria included a gestational sac >20 mm in diameter without a yolk sac or >25 mm in diameter without an embryo. On the basis of these criteria a blighted ovum was diagnosed and was further described as an anembryonic gestation. In contrast, a missed abortion is usually defined as a gestation with a nonviable embryo where there is no detectable fetal cardiac activity. Some studies have shown that chromosomal abnormalities were found more frequently in the early failures defined as blighted ova by the previously described criteria.[6]

With the introduction of transvaginal ultrasonography the ability to get a closer look at the developing gestational sac and embryo has several applications in the assessment of early pregnancy failure and possible determination of future pregnancy outcome. We now understand that in many cases the ultrasonic image of an empty sac is due to a resorption process of a nonviable embryo. Therefore, the most important factor in making a sonographic diagnosis will be the time in the abortion process that the study is performed.

Even though transvaginal sonography has greatly improved the visualization of the early products of conception, the classic criteria for defining blighted ova and missed abortions are still valid and the only ones accepted for effective ultrasonographic differentiation between missed abortions and blighted ova. Different etiologic mechanisms have been suggested to explain early pregnancy failure. These include chromosomal abnormalities, poor implantation, and faulty vascularization of the developing gestational sac.[7]

The advent of color Doppler imaging in combination with vaginal sonography has extended the use of ultrasound imaging to the functional evaluation of the uteroplacental circulation. With this technique small vessels beneath the trophoblast are visualized (Fig. 5-1), and the different flow velocity waveforms derived from uterine, arcuate, and spiral arteries can be evaluated.

As already mentioned, the incidence of structural chromosomal abnormalities is significantly increased with blighted ova.[6] Some chromosomally abnormal embryos, however, will develop long enough to be imaged by transvaginal ultrasound and will potentially be defined as missed abortion when cardiac activity has been lost. Poor or faulty vascularization at the site of implantation and

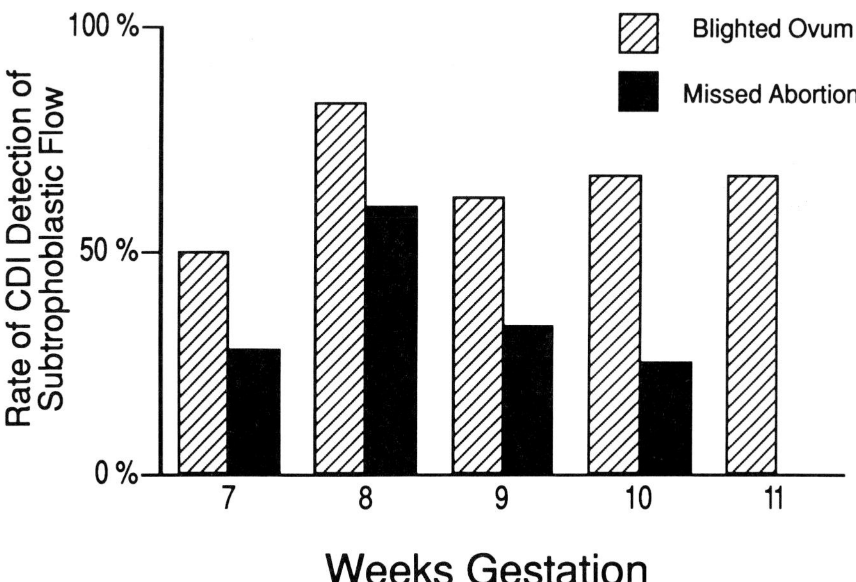

Figure 5-2   Demonstration of the rate of detection of subtrophoblastic flow by CDI in blighted ova and missed abortions.

developing placenta will lead to the death of the developing embryo at different stages, depending on the severity of the circulatory problem. In chromosomally abnormal gestations the trophoblast will often develop even though there is no viable embryo. The early development of the uteroplacental circulation is probably hormone-dependent and therefore is not immediately affected by a chromosomally defective product of conception. A study by the authors confirmed the fact that normal-appearing high diastolic flow was detected more frequently in cases defined as blighted ova as compared with those defined as missed abortion (Figs. 5-2 and 5-3).[8]

This has been demonstrated in other studies as well.[3] The same study[8] also revealed the fact that flow was detected by color Doppler imaging (CDI) in all cases with an abnormal karyotype, possibly pointing to the fact that in these pregnancies the basic problem does not affect the circulation during the early stages of the process. The assessment of the blood flow velocity waveforms derived from cases of early pregnancy failure have also shown that the resistance to flow was lower in blighted ova as compared with that in missed abortions.[9] The mean value of the resistance index (RI) in normal pregnancies was found to be 0.63[2] with very similar values for the abnormal gestations in cases with detected flow by CDI (Fig. 5-4). When the indices of the abnormal gestations were distributed around a cutoff point of a RI of 0.63, most cases of blighted

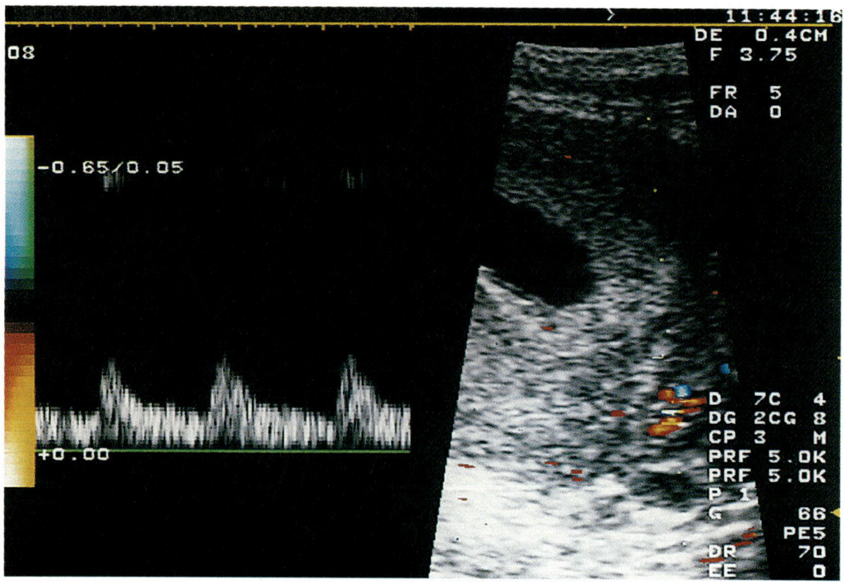

A

Figure 5-3 Detection of trophoblastic flow in two cases of blighted ova (*A, B*) and a missed abortion (*C*). (*Part A is printed with permission from Jaffe R, Warsof SL: Color Doppler imaging in the assessment of uteroplacental blood flow in abnormal intrauterine first trimester pregnancies: an attempt to define etiological mechanisms. J Ultrasound Med 11:41–44, 1992. Part C is printed courtesy of Acuson Ltd, Mountain View, California.*)

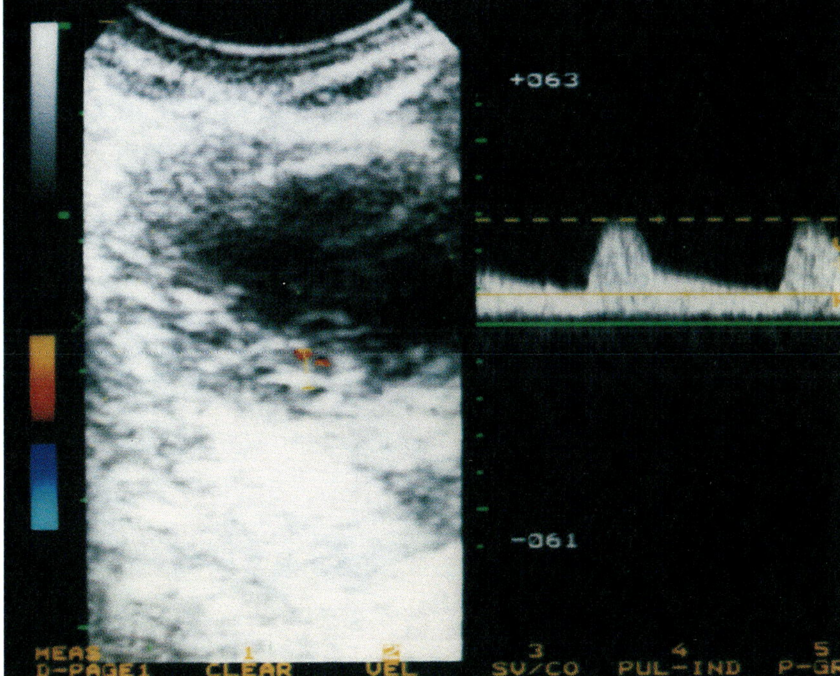

B

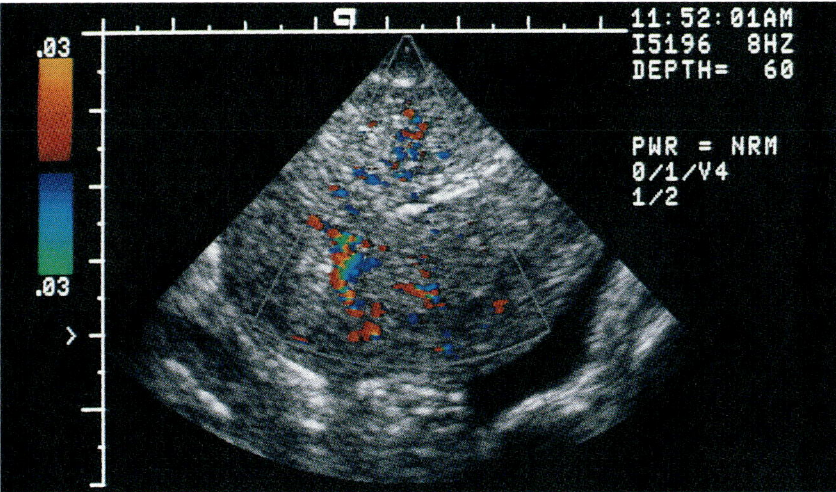

C

Figure 5-3 (*Continued*).

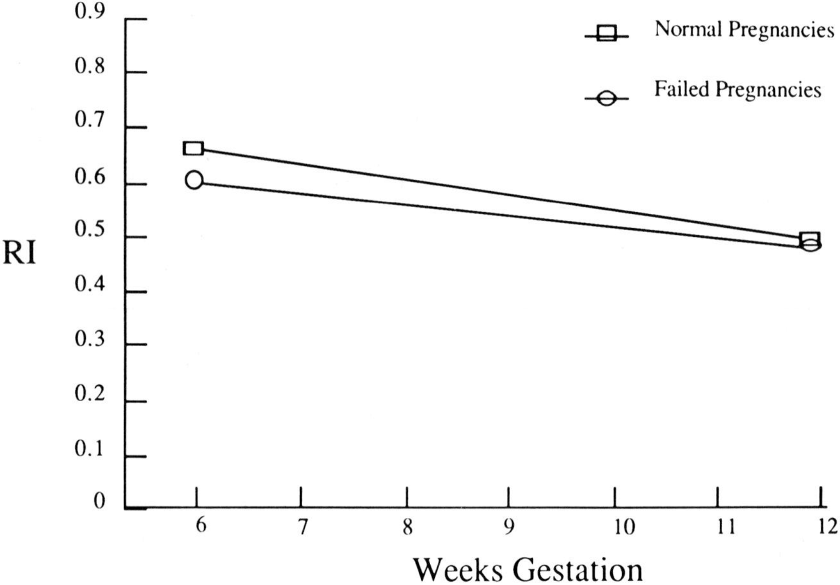

Figure 5-4 Depiction of the RI in early normal and abnormal pregnancies. The calculated RI from early pregnancy failure with detected flow demonstrates values very similar to normal pregnancies with same gestational age.

ovum had indices below that value, whereas the missed abortions had values above it[9] (Table 5-1).

The clear advantage of color Doppler imaging over conventional Doppler is the shorter examination time and the ability to detect flow in vessels too small to recognize on real-time gray scale imaging. The first step in any color Doppler evaluation is the two-dimensional real-time imaging of the gestational sac. When the color system is initiated, color signals will appear in all vessels with flow.

Table 5-1 Distribution of detected flow and calculated RI with a cutoff point of ≤0.63

Detected flow RI ≤ 0.63	Blighted ova (group A)	Missed abortion (group B)
Yes	22	2
No	3	8
Total	25	10

Note: Sensitivity = 88 percent; specificity = 80 percent; positive predictive value = 91.6 percent; negative predictive value = 72.7 percent.

Once a clear color signal is identified, the sample volume of the pulsed Doppler system is directed toward the area of interest. The external and internal iliac arteries are easily identified by their anatomic location and pattern of high resistance with absent diastolic flow (Chap. 4). The uterine arteries are clearly identified along the lateral wall of the uterine cervix and are the only arterial vessels in this area with flow directed cranially (Fig. 5-5).

A hyperechoic area within close proximity of the gestational sac represents the developing trophoblast. In very early gestations this area may surround the whole sac, whereas later on it will be confined to the site of the developing placenta. Color signals from this area, or close to it, will represent subtrophoblastic flow (Fig. 5-1). Flow velocity waveforms from iliac, uterine, and arcuate arteries at the early stages of pregnancy will show characteristics of high pulsatility and no diastolic flow. On the other hand, subtrophoblastic vessels will demonstrate low pulsatility and continuous forward flow during diastole (Fig. 5-6).

The reproducibility of Doppler flow studies has been questioned by several authors. It has been shown that the site of measurement is of great importance because of significant differences in flow velocities obtained from placental and nonplacental sides.[10,11] With color Doppler imaging the precise site of measurement can be defined, and reproducibility of flow velocity waveform analysis will increase significantly.[12]

Bleeding in early pregnancy is a common clinical finding. It has been postulated that if a living embryo is demonstrated on a sonographic examination, the chances of the pregnancy to continue uneventfully are great (85 to 90 percent) and highly dependent on maternal age. Regardless, first trimester uterine bleeding is often an alarming sign preceding early failure, whether it is a blighted ovum or a missed abortion.

Functional assessment of uteroplacental circulation has given us some insight into the development of the normal vascularization of early pregnancy. Initial color Doppler studies of this circulation in abnormal intrauterine first trimester gestations have shown that flow velocity waveforms can be obtained from subtrophoblastic vessels in these pregnancies.[3,8,9] Although the number of cases studied are small and there are no prospective studies of early gestations that eventually fail, this method has given us some indication to the pathophysiology of early pregnancy failure. Hopefully, the understanding of the development of the uteroplacental circulation in normal gestations and the changes occurring in early failures will help us better understand the pathophysiology behind the occurrence of missed abortions and blighted ova.

TROPHOBLASTIC DISEASE

Trophoblastic disease is a general term for a group of disorders that have in common the abnormal development of the trophoblast. The group includes the hydatiform mole, invasive mole, choriocarcinoma, and placental site trophoblastic

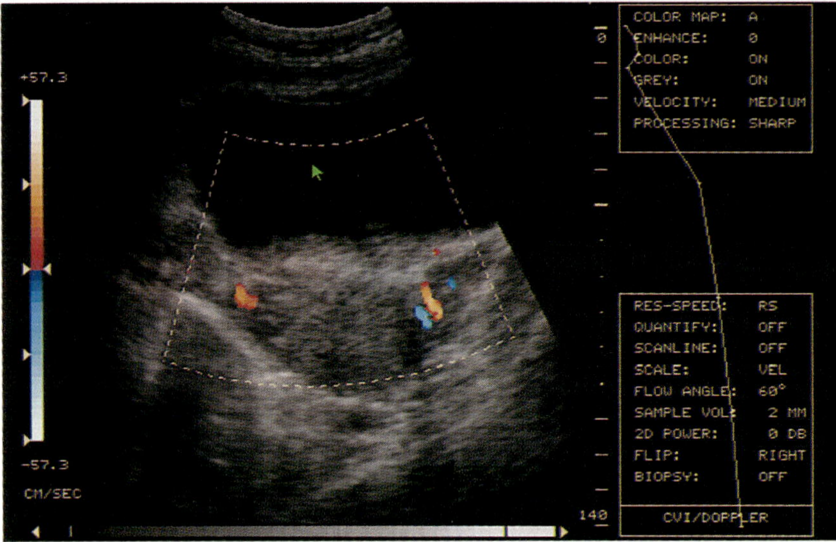

Figure 5-5 Transverse (*A*) and longitudinal (*B*) view of the nonpregnant uterus showing the clear identification of the uterine arteries by CDI. There is no flow detected within the myometrium in a normal nonpregnant uterus.

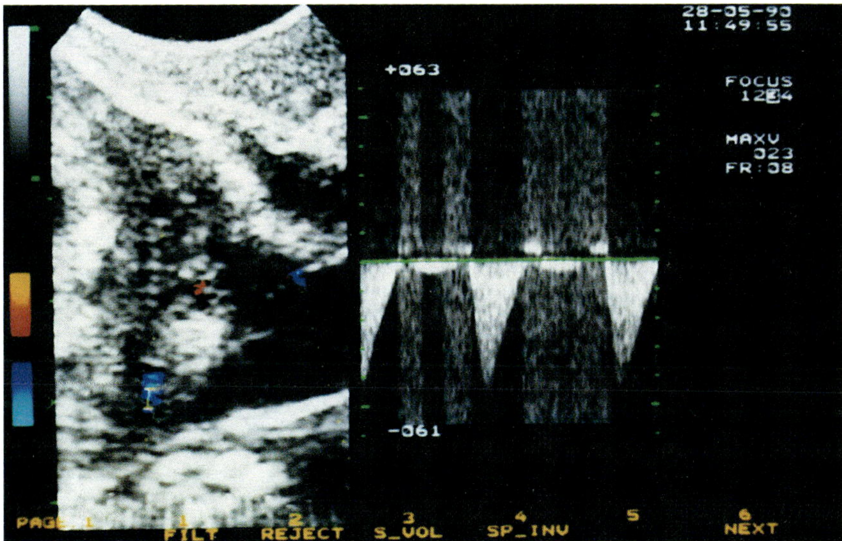

A

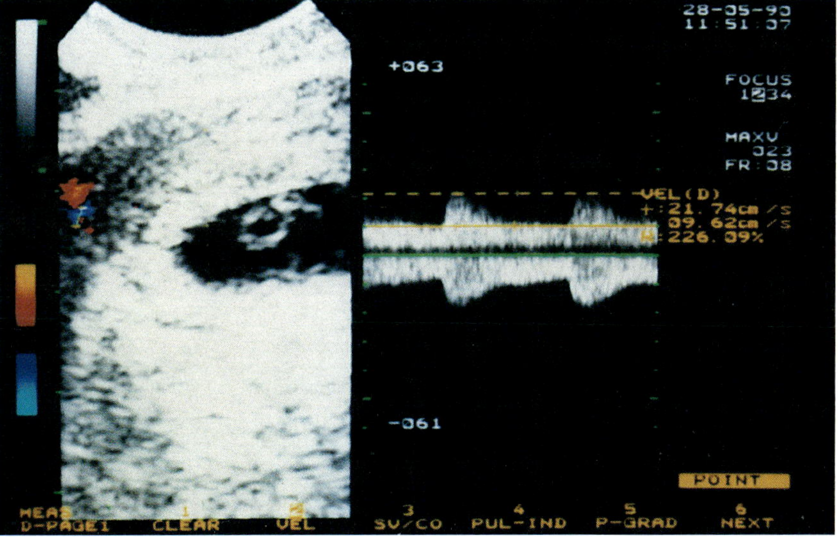

B

Figure 5-6   The flow velocity waveforms from the uterine artery (*A*) and trophoblastic flow (*B*) in a 7-week-old pregnancy. The different characteristics of the waveforms are clearly noted with absent flow during diastole in the uterine artery as compared with a high diastolic component in the trophoblastic vessels *(Printed with permission from Jaffe R, Warsof SL: Transvaginal color Doppler imaging in the assessment of uteroplacental blood flow in the normal first-trimester pregnancy. Am J Obstet Gynecol 164:781–785, 1991.)*

tumor.[13] As a result of the proliferation of the trophoblastic tissue and its invasion of the endometrium and myometrium, the uterine circulation undergoes significant changes. The uterine vasculature proliferates with the development of abundant small vessels that penetrate the invading trophoblast. The hypervascularity transforms the uterus into a low-impedance organ with significant changes in flow patterns of the uterine arteries and its branches. Before the advent of ultrasonography, pelvic angiography was an important tool in the diagnosis of trophoblastic disease.[14,15] The introduction of ultrasonography has given us a noninvasive method for evaluation of the uterus. Ultrasonography is today an established mean for the diagnosis of the presence of abnormal trophoblastic tissue.[16–18] With the introduction of CDI, small vessels with low-velocity flows can be visualized. The use of conventional pulsed Doppler and CDI in the diagnosis of trophoblastic disease has been described[19–20] (Fig. 5-7). In the normal nonpregnant uterus intramyometrial vasculature is usually not demonstrated by CDI, and only the main branches of the uterine artery can be seen (Fig. 5-5). In the normal uterus flow velocity waveforms cannot be obtained from the myometrium by either pulsed Doppler or CDI. In the event of trophoblastic disease that has invaded the myometrium, CDI will show increased vascularity within the walls of the myometrium (Fig. 5-7). The flow velocity waveforms obtained from these vessels will show low resistance to flow, a pattern similar to that of a normal pregnancy, with a significant diastolic component (Fig. 5-7), a finding not detected in a normal nonpregnant uterus. The degree of blood vessel penetration has been shown to correlate with other clinical and pathologic features of the disease as

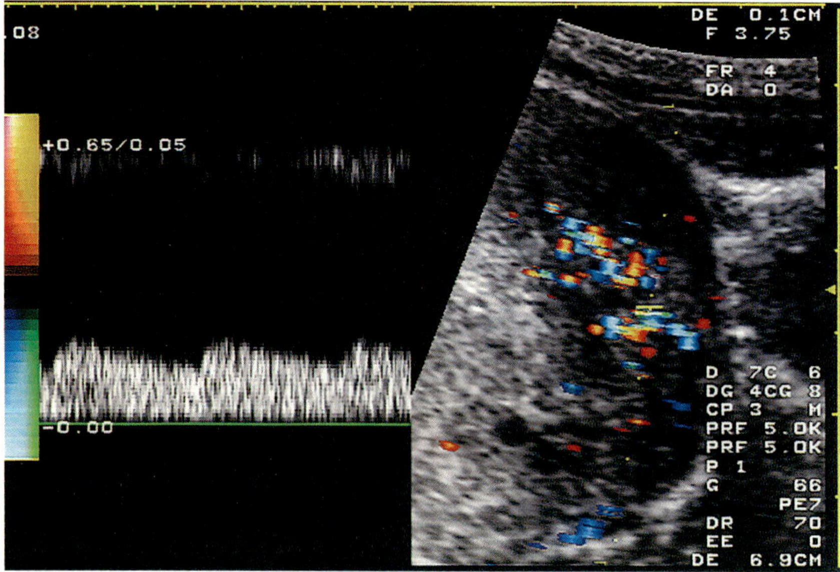

Figure 5-7 Hypervascularization in the uterus of a patient with an invasive mole following a normal gestation.

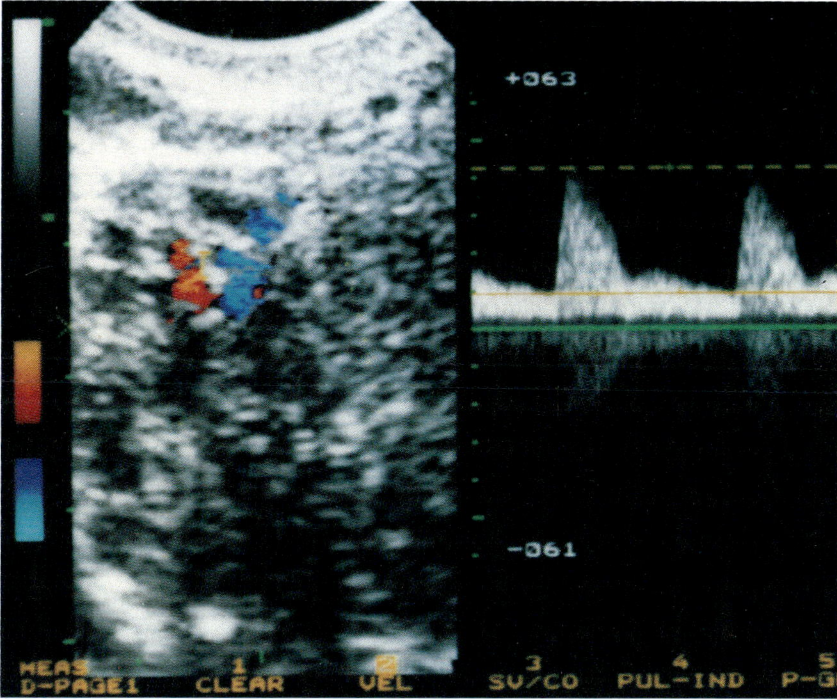

Figure 5-8   Abundant trophoblastic tissue detected by CDI following an incomplete pregnancy termination.

well as with the success of medical or surgical treatment. The area of increased vascularity can be measured, and success or failure of medical treatment can be evaluated with successive CDI examinations[20] in conjunction with serum β-hCG (human chorionic gonadotropin) levels.

Viable trophoblastic tissue can also be present in the uterus following an early abortion not completed by a curettage or after an incomplete curettage for early pregnancy termination (Fig. 5-8). In these cases the real-time gray scale image is often inconclusive, and CDI can be of great importance in the evaluation of the extent of the residual tissue and its disappearance following uterine curettage.

Conventional Doppler and CDI are important noninvasive techniques that have modified our approach to trophoblastic disease. Even though β-hCG is still essential in the diagnosis and follow-up of trophoblastic disease,[21] the Doppler techniques have given us an additional parameter to consider before medical treatment or surgery are instituted.

REFERENCES

1. Goldstein SR: Early detection of pathologic pregnancy by transvaginal sonography. J Clin Ultrasound 18:262–273, 1990.

2. Jaffe R, Warsof SL: Transvaginal color Doppler imaging in the assessment of utero-placental blood flow in the normal first trimester pregnancy. Am J Obstet Gynecol 164:781–785, 1991.

3. Alfirevic Z, Kurjak A: Transvaginal colour Doppler ultrasound in normal and abnormal early pregnancy. J Perinat Med 18:173–180, 1990.

4. Jurkovic D, Jauniaux E, Kurjak A, Hustin J, Campbell S, Nicolaides KH: Transvaginal color Doppler assessment of the uteroplacental circulation in early pregnancy. Obstet Gynecol 77:365–369, 1991.

5. Nyberg DA, Filly RA, Filho DLD, Laing FC, Mahony BS: Abnormal pregnancy: early diagnosis by US and serum chorionic gonadotropin levels. Radiology 158:393–396, 1986.

6. Dewald GW, Michels VV: Recurrent miscarriages: cytogenetic causes and genetic counseling of affected families. Clin Obstet Gynecol 29:865–885, 1986.

7. Pritchard JA, MacDonald PC, Gant N: *Williams Obstetrics,* 17th ed. Norwalk, Connecticut, Appleton-Century-Crofts, 1985, p 467.

8. Jaffe R, Warsof SL: Color Doppler imaging in the assessment of utero-placental blood flow in abnormal first trimester intrauterine pregnancies: an attempt to define etiologic mechanism. J Ultrasound Med 11:41–44, 1992.

9. Jaffe R, Warsof SL: Color Doppler imaging and blood flow velocity waveform analysis of subtrophoblastic vessels in early pregnancy failure. Submitted for publication.

10. Arabin B: "Doppler blood flow measurements in normal pregnancy," in Arabin B (ed), *Doppler Blood Flow Measurement in Uteroplacental and Fetal Vessels. Pathophysiology and Clinical Significance.* Berlin, Springer-Verlag, 1990, pp 37–60.

11. Den Ouden M, Cohen-Overbeek TE, Wladimiroff JW: Uterine and fetal umbilical artery flow velocity waveforms in normal first trimester pregnancies. Br J Obstet Gynaecol 97:716–719, 1990.

12. Arduini D, Rizzo G, Boccolini MR, Romanini C, Mancuso S: Functional assessment of utero-placental and fetal circulations by means of color Doppler ultrasonography. J Ultrasound Med 9:249–253, 1990.

13. Driscoll SG: Gestational trophoblastic neoplasia: surgical pathologic considerations with clinical emphasis. Clin Obstet Gynecol 27:160–171, 1984.

14. Brewis RAL, Bagshawe KD: Pelvic arteriography in invasive trophoblastic neoplasia. Br J Radiol 41:481–495, 1968.

15. Hata H, Sasaki K, Nakano R: Pelvic angiography in malignant trophoblastic disease. Gynecol Obstet Invest 23:28–33, 1987.

16. Munyer TP, Callen PW, Filly RA: Further observations in the sonographic spectrum of gestational trophoblastic disease. J Clin Ultrasound 9:349–358, 1981.

17. Sherer DM, Allen T, Woods J, Jr: Transvaginal sonographic diagnosis of a hydatidiform mole occurring two weeks after curettage for an incomplete abortion. J Clin Ultrasound 19:224–226, 1991.

18. Sakamoto C, Oikawa K, Kashimura M, Egashira K: Sonographic appearance of placental site trophoblastic tumor. J Ultrasound Med 9:533–535, 1990.

19. Long MG, Boultbee JE, Begent RHJ, Hanson ME, Bagshawe KD: Preliminary Doppler studies on the uterine artery and myometrium in trophoblastic tumours requiring chemotherapy. Br J Obstet Gynaecol 97:686–689, 1990.

20. Aoki S, Hata T, Hata K, Senoh D, Miyako J, Takamiya O, Iwanari O, Kitao M: Doppler color flow mapping of an invasive mole. Gynecol Obstet Invest 27:52–54, 1989.

21. Morrow CP: Postmolar trophoblastic disease: diagnosis, management, and prognosis. Clin Obstet Gynecol 27:211–220, 1984.

22. Schiff E, Ben-Baruch G, Moran O, Yahal I, Oelsner G, Mashiach S, Menczer J: Prediction of residual trophoblastic tissue in first-trimester abortions and low levels of human chorionic gonadotropin β-subunit. Am J Obstet Gynecol 162:797–801, 1990.

ULTRASOUND ASSESSMENT OF ECTOPIC PREGNANCY

ASIM KURJAK
IVICA ZALUD

Ectopic pregnancy is still an important problem in clinical practice. Despite the introduction of modern diagnostic methods such as ultrasonography and rapid and specific β-human chorionic gonadotropin (β-hCG) assay, which lead to early surgical intervention, ectopic gestation is still a major cause of maternal mortality in the first trimester of pregnancy. The true incidence is difficult to determine, but the reports indicate that during the last 15 years there has been a marked increase in ectopic gestations. The basic reason for the increase in the rate of ectopic gestation is the fact that more adolescent girls are sexually active, and with this come sexually transmitted diseases as well as pregnancy. The micro-organisms indirectly causing ectopic pregnancy are usually the *Chlamydia* and *Neisseria* gonorrhea, although other microbes may be implicated in the resulting salpingitis.[1] For this reason it is very important to consider ectopic pregnancy in the differential diagnosis of a teenager presenting with abdominal pains and irregular vaginal bleeding. The chance of recurrence varies from 5 to 20 percent.[1] In general, the likelihood of ectopic pregnancy increases with previous tubal disease, ectopic pregnancy, or induced abortion. Intrauterine devices do not prevent ectopic pregnancy from occurring. Some women with a previous ectopic pregnancy develop problems of infertility and will never deliver a living child. According to Curran's projection, by the year 2000 at least 10 percent of all females of reproductive age will become involuntarily sterile as a result of the sequelae of pelvic inflammatory disease and more than 3 percent will experience an ectopic gestation.[2] Ongoing improvements and results of in vitro fertilization programs should not diminish efforts to improve prevention, diagnosis, and treatment of ectopic pregnancy.

TRANSABDOMINAL ULTRASOUND

Early diagnosis of any ectopic pregnancy still remains a challenge. Although diagnostic ultrasound has recently played an increasing role in the assessment of patients suspected of having an ectopic pregnancy, its major role has been to exclude an intrauterine gestation in patients confirmed to be pregnant by biochemical tests.[3–9] The sonographic findings that may be encountered in patients with ectopic pregnancy are divided into those that are considered diagnostic and those that are thought to be suggestive. The diagnostic signs are absence of an intrauterine sac bordered by two layers of decidua, extrauterine and extraovarian adnexal masses, fetal heartbeats, and motion outside the uterus. The suggestive features of ectopic pregnancy are an enlarged uterus with thick, echogenic endometrium in the case of an unruptured extrauterine pregnancy (decidual reaction) and blood or organized clots in the cul-de-sac or pericolic recesses in the case of ruptured ectopic pregnancies. The transabdominal sonographic diagnosis of an ectopic pregnancy can be made with greater confidence if more than one sonographic sign is present (Figs. 6-1 to 6-4).

Because the size of the ectopic pregnancy can be small (less than 1 cm), its sonographic detection as an adnexal mass is variable. In most patients with an unruptured ectopic pregnancy, an adnexal mass separate from the ovary that has a small anechoic center can be identified. Rarely, fetal heart motion of a live

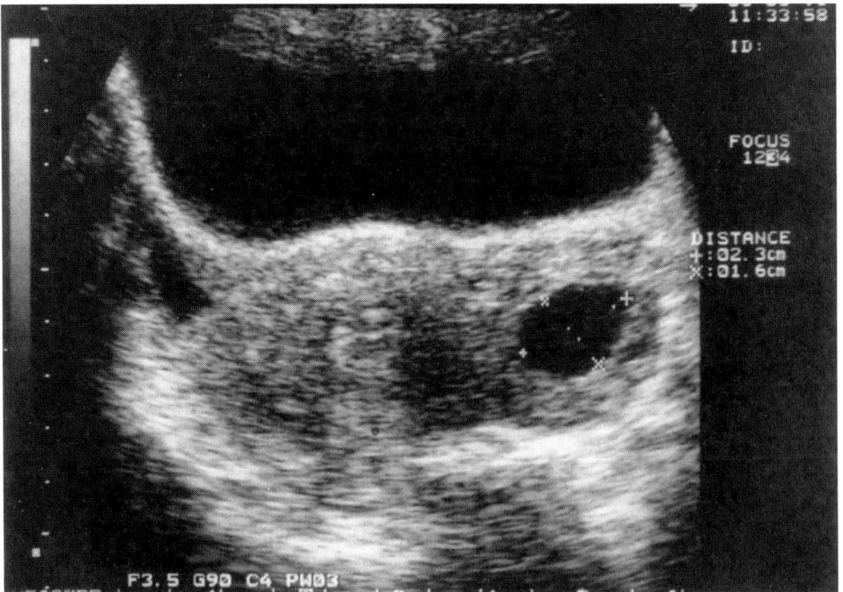

Figure 6-1 Transabdominal ultrasound findings in the case of an ectopic pregnancy. Empty uterus with a decidual reaction and an ectopic gestational sac detected in the left fallopian tube.

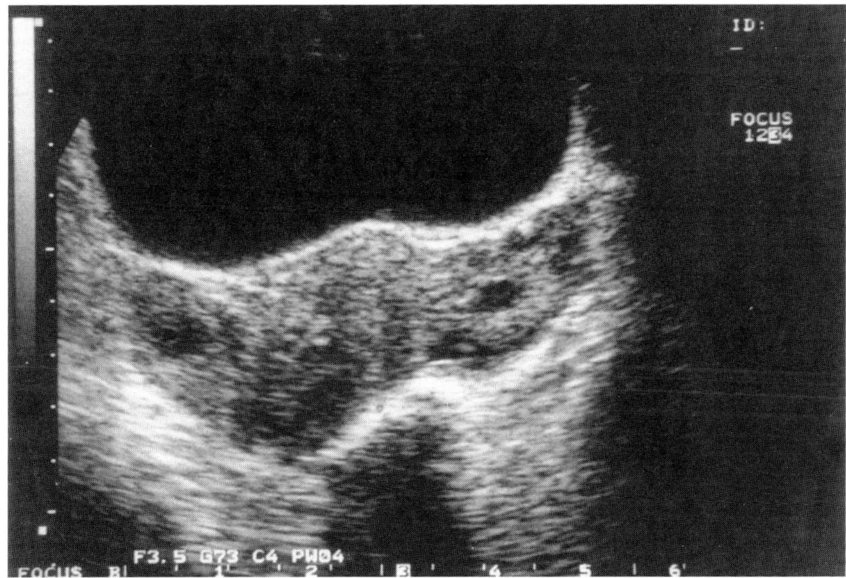

Figure 6-2 A typical B-mode example of an ectopic pregnancy. A gestational sac was visualized in the left fallopian tube and a corpus luteum in the right ovary. Free fluid was detected in the pouch of Douglas.

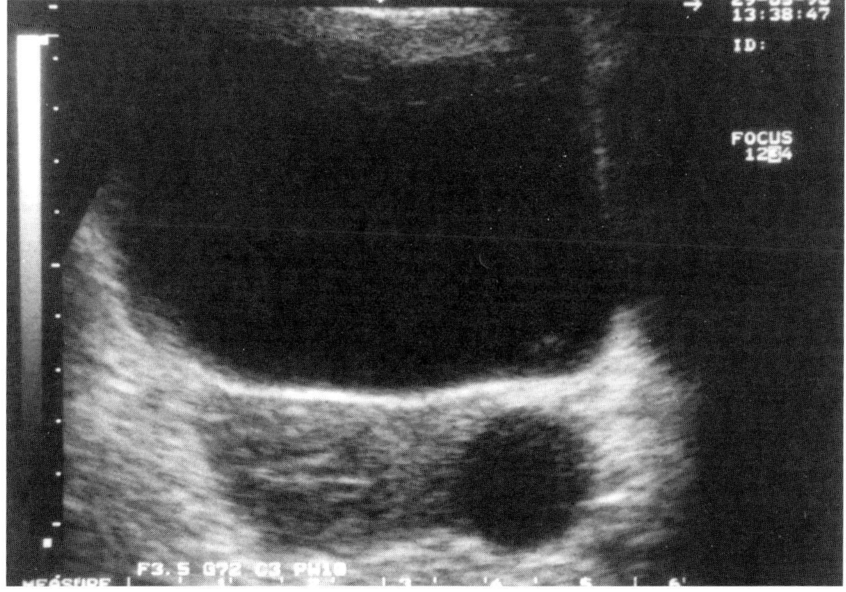

Figure 6-3 Empty uterus and cyst in the left adnexal region. Nonspecific ultrasonic features of ectopic pregnancy. These findings can be of different etiologies.

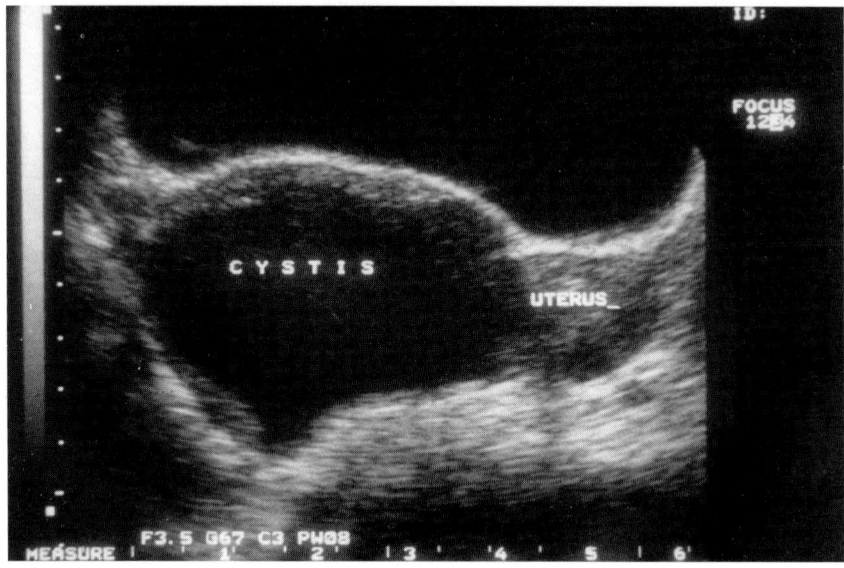

Figure 6-4 Another example of nonspecific ultrasonic findings in the case of a suspected ectopic pregnancy. However, hydrosalpinges was found on laparoscopy.

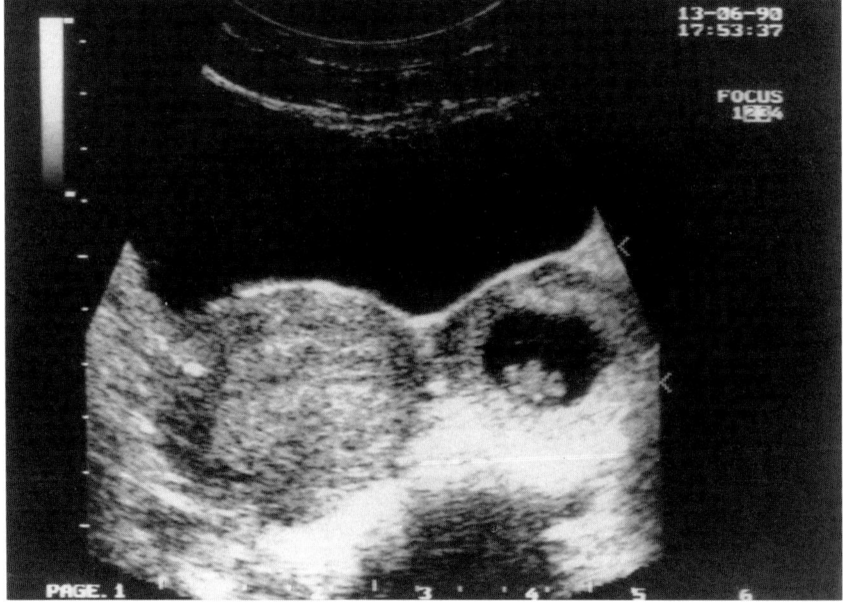

Figure 6-5 An abdominal ultrasound of a 7-week gestation with an embryo in a tubal sac. Fetal heartbeats were detected.

fetus can be detected within the ectopic gestational sac (Fig. 6-5). In addition, the uterus in a patient with an ectopic pregnancy typically has an hyperechoic endometrium, a sign of a decidual thickening associated with ectopic pregnancy. This finding is described as a ''pseudogestational sac.'' In contrast to the two concentric rings of decidua identified in an early intrauterine pregnancy, the decidual ring of an ectopic pregnancy has only one layer of decidua. A double decidual sac can occasionally be mimicked by separation of the decidua from the myometrium prior to expulsion of a decidual cast associated with an ectopic pregnancy. A double decidual sac can also be encountered in patients with an incomplete abortion. Furthermore, some of the patients with a single decidual layer have a viable intrauterine pregnancy. Obviously, pseudogestational sacs may be a source of a false diagnosis, both positive and negative. The sonographic detection of the double decidua is highly dependent on the resolution of the scanner used and the scanning ability and experience of the individual performing the examination.

TRANSVAGINAL ULTRASOUND

High-frequency transvaginal probes with better resolution generate higher quality images than traditional abdominal probes. The improved images obtained involve all the target organs and spaces which are scanned in the workup of an ectopic pregnancy.[10–18] The detection of an intrauterine gestational sac can be achieved by the transvaginal approach earlier (as early as 16 days postconception) and easier than by the transabdominal route. When using a transabdominal probe, one may find it difficult to differentiate a pseudogestational sac from a true gestational sac. Employing transvaginal sonography, these echoes were found to originate from local blood clots or from a central sonolucent area outlined by a thick endometrium. If an intrauterine gestation cannot be identified, one should proceed to scan the fallopian tubes (Fig. 6-6 to 6-8).

The fallopian tube may be identified if outlined by fluid or if its lumen contains a fluid phase. The diagnosis of tubal pregnancy by transvaginal ultrasound can be based on three different characteristic patterns.[10] The first depends on the capability of transvaginal ultrasound to recognize gestational structures in the fallopian tube using the same criteria as in an intrauterine pregnancy. Therefore, one may rely on the detection of structures such as a gestational sac, yolk sac, or embryo within the fallopian tube when making the diagnosis. The second pattern is based on the recognition of a fallopian tube containing an amorphous content. At surgery this content is usually found to be composed of blood clots and gestational material. The third pattern is based on indirect signs such as an empty uterus, a positive serum β-hCG test, and detection of blood and/or clots in the cul-de-sac. Rottem et al. have found the first pattern in nearly 50 percent of investigated suspected ectopic pregnancies, the second pattern in nearly 40

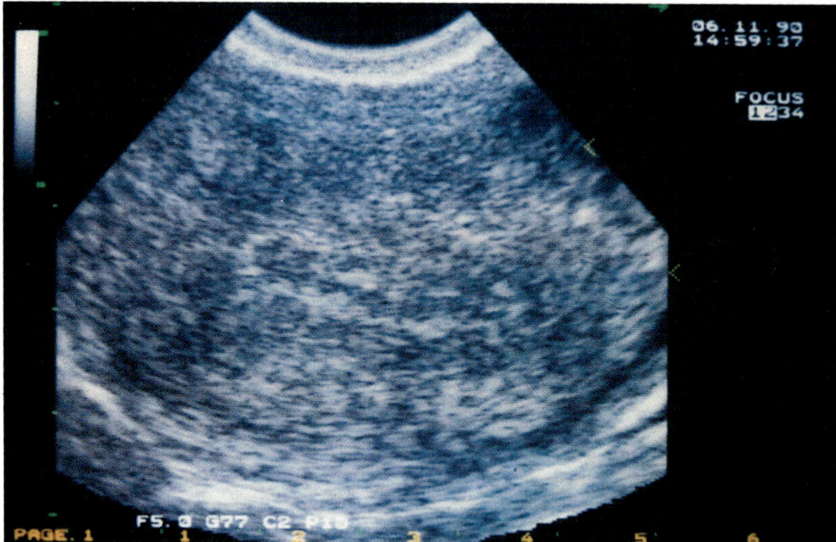

Figure 6-6 Transvaginal scan of empty uterus in the case of a suspected ectopic pregnancy. The decidual reaction is clearly visualized and should not be mistaken for a gestational sac.

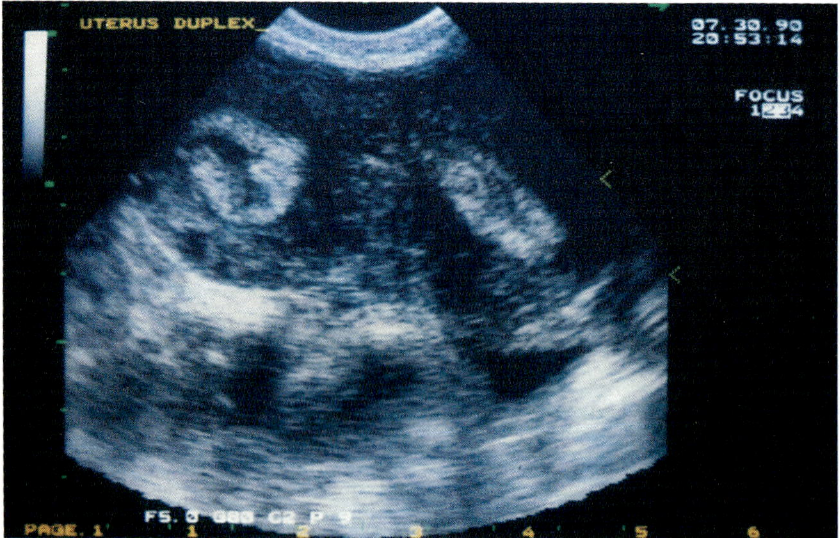

Figure 6-7 Uterus duplex detected by transvaginal ultrasound. Decidual reaction in both uteri is obvious. Free fluid in the pouch of Douglas was visualized. An ectopic gestation was found in the right fallopian tube.

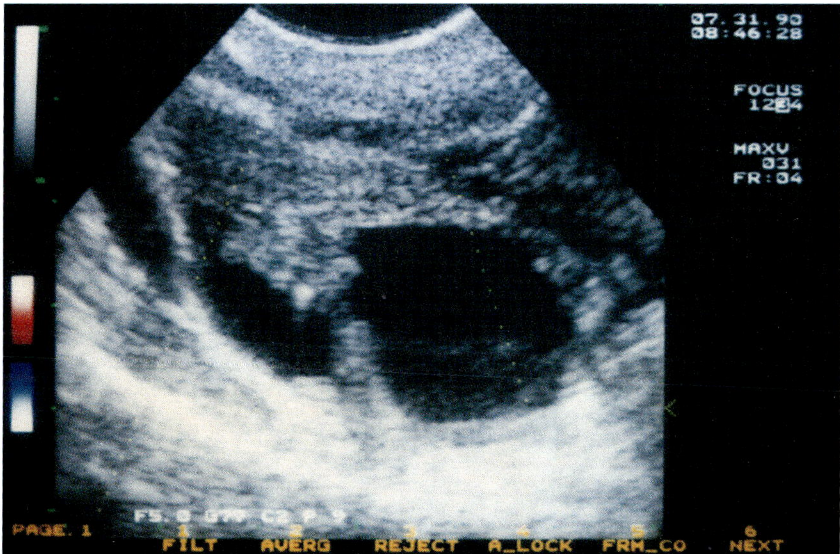

Figure 6-8   Complex adnexal mass detected by transvaginal ultrasound. Nonspecific ultrasonic findings by ectopic pregnancy. Tubal abortion was diagnosed on laparoscopy.

percent, and the third pattern in about 10 percent of the patients.[10] Fetal heartbeats were observed in nearly 23 percent of the cases.

Even though transvaginal sonographic examination has become the most reliable instrument in the diagnosis of normal and abnormal intrauterine pregnancies, unfortunately it has not reached such a level of success in the diagnosis of ectopic pregnancy. Demonstration of the ectopic pregnancy with transvaginal ultrasound allows a more precise preoperative diagnosis and is likely to allow earlier surgical intervention and minimization of tubal damage. Many ectopic pregnancies do not develop an embryo, so these specific findings will not be demonstrated and the presence of an adnexal mass may be ambiguous. A prudent approach to the management of ectopic pregnancies should take into consideration a number of limitations of transvaginal sonography in the workup of this condition. The main limitation is the risk of obtaining a false-positive diagnosis of the corpus luteum. A false-negative diagnosis may be made in the case of an ectopic gestation that is located outside the true pelvis or in the event of a very small tubal gestation. For these reasons other means for identification of the nature of an adnexal mass become important, and some of them are still controversial.

DOPPLER ULTRASOUND

The first transabdominal Doppler study of ectopic pregnancies was reported in 1989.[19] A viable ectopic embryo was documented in only 14 percent of the cases.

High velocity flow, suggesting the presence of an ectopic pregnancy, was documented in 54 percent of the patients. The positive predictive values were 47 percent for B-mode imaging alone and 85 percent for Doppler sonography. The negative predictive values were 60 percent for imaging alone and 81 percent for Doppler. The limitations of transabdominal Doppler imaging in the diagnosis of ectopic pregnancy currently include the need for a full bladder and the necessity of considerable operator experience in locating the trophoblastic flow and optimizing the signals. Taylor and coworkers[19] concluded that these difficulties and high false-positive rates should be reduced by the addition of color and pulsed Doppler imaging to the transvaginal probe. This would combine the advantages of transvaginal sonography with the tissue-characterizing ability of color Doppler imaging. Such sensitive equipment has recently been produced, and transvaginal color and pulsed Doppler ultrasonography have been tested for the assessment of ectopic pregnancy.[3,20–23] Transvaginal color Doppler can help to characterize the nature of the adnexal mass, thus permitting preoperative diagnosis when the ectopic embryo and its heartbeat cannot be visualized by conventional sonography. We have studied the value of transvaginal color Doppler in the detection of blood flow in the ectopic pregnancy. A vaginal ultrasound and color Doppler imaging were performed, and blood was drawn for a quantitative β-hCG serum level in 184 amenorrheic women. The sonographer was not aware of the results of the biochemical test at the time of the scan. The equipment used was Aloka Color Doppler SSD-680 with a 5-MHz transvaginal convex probe. Suspected adnexal masses were carefully examined for color flow and if found, a resistance index was calculated. On each examination, a minimum of five cardiac cycles were measured to calculate a mean value for the RI. Before any assessment of a suspected ectopic pregnancy is made, the normal uterine and ovarian perfusions have to be evaluated. All women were followed for clinical outcome, and all operative reports were reviewed. Ectopic pregnancy was confirmed by histologic examination of tissue removed at time of surgery.

Ectopic pregnancy was diagnosed if ectopic color flow, usually prominent and randomly dispersed within a solid part of an adnexal mass, was demonstrated, and it was clearly separated from ovarian tissue and corpus luteum (Figs. 6-9 to 6-11). Pulsed Doppler waveform analysis showed a very low impedance signal and calculated RIs were always below 0.40 because of increased end-diastolic flow (Figs. 6-12 to 6-14).

Taylor[24] hypothesized that such low impedance flow around the ectopic gestation results from the hemodynamics of early placentation. The trophoblast actively invades the maternal tissue, eroding blood vessels which bleed into the intervillous space and thereby starting a primitive trophoblastic circulation. The hemodynamics involved in this process provide the basis for the characteristic flow observed. The fact that the intervillous space lacks muscle layers could explain the low resistance to flow. The brightness of color is usually high, indicating high velocity flow in the ectopic gestation.

Among 184 women, 6 had a normal intrauterine pregnancy, 103 had an

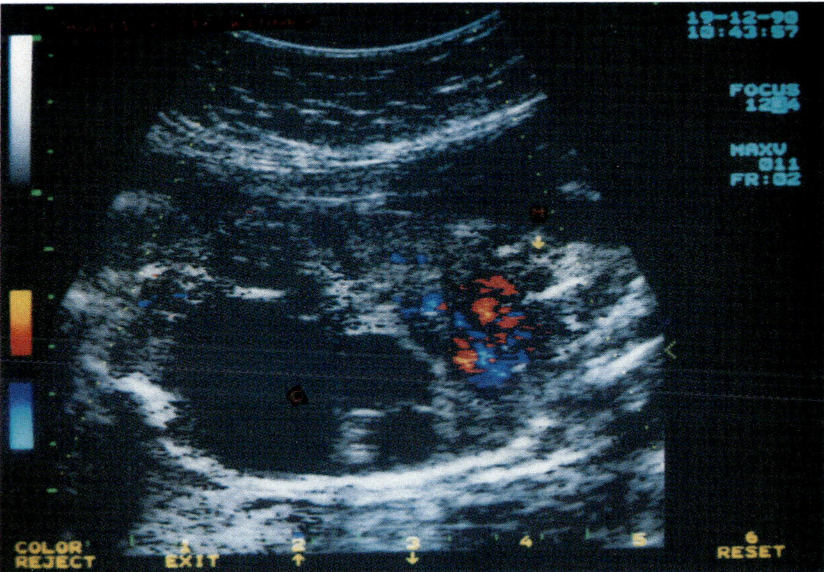

Figure 6-9   Typical transvaginal color Doppler signals in the case of nonspecific B-mode ultrasound findings. Color-coded areas represented ectopic implantation of the trophoblast. Ectopic gestation was confirmed on histopathology.

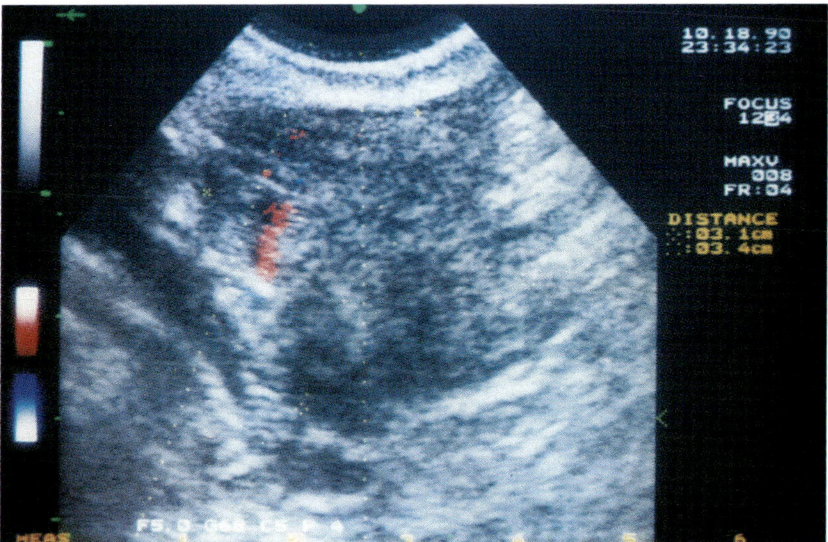

Figure 6-10   Another example of an ectopic gestation detected only by transvaginal color Doppler. B-mode ultrasound findings were nonspecific, demonstrating an empty uterus and a solid adnexal mass.

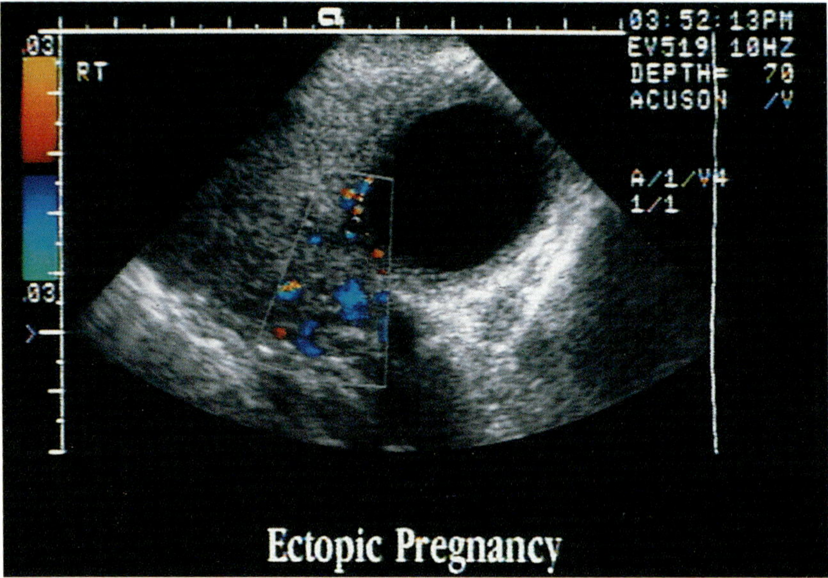

Figure 6-11 A cystic adnexal mass with ectopic blood flow detected by color Doppler. A tubal pregnancy was diagnosed during laparoscopy.

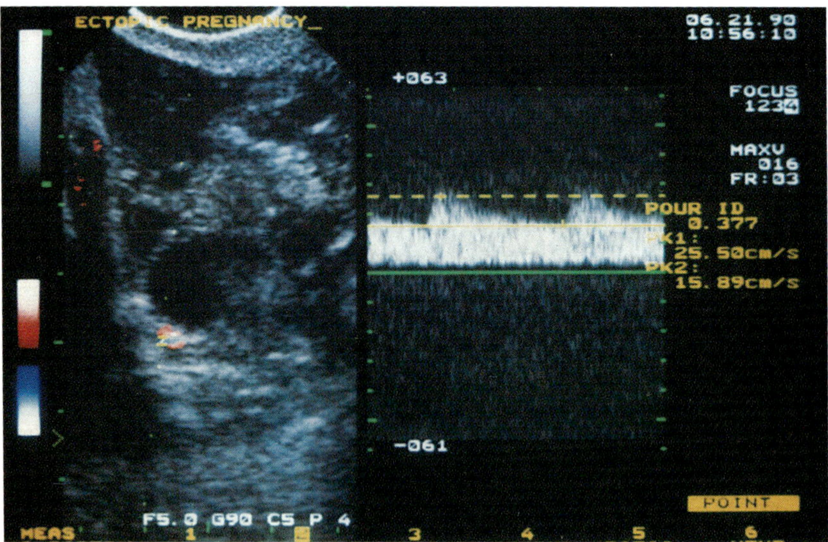

Figure 6-12 Complex adnexal mass. Transvaginal color Doppler showed ectopic blood flow, and pulsed Doppler (*right*) permitted waveform analysis. Increased diastolic blood flow and very low resistance to flow were noted (RI = 0.377). Typical transvaginal Doppler findings of an ectopic pregnancy.

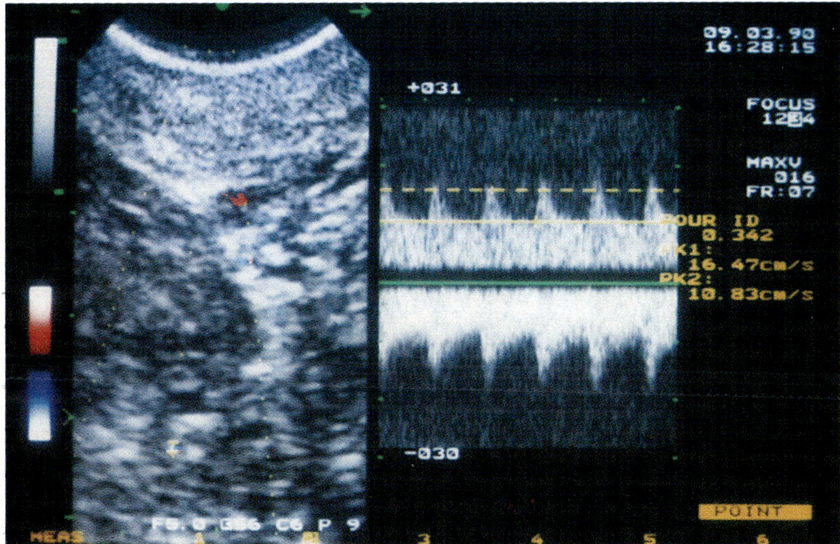

Figure 6-13 An additional example of ectopic gestation detected by transvaginal color and pulsed Doppler.

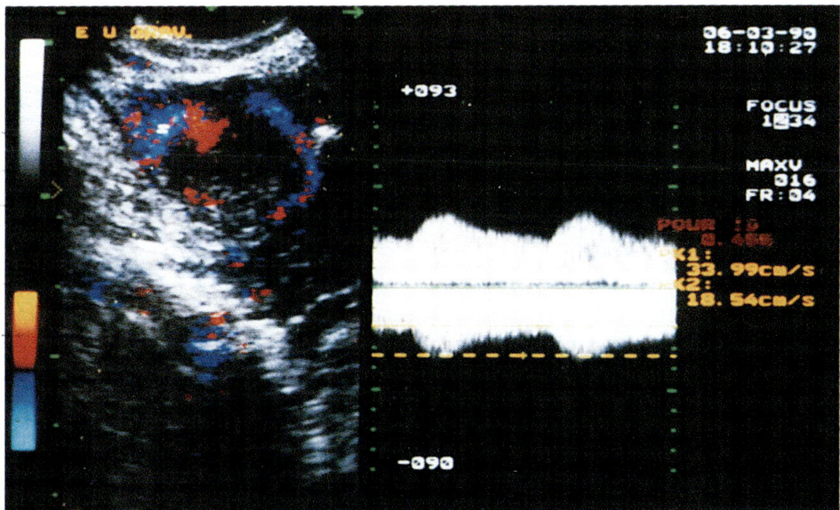

Figure 6-14 An additional example of ectopic gestation detected by transvaginal color and pulsed Doppler.

ectopic pregnancy, and 75 were not pregnant. Of the 103 ectopic pregnancies, 18 had cystic adnexal structures suggestive of a gestational sac, and 7 of these had a living embryo. The remaining 85 patients had solid cystic or complex adnexal masses.

Color flow was seen in 95 patients. Adnexal color flow patterns with an RI of 0.40 or less were seen in 92 documented ectopic pregnancy masses and in three nonectopic adnexal masses. Eleven ectopic pregnancies did not demonstrate any color flow, and 78 nonpregnant or intrauterine pregnancies did not show any adnexal color flow. High predictive values, sensitivity, specificity, and accuracy of this diagnostic method were obtained (Table 6-1).

The RIs were plotted against the β-hCG levels, excluding those that demonstrated no flow. In general, the higher the concentration of the hormone, the lower the RI. In the 11 cases in which there was no flow, the β-hCG was below 500 mIU/mL. Next, the RI was plotted against the last menstrual period, but no significant relationship was found. When the last menstrual period was plotted against the β-hCG, a strong correlation emerged.

The results obtained by transvaginal color Doppler diagnosis of ectopic pregnancy are good enough to encourage its clinical application. We suggest that the current policy should be to wait with surgical intervention if there is no ectopic blood flow outside an empty uterus in amenorrheic patients. On the contrary, if there is color flow in the adnexal region with a resistance index of ≤ 0.40, the patient should be scheduled for laparoscopy regardless of the clinical signs. The hypothesis is that the absence of color flow from the ectopic pregnancy and corpus luteum may indicate that the ectopic pregnancy is no longer viable. There is no doubt that some ectopic embryos die and are resorbed. Color Doppler signals may therefore prove helpful in predicting which ectopic embryos could be treated expectantly.

Table 6-1   Diagnostic value of transvaginal color Doppler in the detection of ectopic pregnancy ($N = 184$)

Color flow and	Ectopic pregnancy		
RI $\leq$ 0.40	Yes	No	Total
Yes	92	3	95
No	11	78	89
Total	103	81	184

Note: PPV (positive predictive value) = 96.8 percent; NPV (negative predictive value) = 87.6 percent; sensitivity = 89.3 percent; specificity = 96.3 percent; accuracy = 92.4 percent.

CONCLUSION

Transvaginal color Doppler is expected to have direct implications for the diagnosis and therapy of ectopic pregnancies, particularly when typical ultrasound morphology (gestational sac and embryonic heart activity) are absent. Since Doppler appears to identify the viability, and perhaps the invasiveness of the trophoblast, more accurately than any other available diagnostic method, it may provide a foundation for a more selective management of ectopic pregnancy.

REFERENCES

1. Rottem S, Timor-Tritsch IE: "Think ectopic," in Timor-Tritsch IE, Rottem S (eds), *Transvaginal Sonography*, 2d ed. New York, Elsevier, 1991, p 373.
2. Curran JW: Economic consequences of pelvic inflammatory disease in the United States. Am J Obstet Gynecol 138:848–851, 1980.
3. Kurjak A, Zalud I, Volpe G: Conventional B-mode and transvaginal color Doppler in ultrasound assessment of ectopic pregnancy. Acta Med Iugosl 44:91–95, 1990.
4. Fleischer AC, Cartwright PS, DiPetro DL, James AE: "Sonographic evaluation of ectopic pregnancy," in Sanders RC (ed), *The Principles and Practice of Ultrasonography in Obstetrics and Gynecology*. Norwalk, Conn., Appleton-Century-Crofts, 1985, p 399.
5. Gleicher N, Giglia RV, Deppe G, Elrad H, Friberg J: Direct diagnosis of unruptured ectopic pregnancy by real-time ultrasonography. Obstet Gynecol 61:425–427, 1983.
6. Mahony BS, Filly RA, Nyberg DA, Callen PW: Sonographic evaluation of ectopic pregnancy. J Ultrasound Med 4:221–223, 1985.
7. Kadar N, Romero R: The timing of a repeat ultrasound examination in the evaluation for ectopic pregnancy. J Clin Ultrasound 10:211–215, 1987.
8. Romero R, Kadar N, Jeanty P, Copel JA, Chervenak FA, DeCherney A, Hobbins J: Diagnosis of ectopic pregnancy: value of the discriminatory human chorionic gonadotropin zone. Obstet Gynecol 66:357–360, 1985.
9. Nyberg DA, Filly RA, Laing FC, Mack LA, Zarutskie PW: Ectopic pregnancy: diagnosis by sonography correlated with quantitative hCG levels. J Ultrasound Med 6:145–148, 1987.
10. Rottem S, Thaler I, Levron J, Peretz B, Istkowitz J, Brandes J: Criteria for transvaginal sonographic diagnosis of ectopic pregnancy. J Clin Ultrasound 18:274–276, 1990.
11. DeCrespigny LC: Demonstration of ectopic pregnancy by transvaginal ultrasound. Br J Obstet Gynaecol 95:1253–1255, 1988.
12. Fleischer AC, Pennell RG, McKee MS, Worrell JA, Keefe B, Herbert CM, Hill GA, Cartwright PS, Kepple DM: Ectopic pregnancy: features at transvaginal sonography. Radiology 174:375–378, 1990.
13. Nyberg DA, Mack LA, Jeffrey RB, and Laing FC: Endovaginal sonographic evaluation of ectopic pregnancy: a prospective study. Am J Roentgen 149:1181–1183, 1987.
14. Shapiro B, Cullen M, Taylor KJW, DeCherney AH: Transvaginal ultrasonography for the diagnosis of ectopic pregnancy. Fertil Steril 50:425–428, 1988.
15. Cacciatore B, Stenman UH, Ylostalo P: Comparison of abdominal and vaginal sonography in suspected ectopic pregnancy. Obstet Gynecol 73:770–773, 1989.
16. Kadar N: Transvaginal ultrasound for ectopics. Fertil Steril 51:909–912, 1989.
17. Neiger R, Bailey S, Wall AM, Palmisano G: Diagnosis of ectopic pregnancy using transvaginal ultrasound scanning. J Reprod Med 34:52–55, 1989.
18. Enk L, Wikland M, Hammarberg K, Lindblom B: The value of endovaginal sonography and

urinary human chorionic gonadotropin tests for differentiation between intrauterine and ectopic pregnancy. J Clin Ultrasound 18:73–78, 1990.
19. Taylor KJW, Ramos IM, Feyock AL, Snower DP, Carter D, Shapiro BS, Meyer WR, DeCherney AH: Ectopic pregnancy: duplex Doppler evaluation. Radiology 173:93–96, 1989.
20. Kurjak A, Zalud I, Alfirevic Z, Jurkovic D: The assessment of abnormal pelvic blood flow by transvaginal color Doppler. Ultrasound Med Biol 16:437–441, 1990.
21. Kurjak A, Miljan M, Jurkovic D, Alfirevic Z, Zalud I: Color Doppler in the assessment of fetomaternal circulation. Rech Gynecol 1:269–275, 1989.
22. Kurjak A: *Transvaginal Color Doppler*. Carnforth, N.J., Parthenon Publishing, 1990.
23. Kurjak A, Jurkovic D, Alfirevic Z, Zalud I: Transvaginal color Doppler imaging. J Clin Ultrasound 18:227–232, 1990.
24. Taylor KJW: New techniques for the diagnosis of ectopic pregnancy—transvaginal sonography and Doppler. Naples, Italy, ECO Italia '89, 1989, October 5–7, p 13.

UMBILICAL AND UTEROPLACENTAL CIRCULATIONS IN LATE PREGNANCY

JOAQUIN SANTOLAYA-FORGAS

FitzGerald and Drumm[1] were the first to describe the use of Doppler ultrasound for the evaluation of the fetal circulation. It has been demonstrated that throughout the normal pregnancy the morphology of the blood velocity waveforms of the uterine and umbilical arteries changes and that in these arteries the relative proportion of the diastolic component of the waveforms increases as the pregnancy advances. Some abnormal pregnancies, on the other hand, have abnormal blood velocity waveforms in these and other fetal vessels. Experimental models have been developed to determine the meaning of normal and abnormal Doppler measurements. Abnormal waveforms have been related to human fetal blood gases, metabolic disturbances, and clinical outcome. Histologic changes of the placenta have been found to correlate with abnormal Doppler waveforms. Color flow mapping has added additional value to the Doppler technique by allowing a precise recognition of the sampled vessel which is required for (1) accurate placement of the sample volume, (2) angle of insonation determination for cosine factor correction, (3) better determination of the vessel cross-sectional area, and (4) precise recognition of the site of sampling to allow repetition of examinations. Color flow Doppler also offers the possibility of structural evaluation of the fetus, cord, and placenta and shortens the time needed to obtain good blood velocity waveforms from any vessel.[2]

This chapter presents a brief review of the vascular development and methods of measurement of the blood flows on both sides of the placenta. It also outlines the differentiation between normal and abnormal blood velocity waveforms, the correlations and utility of Doppler studies at these particular sites, and some mechanical applications of the color flow Doppler technique.

UTEROPLACENTAL AND FETOPLACENTAL VASCULATURE DEVELOPMENT

The maternal circulation must be able to adapt to allow a normal pregnancy and healthy fetus to develop. The uterine, arcuate, radial, basal, and spiral arteries dilate during pregnancy. At 6 to 12 weeks of pregnancy, the spiral arteries are first invaded at the level of the decidua with hormone-dependent vasodilatation. By 16 to 22 weeks, the endovascular trophoblast reaches the myometrial portion of the spiral artery with disappearance of the smooth muscle and consequent dilatation. By this time, these arteries receive the name of uteroplacental or intervillous arteries, and there are 100 to 150 in each placenta.[3] The products of conception also develop a cardiovascular system capable of progressive adjustments to allow diffusion of carrying substances for fetoplacental metabolism and growth. At the placental level, this process continues throughout pregnancy and is related to proliferation and maintenance of small vessels in the secondary and tertiary villi.[4]

BLOOD FLOW MEASUREMENT

In vitro, accurate measurement of flow can be done by collecting, in a graduated cylinder, all the fluid passing through a vessel over a measured unit of time. In live animals, electromagnetic flowmeters, thin film anemometers, and dye dilution techniques can be used.[5] Human fetal blood flow is measured noninvasively by ultrasonic flowmeters using the Doppler principle. Briefly, this principle states that if a probe that is emitting ultrasound waves at a fixed frequency is applied to the skin surface over a vessel, the sound will be backscattered by the moving red blood cell in the vessel and can be received by the probe. A Doppler frequency shift occurs in the reflected sound, and the frequency change is directly proportional to the blood velocity. Knowing this velocity and the cross section of the vessel, the volume of flow can theoretically be measured. However, because of the characteristics of flow in the umbilical and uterine vessels and technical limitations in maintaining a constant relationship between sample volume and vessel as well as difficulties related to determination of angle of insonation, this spectral waveform analysis has too much inter- and intraobserver variability to allow for accurate estimation of absolute velocities or blood flow volumes (Chap. 1). These limitations have brought about the development of qualitative, or subjective, interpretations of the Doppler blood velocity waveforms.

INTERPRETATIONS OF THE FETOPLACENTAL-UTERINE DOPPLER WAVEFORMS

The Doppler spectrum of velocities is related to the Doppler sound and, therefore, audio and visual display of the Doppler signal improves quality control during the examination. Three graphic dimensions must be visualized to interpret blood velocity waveforms: time (abscissa); peak velocities (ordinate); and spectrum determined between the zero and the peak velocities. Spectral broadening occurs in any vessel with laminar flow where the sample volume approaches the diameter of the vessel. This explains why continuous Doppler, which has an infinite sample size, detects the high velocities in the center of the vessel and the entire continuum of velocities down to zero at the vessel wall.

The basis for qualitative analysis of the Doppler waveforms is that each artery has its own specific waveform pattern, and these waveforms provide important physiologic information about the pumping heart, condition of the vessel wall, and downstream peripheral resistance.[6] Three qualitative indices are used to express the relation between the systolic and diastolic components of the waveforms: (1) systolic-to-diastolic ratio (A/B or S/D), (2) resistance index (RI), and (3) pulsatility index (PI) (Chap. 1). Qualitative measurements of the blood velocity waveforms of the umbilical and uterine circulations are required to reduce the variability of the Doppler measurements because: (1) These vessels are coiled and rarely straight. Blood flow in these vessels is modified laminar, and the maximum velocity within the vessel may not be in the center of the stream; therefore, peak velocities will not equal twice the mean velocity. (2) The vascular tree has elastic properties to prevent large pressure changes during the cardiac cycle, causing alterations of the cross-sectional area of the vessel.

Fluctuations in heart rate will change the length of the cardiac cycle. This will affect the resistance and volume of blood flow through the vessels, thus altering the end-diastolic frequencies of the Doppler waveform.[7,8] To minimize the variations in diastolic flow due to heart rate fluctuations, a mean value of at least three waveform indices should be calculated.[9]

Categorization of the blood velocity waveforms by visual impression can also be done. In the umbilical artery, abnormal waveforms are those with absent end-diastolic flow, and borderline are those with minimum amount of diastolic flow but with a measured index outside the limits of normal. Normal waveforms are those with significant diastolic flow and indices within the normal limit. In the uteroplacental circulation, abnormality will be described in the presence of a diastolic notch.[10]

CORRELATION BETWEEN BLOOD VELOCITY WAVEFORM INDICES AND CLINICAL, MECHANICAL, AND ANIMAL STUDIES

All Doppler indices correlate clinically with each other and are consistent for each examiner, independent of the technique (continuous or pulsed Doppler) and population studied.[11–13]

Mechanical models, in which volume and pressure of flow can be controlled while Doppler velocimetry is determined, have proven that the waveform indices correlate with volume of flow and that the shape of the waveform is in part a function of downstream resistance. The increase in waveform ratios probably occurs earlier than the calculated vascular resistance owing to the impact of the reflected waveform on the end-diastolic flow. In complex waveforms or in cases where there are no end-diastolic velocities, a better assessment of changes will be obtained using the pulsatility index. The pulsatility index increases as vascular resistance increases, and it is better correlated with distal impedance than the other indices, as they cannot be calculated when diastolic flow is very low or absent.[14–16]

In animal studies, acute embolization of the fetoplacental circulation has shown that the umbilical artery velocity waveforms and their indices are directly related to the integrity of the placental vessels. Different degrees of placental embolization produce progressive loss of end-diastolic flow, acidosis, hypercapnia, and decreased oxygen content.[17–19] Embolization of the uterine circulation produces fetal growth retardation and similar metabolic changes.[20] Animal models have also shown that prolonged fetal hypoxemia and acidosis or increasing fetal hematocrits and viscosity have very little effect on the blood velocity waveform patterns.[21]

UTERINE ARTERY BLOOD VELOCITY WAVEFORMS

Uterine artery blood flow is easily differentiated from other vascular flows in the pelvis by any type of Doppler equipment because this is the only flow in the pelvis directed toward the patient's head. As mentioned earlier, with pulsed Doppler ultrasound major blood vessels are visualized and can be evaluated. Color flow mapping increases the visualization of minor vessels.

In the spontaneous normal menstrual cycle the resistance to uterine artery blood flow decreases following ovulation. This decrease in resistance is more prominent on the side of ovulation (Fig. 7-1).[22]

In the uterine arteries a notch at the beginning of the diastolic phase is typical, and lack of end-diastolic flow is a common finding during the follicular phase. In contrast, absent end-diastolic velocities should not be expected during a normal pregnancy. Doppler application and evaluation of the first trimester uteroplacental circulation are described in Chaps. 4 to 6. It is known that the development of the uteroplacental arteries decreases the vascular impedance to the uterine artery blood flow.[23] It has also been shown that the lower in the endometrium the blood velocity waveforms are obtained, the less peripheral resistance will be recorded. The uterine artery demonstrates significant changes in the waveform indices from 12 to 26 weeks gestation. In early pregnancy those on the side of placentation yield lower flow velocity indices than those from the contralateral uterine artery, but they will change minimally after 24 weeks, whereas the contralateral indices fall continuously with advancing gestation.[24,25]

The prevalence of abnormal uterine artery indices in the general obstetrical population is 1 to 2 percent, and they are usually dependent on high resistance

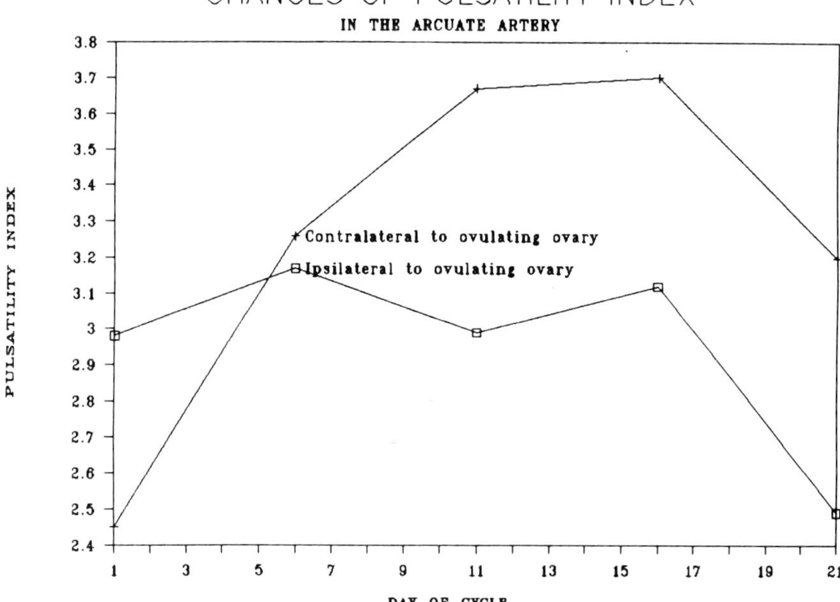

Figure 7-1   Mean value of the pulsatility index (PI) determined separately from both uterine arteries throughout 20 menstrual cycles in 16 healthy women.

to flow in only one of the two uterine arteries.[26] Abnormally high Doppler indices in the uteroplacental circulation predict more severe forms of pregnancy-induced hypertension or intrauterine growth retardation (IUGR).[27-30] Lack of trophoblastic invasion of the spiral arteries and fibrinoid necrosis with lipolytic macrophage infiltration are seen closing the lumen of the spiral artery in some of these pregnancies with IUGR fetuses. These findings have not been observed in the spiral arteries of the nonplacental bed explaining the reported diversity of blood velocity waveforms from each uterine artery in clinically diagnosed IUGR fetuses.[3] Since uterine artery blood velocity waveforms are slightly different depending on whether they were obtained from the placental or nonplacental site, four markers have been suggested to detect pregnancy complications: (1) a utero placental blood flow from either side with RI > 0.58[27]; (2) a mean A/B ratio between both uterine arteries >2.6; (3) the presence of a diastolic notching after 26 weeks; (4) a marked difference in the indices between the placental and nonplacental sites.[10,28]

UMBILICAL ARTERY BLOOD VELOCITY WAVEFORMS

The umbilical artery is an optimal vessel for Doppler evaluation because it is long, unbranched, and surrounded by amniotic fluid, it has a parallel vein with flow in the opposite direction and, with the exception of the entrance into the fetal abdomen, the site of measurements is not of great importance.[31] Different authors have assessed the umbilical artery Doppler's potential as a screening test for pregnancy complications. Results, however, show poor performance due to the low incidence (3 to 5 percent) of abnormal ratios in fetuses of a middle-class, low-risk population.[26] Umbilical artery end-diastolic velocities appear around 12 to 13 weeks gestation.[32] From the beginning of the second trimester, until term, the diastolic flow increases and the indices of umbilical artery flow velocity waveforms decrease (Fig. 7-2).[33,34]

It is important to accept umbilical artery Doppler signals only when both the umbilical artery and the vein are represented on the screen, as this will significantly improve the reproducibility of the results.[12] Nomograms of the Doppler indices from the umbilical artery have been done during fetal quiet and apneic states. Fetal apnea can be documented by lack of ultrasonographic observation of fetal chest and diaphragmatic excursions and by absent undulation of umbilical venous blood flow. However, if we increase the number of measured waveforms, the mean value of the indices remains reasonably constant even in the presence of fetal breathing or spontaneous movements. Averaging a number of waveform calculations is also important to reduce to minimal the variance

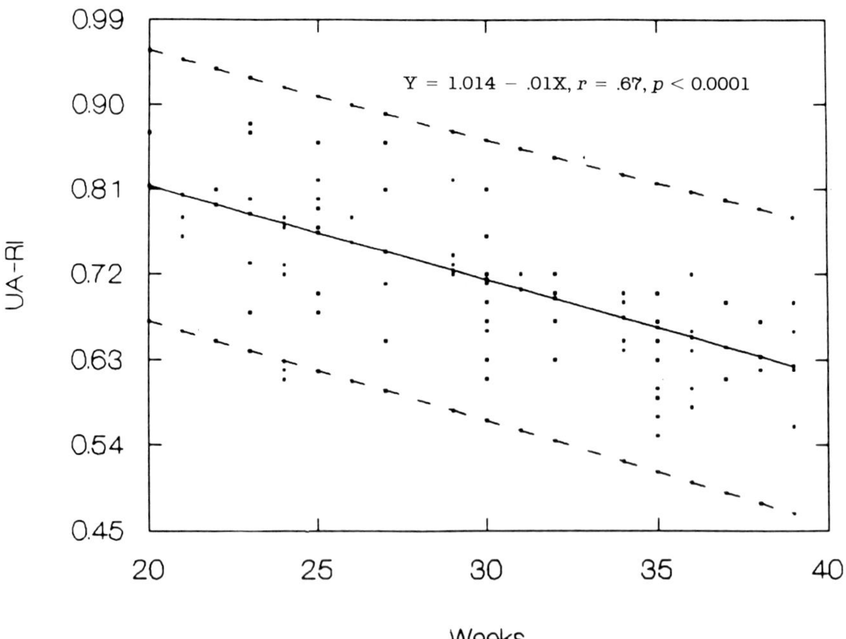

Figure 7-2 Nomogram (mean and 95 percent confidence intervals) of the resistance index (RI) derived from 70 measurements of the umbilical artery in well-dated normal pregnancies with term deliveries.

between longitudinal measurements of the indices.[35] Doppler analysis of the venous circulation can be used to evaluate fetal cardiac function and, perhaps, fetal hemodynamics should be assessed by the simultaneous evaluation of both the arterial and venous circulations (Chaps. 9 and 10). Cyclic analysis of these circulations, accounting for periods of apnea and breathing movements, may allow noninvasive hemodynamic insights into the pathophysiology of specific fetal diseases.

Abnormally reduced end-diastolic velocities in the umbilical artery can be found in presence of IUGR due to primary fetal disorder or secondary to an inadequate uteroplacental circulation. Fetuses demonstrating abnormal waveforms have worse prognosis than the general population.[18] Umbilical artery velocimetry has a sensitivity two to three times higher than fetal heart rate monitoring for detection of fetal outcome, and abnormal indices are associated with higher (1) perinatal mortality, (2) small for gestational age fetuses, (3) operative delivery for fetal distress, and (4) admissions to the neonatal intensive care unit.[13,36–39] Antepartum abnormal umbilical artery waveforms in IUGR fetuses are significantly associated with fetal hypoxia, acidosis, and thrombocytopenia.[40–43] However, the association of an iatrogenic fetal metabolic acidosis and a decreased cardiac inotropism, with normal heart rate and rhythm maintained, did not change the umbilical artery resistance index.[44] Other studies of the umbilical artery velocimetry performed before cesarean section in fetuses in which the majority were not IUGR have also shown lack of correlation between cord pH and Doppler findings.[45]

The placentas of fetuses with high umbilical artery Doppler indices may show a normal quantity of tertiary stem villi, whereas the small arterioles are either obliterated or have never developed.[46–49]

CLINICAL UTILIZATION OF DOPPLER STUDIES

Hypertension

Not all hypertensive pregnant women have abnormal Doppler findings or adverse outcome. However, patients with chronic hypertension or pregnancy-induced hypertension with abnormal umbilical artery blood velocity waveforms have worse perinatal outcome.[28] Subplacental arcuate arteries show reduced blood flow in some hypertensive pregnancies.[27,50] In some preeclamptic patients, the second trophoblastic invasion may not occur, and the caliber of the spiral arteries is smaller. These arteries also maintain the musculoelastic layer which is capable of undergoing vasospasm in reaction to circulating vasoactive agents, a fact that could explain the persistence of diastolic notching in the uterine artery waveforms beyond the 26th week of gestation.[3]

A classification scheme of hypertensive pregnancies based on uterine and umbilical artery Doppler velocimetry has been proposed.[12,51] In this classification, women with decreased uterine, but normal umbilical flow, delivered prematurely but appropriate for gestational age fetuses. Women with normal uterine but reduced umbilical flow gave birth to growth-retarded infants. Women with reduced flow in both vessels have the worst prognosis because of early onset of the disease. In this situation, the short-term predictor of fetal well-being is dependent on the pattern of fetal circulation. It has been postulated that in some women the reduced umbilical flow velocities may induce a hypertensive response.[52] In general, in hypertensive pregnant women, examination of the uteroplacental vessels will indicate if there is evidence of high impedance in the placental vascular bed. If such is the case, studies of fetal circulation should be carried out regularly to observe any of the known alterations that are associated with fetal hypoxia, acidosis, and adverse perinatal outcome.

Diabetes

Diabetes mellitus remains a significant complication of pregnancy with high fetal morbidity due to suboptimal glycemic control. Current obstetrical management includes maternal glucose control, ultrasonography to rule out fetal anomalies and to estimate growth, and intensive fetal surveillance with fetal cardiotocography beyond the 30th week. This control scheme does not detect all fetuses at risk for an adverse outcome. Several authors have used Doppler velocimetry in diabetic pregnancies showing that abnormal findings before delivery predict a worse perinatal outcome. However, there is no convincing evidence that the technique has any advantage over the standard management of these pregnancies.[53–55] In a longitudinal study performed on fetuses of obese pregnant women, the umbilical artery RI was lower for a given gestational age in those cases in which the mother eventually developed gestational diabetes. This decrease in umbilical artery RI was associated with the presence of fetal macrosomia (Fig. 7-3 *top, center*). The difference in umbilical artery RI disappeared if these macrosomic fetuses were matched with a control group for estimated fetal weight (Fig. 7-3 bottom).[56] Placentas of gestational diabetic pregnancies have excessive weight. Studies of placental histologic differentiation are conflicting and show different degrees of vascularization.[57,58] In macrosomic fetuses, larger placental vascular insults may be needed before abnormal umbilical artery Doppler indices develop.

Intrauterine Growth Retardation

Real-time ultrasonography has been used in the diagnosis of clinically suspected small-for-gestational-age fetuses for over a decade. IUGR fetuses are those whose estimated weight falls two standard deviations below the mean weight when adjusted for gestational age. This definition, however, remains suboptimal owing to biologic variations of fetal growth and, often, lack of accurate dating for evaluation of fetal weight or interval growth. All ultrasonographically recognized

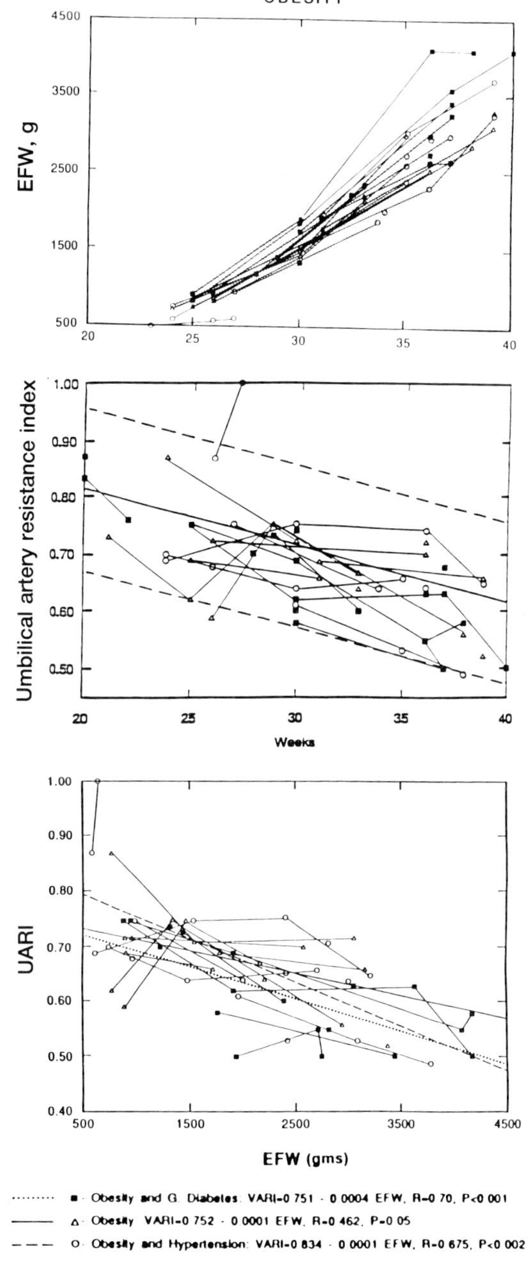

Figure 7-3   Fetal biometrical and umbilical artery Doppler evaluations (RI) were performed in 28 obese patients (mean maternal weight 255 lb, SD 52.2 lb). The patients either developed no medical complications (group 1), developed pregnancy-induced hypertension (PIH) (group 2) or developed gestational diabetes (GD) (group 3). The obese patients with GD developed macrosomia (*top*). The macrosomic fetuses had a tendency to have lower RI for gestational age (*center*), a difference that was not noted when the RI values were plotted against the estimated fetal weight (*bottom*).

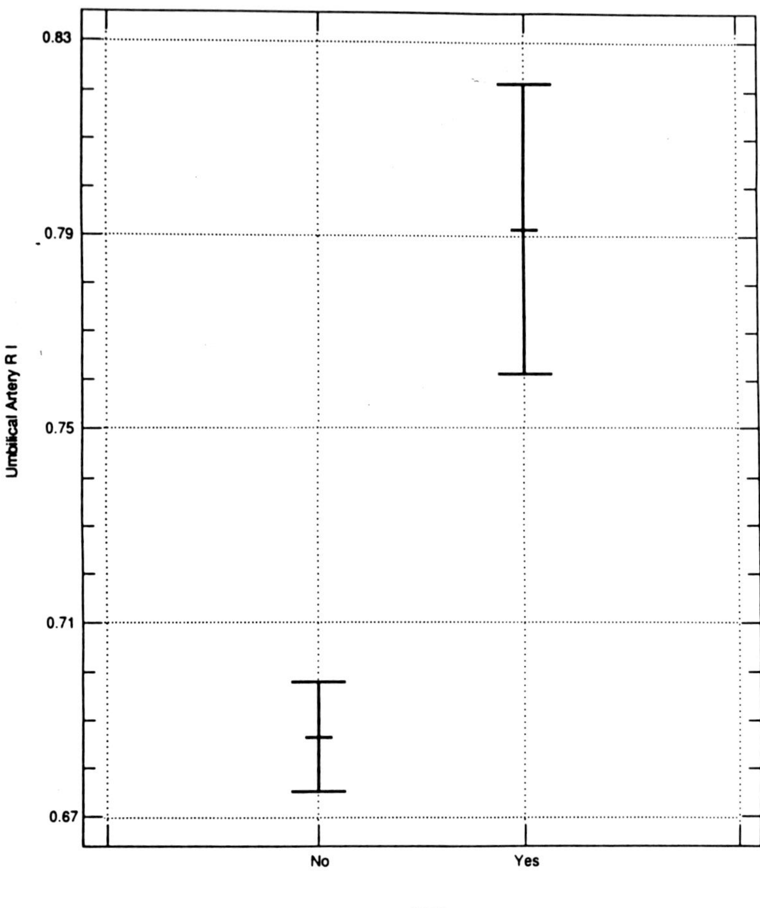

Figure 7-4 Umbilical artery resistance indices (RI) were determined 135 times at different gestational ages in 55 well-dated normal pregnancies and 26 times in 12 growth-retarded fetuses (IUGR). Linear regression was used to show by the T′ and GT2 methods that the slopes of the RI as a function of gestational age did not differ between the normal and IUGR fetuses. The group means were then compared with analysis of the covariance, using the gestational age as a covariate to correct for its effect on the umbilical artery RI, with IUGR as a factor. Scheffe's test with a significant cutoff point of $p < 0.05$ was used for post-hoc comparison.

IUGR fetuses do not have abnormal umbilical artery blood velocity waveforms. However, IUGR is known to be a significant factor for increasing umbilical artery Doppler indices (Fig. 7-4).[59] IUGR fetuses with abnormal umbilical artery waveforms have progressive hematologic and metabolic alterations which may lead to their intrauterine death.[40,43] Since abnormal umbilical artery blood velocity waveforms are clearly associated with an adverse perinatal outcome, Doppler velocimetry has a role in determining which of the ultrasonically determined small-for-gestational-age fetuses need a closer antepartum monitoring (Chap. 11).

Chromosomal and Congenital Anomalies

Some aneuploid fetuses are associated with IUGR, stillbirth, and abnormal Doppler studies.[52,49] These abnormal Doppler indices may result from decreased placental angiopoiesis or may be due to obliteration of small arteries triggered by the presence of a fetus with a major malformation.[60,61] The malformation rate in fetuses with appropriate-for-gestational-age weights and abnormal S/D ratios is higher than in those fetuses with normal S/D ratios.[62] Abnormal Doppler velocimetry in the umbilical artery may be prognostic of the short-term outcome in fetuses with major anomalies and nonimmune hydrops of different etiologies.[63–65] Therefore, abnormal Doppler findings can improve our ability to identify fetoplacental dysfunctions and fetal structural abnormalities. It is postulated that in a compromised fetus, loss of umbilical artery diastolic blood flow will precede death.

Twin Gestations

In twin pregnancies, Doppler velocimetry can be useful in the evaluation of prenatally diagnosed discordant fetal growth. Color Doppler can be used in discordant twins to trace both fetal circulations. Monochorionic twins with the twin-twin transfusion syndrome have an unbalanced arteriovenous shunting associated with concordant umbilical artery blood velocity waveforms[66] or abnormal findings in the donor twin.[67] Doppler velocimetry enables us to study the spectrum of changes and severity in this altered hemodynamic state. Since abnormal umbilical artery blood velocity waveforms are highly predictive of an IUGR fetus and bad perinatal outcome, the combination of Doppler screening and real-time measurements at the beginning of the third trimester of pregnancy has been proposed to identify twin pregnancies at risk for adverse outcome.[67]

Oligohydramnios

Quantification of the amount of amniotic fluid is necessary for determination of the biophysical profile. Color flow Doppler could be useful to differentiate umbilical cord from a small pocket of amniotic fluid (Fig. 7-5).

Doppler velocimetry can also assist in the differentiation between severe IUGR fetuses and cases of preterm premature rupture of membranes, since the latter condition does not affect the umbilical artery velocimetry.[68] Postdatism is still the most common indication for induction of labor; however, a conservative management of prolonged pregnancy using a combination of the biophysical profile and Doppler velocimetry as a method of determining fetal well-being has been proposed.[69]

(Text continues on page 114.)

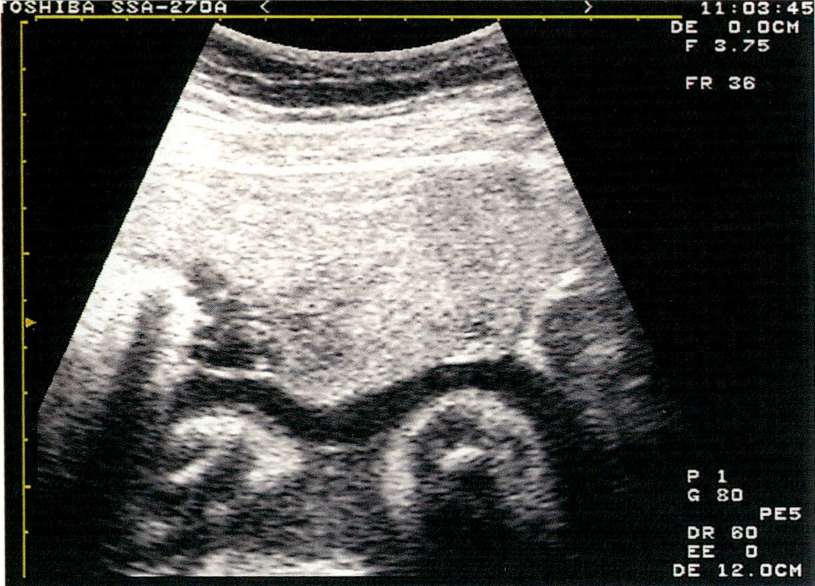

A

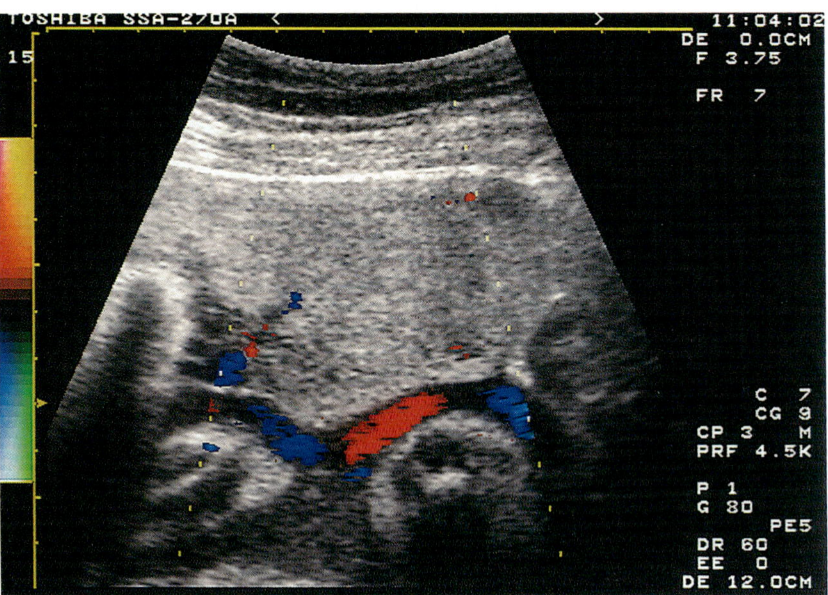

B

Figure 7-5   A sonogram of a 35-week-old fetus. The gray scale image showed a small area of fluid between the fetus and the placenta (*A*). When color was superimposed, it was immediately realized that the ''fluid'' was a loop of umbilical cord (*B*).

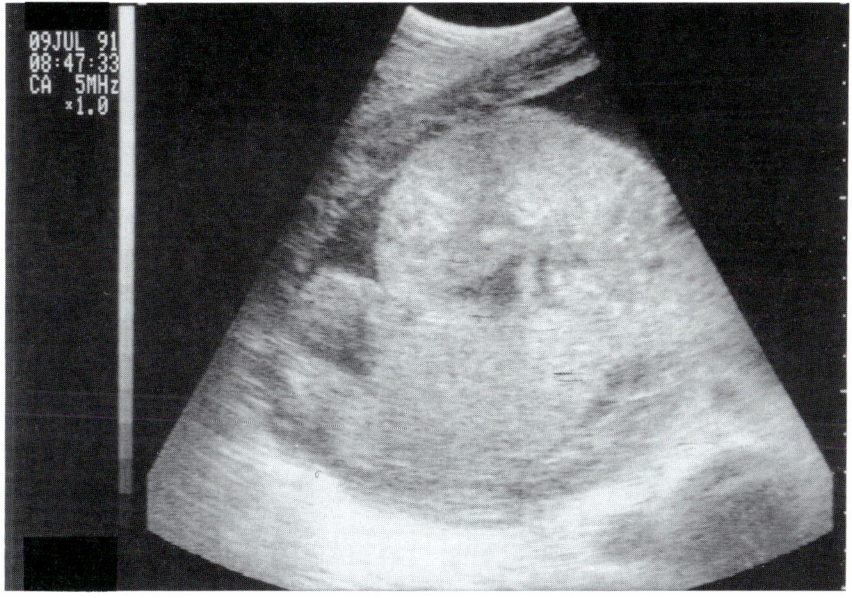

A

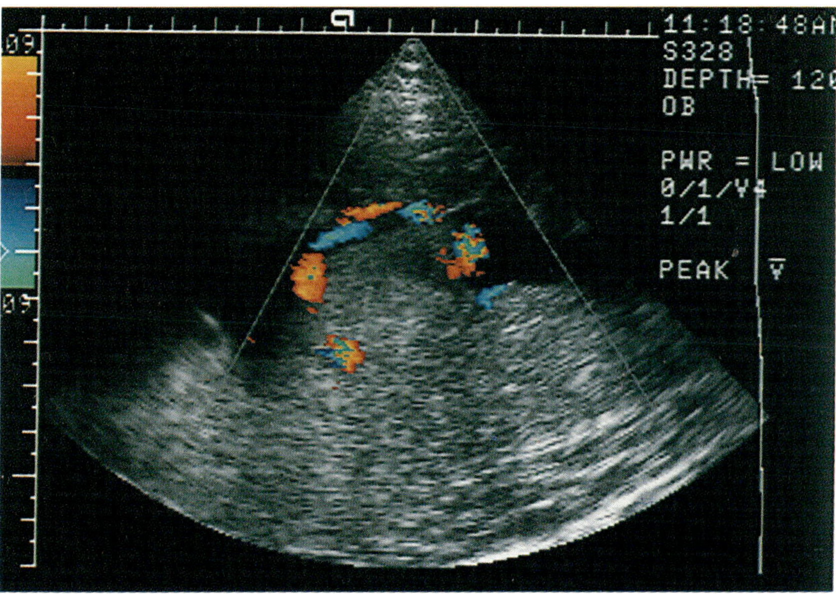

B

Figure 7-6 The gray scale image of a 30-week gestation revealed a mass protruding from the placenta into the amniotic cavity (*A*). Color imaging showed that the tumor was not vascular, and the cord was seen lying over the tumor (*B*).

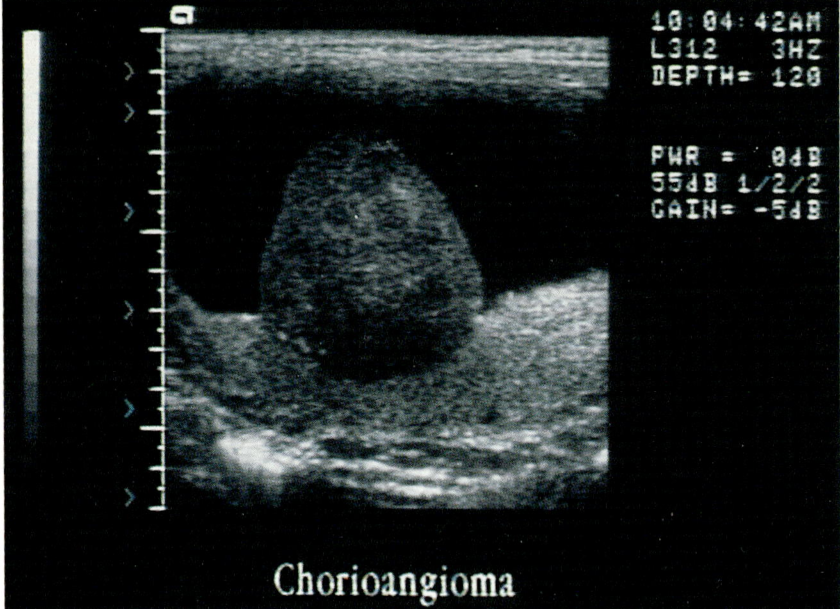

A

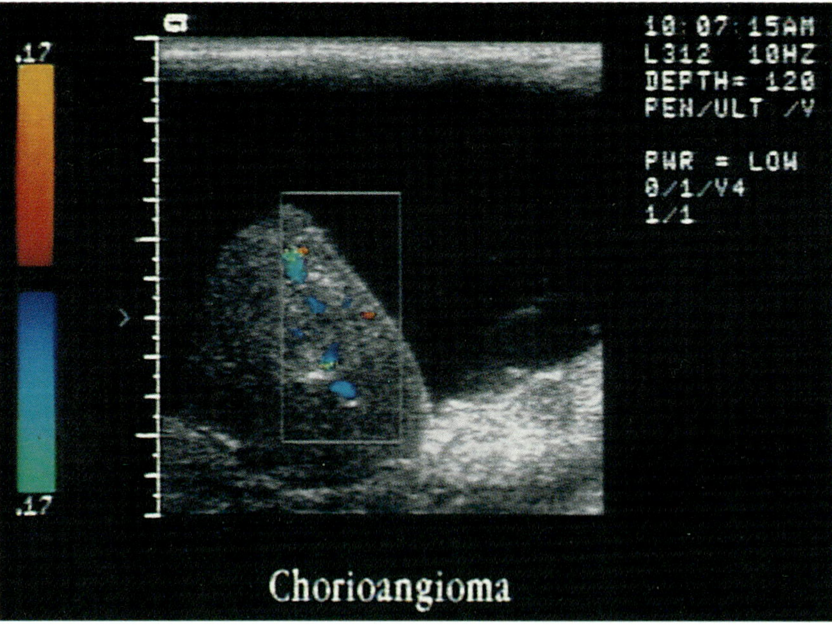

B

Figure 7-7   In a case similar to that in Fig. 7-6, a mass was seen protruding from the surface of the placenta into the amniotic cavity (*A*). When color imaging was superimposed, the hypervascularization of the tumor was immediately recognized (*B*). The diagnosis of a chorioangioma was made, and it was confirmed by histopathology following delivery. *(Courtesy of Acuson Ltd, Mountain View, California.)*

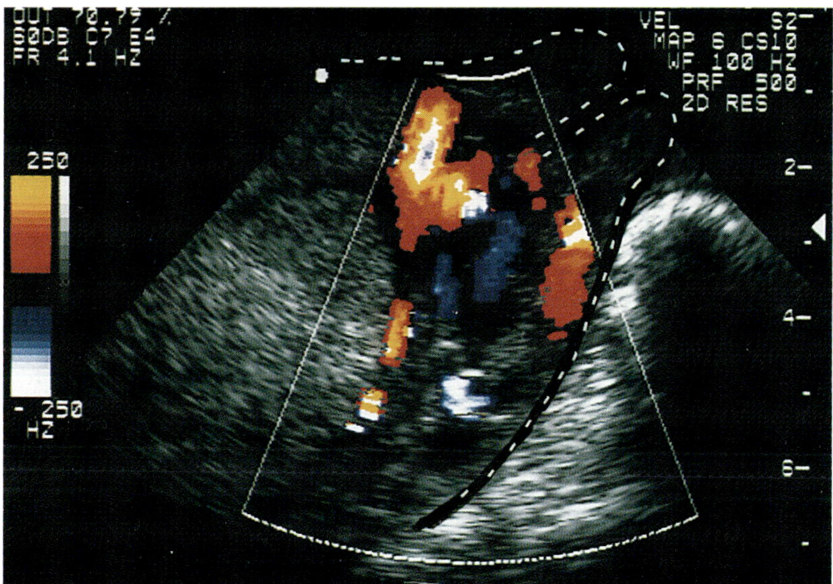

Figure 7-8 A transvaginal ultrasonographic sagittal view of the cervix and lower segment of the uterus at 32 weeks gestation. The superimposed color imaging demonstrates the lacunar blood flow within sonolucencies of the placenta. This pattern is highly suggestive of an adherent placenta. A cesarean section was performed at 35 weeks gestation. The pathology confirmed the diagnosis of placenta previa accreta, and a cesarean hysterectomy was done. The patient was transfused with nine units of blood. *(Courtesy of Dr. I. E. Timor, New York.)*

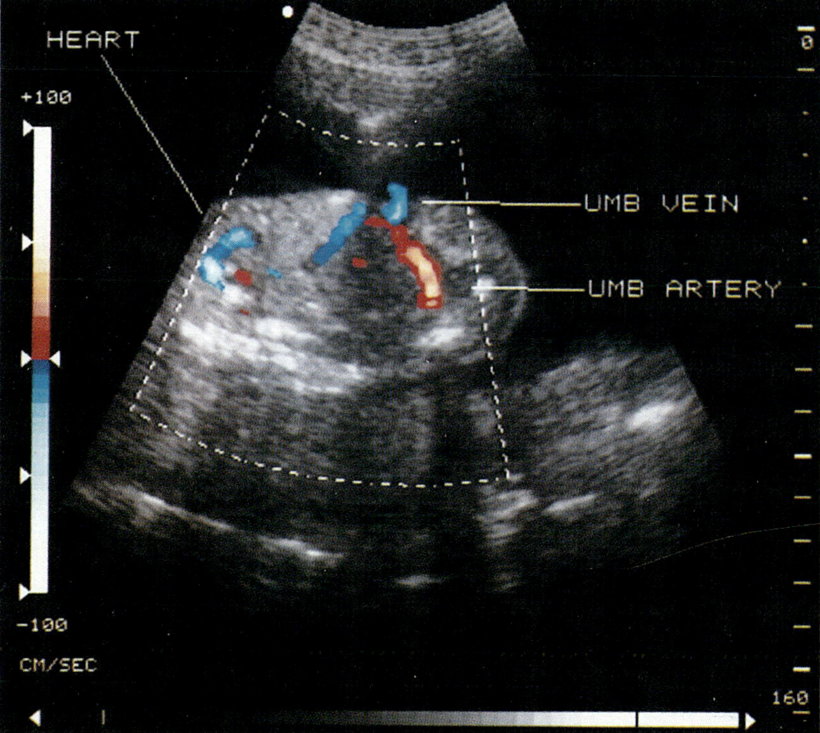

Figure 7-9 A color imaging of a 20-week-old fetus. The umbilical arteries are clearly visualized (red), and the umbilical vein (blue) can be seen as it enters the fetus and traverses the liver toward the vena cava and right heart.

Fetal Blood Sampling

The technique of *fetal blood sampling* (PUBS) imposes some risks to the fetus.[70] Severe intrauterine growth retardation is one of the second- and third-trimester indications for rapid fetal karyotyping and possible evaluation of its blood gases and biochemical and metabolic status.[40,71] IUGR is frequently associated with severe oligohydramnios, which hampers cord visualization. If other sites of fetal blood sampling are not considered, color Doppler imaging of blood flow can be invaluable in finding a cord sampling site. Doppler can also document and time umbilical artery vasoconstrictions secondary to fetal blood samplings and clarify the risk that this imposes to the fetus. Acute vasoconstriction may not alter the blood velocity waveforms significantly until the reduction in umbilical blood flow and fetal oxygenation is severe. An angiotensin II infusion model that acts selectively on the umbilical artery and its major tributaries, and not on the placental low-resistance vessels, was associated with a large increase in umbilical artery resistance and decreased umbilical blood flow, but it did not alter the blood velocity waveforms.[19] Perhaps, the combination of severe fetal hypoxemia and acidosis may be required for occurrence of abnormal Doppler indices, which will then become normal with restoration of fetal oxygenation.[71]

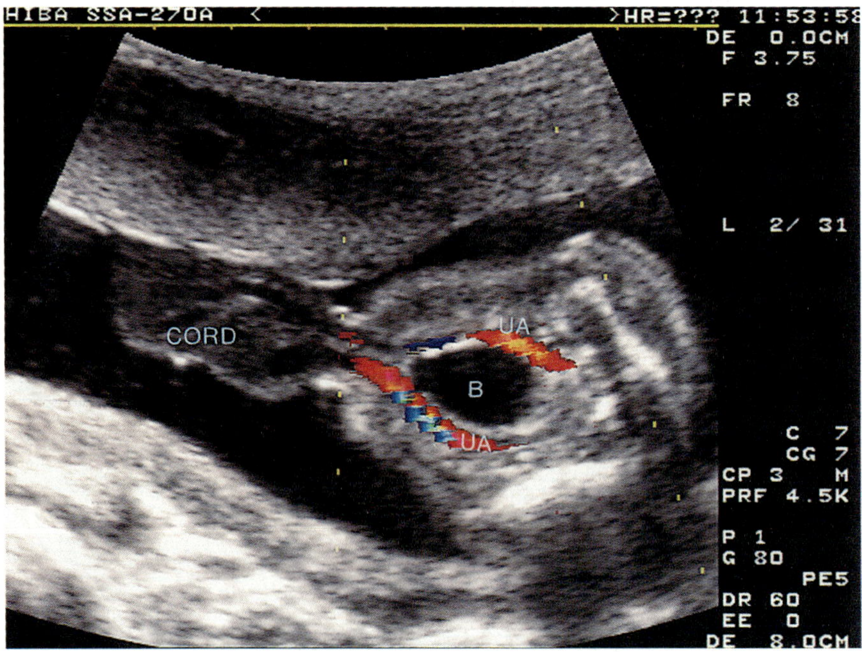

Figure 7-10 An oblique sonogram of the lower body of a 28-week-old fetus. The bladder is seen (B) with both umbilical arteries (UA) surrounding it before they enter the umbilical cord.

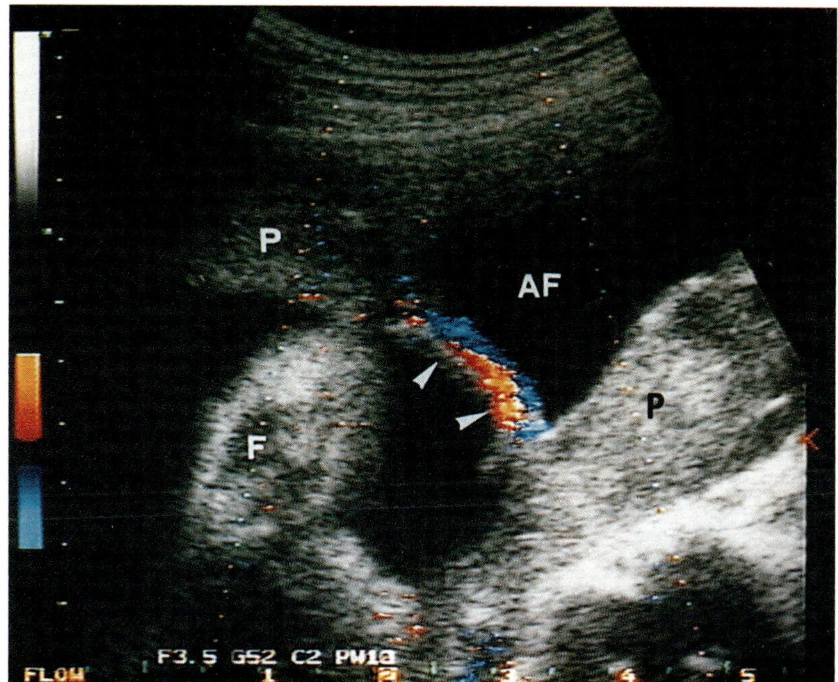

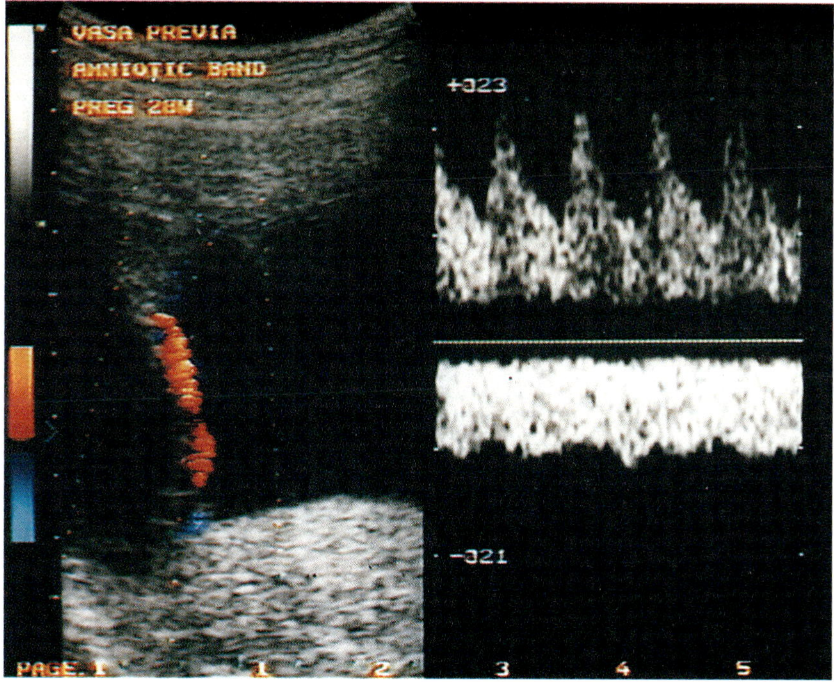

Figure 7-11 *A.* The coiling umbilical artery (red) and vein (blue) running along the medial edge of the amniotic band (*arrowhead*), which connects the anterior and posterior placenta. P = placenta; AF = amniotic fluid, F = fetal part. *B.* Flow velocity waveform from the coiling umbilical vessels. The waveform pattern indicates that there is an umbilical artery running from the posterior placenta to the anterior placenta and an umbilical vein running in the reverse direction. *(Reprinted with permission from Fon-Jou Hsieh, Hsin-Fu Chen, Tsang-Ming Ko, Chang-Yao Hsieh, Hsi-Yao Chen: Antenatal diagnosis of vasa previa by color-flow mapping. J Ultrasound Med 10:397–399, 1991.)*

Anomalies of Placenta and Cord

The intraplacental blood flow can be visualized by color flow Doppler. Although quantification of this blood flow is not yet possible, anatomic interpretations can be done helping in the diagnosis of placental tumors, placental lakes, abnormally adherent placentas, and abruptio placenta.[72] Placental tumors can be either solid or very vascular, and color Doppler can help define the nature of a specific tumor (Figs. 7-6 and 7-7). Placental position in relation to the uterine cervix can be readily visualized by vaginosonography.[73] Although not essential for diagnosis, the association between placenta previa and acreta can be suspected by looking at the lacunar flow within sonolucent areas occupying almost the entire thickness of the placenta (Fig. 7-8).[74]

Color Doppler imaging facilitates tracing of the umbilical arteries and veins within the fetus. The umbilical vein can be seen entering the fetus and linking with the intrahepatic vein, inferior vena cava, and right atrium (Fig. 7-9). Both umbilical arteries can be seen on both sides of the bladder just before they become part of the cord (Fig. 7-10). Diagnoses of a single umbilical artery in severely malformed singletons and in twin pregnancies have been reported.[75] This same author also showed the value of color flow Doppler in the differential diagnosis

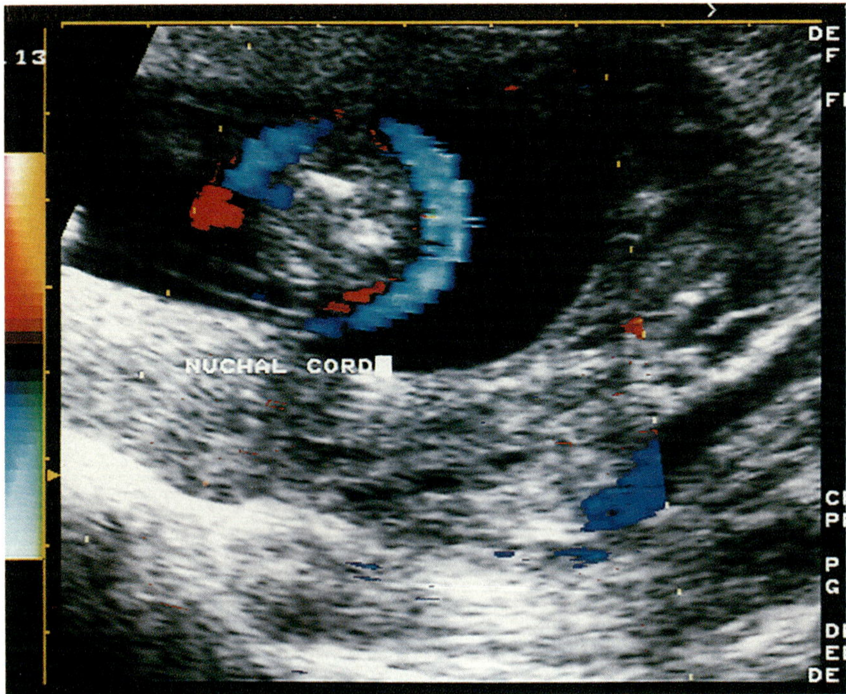

Figure 7-12 A sonogram of a 30-week-old fetus. The umbilical cord is tangled around the fetal neck.

of umbilical cord masses. Several reports have also shown that transvaginal ultrasound and color Doppler can demonstrate the direction and route of umbilical blood flow in cases in which vasa previa is suspected because of a succenturiate placenta or low umbilical cord insertion (Fig. 7-11).[76,77] Although not clinically indicated for every patient, color Doppler imaging can be employed during labor in fetuses with severe variable decelerations as it may demonstrate tangled arrangements of the cord or a tight cord around the neck or shoulder (Fig. 7-12).

REFERENCES

1. FitzGerald DE, Drum JE: Non-invasive measurements of human fetal circulation using ultrasound: a new method. Br Med J 2:1450–1451, 1977.
2. Arduini D, Rizzo G, Boccolini MR, Romanini C, Mancuso S: Functional assessment of utero-placental and fetal circulations by means of color Doppler ultrasonography. J Ultrasound Med 9:249–253, 1990.
3. Khong TY: Pathological correlation of blood flow in preeclampsia. Conference in Postgraduate Course in Obstetrics and Gynecology, Queen Charlotte's Maternity Hospital, London, 1988.
4. Kaufman P, Sen DK, Schweikhert G: Classification of human placental villi. I Hist Cell Tiss Res 200:409–423, 1979.
5. Roach MR, Boughner DR: "Biophysical principles in the cardiovascular system," in Goodwin JW, Godden JO, Chance GW (eds), *Perinatal Medicine: The Basic Science Underlying Clinical Practice*. Baltimore, Williams and Wilkins, 1976, pp 119–133.
6. Skidmore R, Woodcock JP: Physiological interpretation of Doppler-shift waveforms, I. Theoretical considerations. Ultrasound Med Biol 6:7–10, 1980.
7. Brar HS, Medearis AL, Platt RD: Relationship of systolic/diastolic ratios from umbilical velocimetry of fetal rate. Am J Obstet Gynecol 160:188–191, 1989.
8. Mires G, Dempster J, Patel NB, Crawford JW: Effect of fetal heart rate on umbilical artery flow velocity waveforms. Br J Obstet Gynaecol 94:665–669, 1987.
9. Erskine RLA, Richie JWK: Umbilical artery blood flow characteristics in normal and growth retarded fetuses. Br J Obstet Gynaecol 151:605–610, 1985.
10. Schulman H: The clinical implications of Doppler ultrasound analysis of the uterine and umbilical arteries. Am J Obstet Gynecol 156:889–893, 1987.
11. Mehalek KI, Berkowitz GS, Chitkara U, Rosenberg A, Berkowitz R: Comparison of continuous-wave and pulsed Doppler S/D ratios of umbilical and uterine arteries. Obstet Gynecol 72:603–606, 1988.
12. Cohen-Overbeek TE, Campbell S: "Doppler ultrasound techniques for the measurement of uterine and umbilical blood flow," in Rosenfield CR (ed), *The Uterine Circulation. Reproductive and Perinatal Medicine*, vol X. New York, Perinatology Press, 1989, pp 76–107.
13. Divon MY: Intrauterine growth retardation: evaluation of the umbilical vasculature. The 35th annual convention of the American Institute of Ultrasound in Medicine (AIUM), Atlanta, Ga. February 1991. Color Doppler: ultrasonography course. pp 109–112.
14. Skidmore R, Woodcock JP, Wells PNT, Bird D, Baire RN: Physiologic interpretation of Doppler shift waveforms–III. Ultrasound Med Biol 6:227–231, 1980.
15. Noordam MJ, Wladimiroff JW, Lotgering FK, Struijk PC, Tonge HM: Fetal blood flow velocity waveforms in relation to changing peripheral vascular resistance. Early Hum Dev 15:119–127, 1987.
16. Spencer JAD, Giussani DA, Moore PJ, Hanson MA: In vitro validation of Doppler indices using blood and water. J Ultrasound Med 10:305–308, 1991.
17. Trudinger BJ, Stevens D, Connelly A, Hales JRS, Alexander G, Bradley L, Fawcett A, Thompson

RS: Umbilical artery flow velocity waveforms and placental resistance: the effects of embolization of the umbilical circulation. Am J Obstet Gynecol 157:1443–1448, 1987.

18. Morrow RF, Adamson SL, Bull SB, Ritchie JWK: Effect of placental embolization on the umbilical arterial velocity waveform in fetal sheep. Am J Obstet Gynecol 161:1055–1060, 1989.

19. Adamson SL, Morrow RJ, Langille BL, Bull SB, Ritchie JWK: Site-dependent effects of increases in placental vascular resistance on the umbilical arterial velocity waveform in fetal sheep. Ultrasound Med Biol 16:19–27, 1990.

20. Clapp JF, Szeto HH, Larrow R, Hewitt J, Mann LI: Umbilical blood flow response to embolization of the uterine circulation. Am J Obstet Gynecol 138:60–67, 1980.

21. Morrow RJ, Adamson SL, Bull SB, Ritchie JWK: Hypoxic acidemia, hyperviscosity, and maternal hypertension do not affect the umbilical arterial velocity waveform in fetal sheep. Am J Obstet Gynecol 163:1313–1320, 1990.

22. Santolaya J, Warsof S, Ramakrishnan V, Abramowicz J, Archer D: Vaginosonographic determination of the pulsatility index throughout the normal cycle in the ipsilateral and contralateral uterine artery to the site of ovulation: preliminary report. J Ultrasound Med 10:S57, 1991.

23. Jurkovic D, Jauniaux E, Kurjak A, Hustin J, Campbell S, Nicolaides KH: Transvaginal color Doppler assessment of the uteroplacental circulation in early pregnancy. Obstet Gynecol 77:365–369, 1991.

24. Trudinger BJ, Giles WB, Cook CM: Flow velocity waveforms in the maternal uteroplacental and fetal umbilical placental circulations. Am J Obstet Gynecol 152:155–163, 1985.

25. Pearce JM, Campbell S, Cohen-Overbeek TE, Hernandez J, Royston JP: References ranges and sources of variation for indices used to characterize flow velocity waveforms obtained by duplex, pulsed Doppler ultrasound from the uteroplacental and fetal circulation. Br J Obstet Gynaecol 95:248–256, 1988.

26. Schulman H, Winter D, Farmakides G, Ducey J, Guzman E, Coury A, Penny B: Pregnancy surveillance with uterine umbilical Doppler velocimetry. Am J Obstet Gynecol 160:192–196, 1989.

27. Campbell S, Pearce JMF, Hackett G: Qualitative assessment of uteroplacental blood flow: early screening test for high-risk pregnancies. Obstet Gynecol 68:649–653, 1986.

28. Fleischer A, Schulman H, Farmakiedes G, Bracen L, Grunfeild L, Rocheslon B, Koenigsberg M: Uterine artery Doppler velocimetry in pregnant women with hypertension. Am J Obstet Gynecol 154:806–813, 1986.

29. Soothill PW, Nicolaides KH, Bilardo K, Hackett GA, Campbell S: Uteroplacental blood velocity resistance index and umbilical venous pO_2, pCO_2, pH, lactate and erythroblast count in growth-retarded fetuses. Fetal Ther 1:176–179, 1986.

30. Steel SA, Pearce JMF, Chamberlain GVP: Doppler ultrasound of the uteroplacental circulation as a screening test for severe preeclampsia with intrauterine growth retardation. Eur J Obstet Gynecol Reprod Biol 28:279–287, 1988.

31. Abramowicz JS, Arrington J, Levy DL, Warsof SL: Doppler study of umbilical artery blood flow waveforms; should we use an instrument adapted nomogram? J Ultrasound Med 8:183–185, 1989.

32. Fisk NM, MacLachlan N, Ellis C, Tannirandorn Y, Tonge HM, Rodeck CH: Absent end-diastolic flow in first trimester umbilical artery. Lancet 2:1256–1257, 1988.

33. Arduini D, Rizzo G, Mancuso S, Romanini C: Longitudinal assessment of blood flow velocity waveforms in the healthy human fetus. Prenat Diag 7:613–617, 1987.

34. Hendricks SK, Sorenson TK, Wang KY, Bushnell JM, Sequin EM, Zingheim RW: Doppler umbilical artery waveform indices—normal values from fourteen to forty-two weeks. Am J Obstet Gynecol 161:761–765, 1989.

35. Spencer JAD, Price J, Lee A: Influence of fetal breathing and movements on variability of umbilical Doppler indices using different numbers of waveforms. J Ultrasound Med 10:37–41, 1991.

36. Trudinger BJ, Cook CM, Jones L, Giles WB: A comparison of fetal heart rate monitoring and

umbilical artery waveforms in the recognition of fetal compromise. Br J Obstet Gynaecol 93:171–175, 1986.

37. Trudinger BJ, Cook CM, Giles WB, Connelly A, Thompson RS: Umbilical artery flow velocity waveforms in high-risk pregnancy. Randomized controlled trial. Lancet i:188–190, 1987.

38. Berkowitz GS, Mehalek KE, Chitkara U, Rosenberg J, Cogswell C, Berkowitz RL: Doppler umbilical velocimetry in the prediction of adverse outcome in pregnancies at risk for intrauterine growth retardation. Obstet Gynecol 71:742–746, 1988.

39. Pearce JM: ''Doppler ultrasound blood velocity waveforms,'' in Spencer JAD (ed), *Fetal Monitoring: Physiology and Techniques of Antenatal and Intrapartum Assessment*. Philadelphia, F.A. Davis Company, 1989, pp 78–84.

40. Nicolaides KH, Bilardo CM, Soothil PW, Campbell S: Absence of end diastolic frequencies in umbilical artery: a sign of fetal hypoxia and acidosis. Br Med J 297:1026–1027, 1989.

41. Ferrazzi E, Pardi G, Bauscaglia M, Marconi AM, Gementi B, Bellotti M, Makowski EL, Battaglia FC: The correlation of biochemical monitoring versus umbilical flow velocity measurements of the human fetus. Am J Obstet Gynecol 159:1081–1087, 1988.

42. Wilcox GR, Trudinger BJ, Cook CM, Wilcox WR, Connelly AJ: Reduced fetal platelet counts in pregnancies with abnormal Doppler umbilical flow waveforms. Obstet Gynecol 73:639, 1989.

43. Nicolini U, Nicolaidis P, Fisk NM, Vaughan JI, Fusi L, Gleeson R, Rodeck CH: Limited role of fetal blood sampling in prediction of outcome in intrauterine growth retardation. Lancet 336:768–772, 1990.

44. Santolaya J, Warsof S: Normal umbilical artery blood velocity waveforms in a severely hemodynamically compromised fetus. The Fetus 1:5, 1–3, 1991.

45. Vintzileos AM, Campbell WA, Rodis JF, McLean DA, Fleming AD, Scorza WE: The relationship between fetal biophysical assessment, umbilical artery velocimetry, and fetal acidosis. Obstet Gynecol 77:622–626, 1991.

46. Giles WB, Trudinger BJ, Baird PJ: Fetal umbilical artery flow velocity waveforms and placental resistance: pathological correlation. Br J Obstet Gynecol 92:31–38, 1985.

47. MacCowan M, Mullen BM, Ritchie K: Umbilical artery flow velocity waveforms and the placental vascular bed. Am J Obstet Gynecol 1157:900–902, 1987.

48. Rochelson B, Kaplan C, Guzman E, Arato M, Hansen K, Trunca C: A qualitative analysis of placental vasculature in the third trimester fetus with autosomal trisomy. Obstet Gynecol 75:59–63, 1990.

49. Kuhlman RS, Werner AL, Abramowicz J, Warsof SL, Arrington J, Levy DL: Placental histology in fetuses between 18 and 23 weeks gestation with abnormal karyotype. Am J Obstet Gynecol 163:1264–1270, 1990.

50. Trudinger BJ, Giles WB, Cook C: Uteroplacental blood flow velocity-time waveforms in normal and complicated pregnancy. Br J Obstet Gynecol 92:39–45, 1985.

51. Ducey J: Velocity waveforms in hypertensive disease. Clin Obstet Gynecol 32:679–686, 1989.

52. Rochelson B: The clinical significance of absent end diastolic velocity in the umbilical artery waveforms. Clin Obstet Gynecol 32:692–702, 1989.

53. Bracero LA, Bereck D, Kirshenbaum N, Pfeiffer M, Stalter P, Schulman H: Doppler velocimetry and placental disease. Am J Obstet Gynecol 161:388–393, 1989.

54. Bracero L, Schulman H, Fleischer A, Farmakides G, Rochelson B: Umbilical artery velocimetry in diabetes and pregnancy. Obstet Gynecol 68:654–658, 1986.

55. Bracero LA, Jovanovic L, Rochelson B, Bauman W, Farmakides G: Significance of umbilical and uterine artery velocimetry in the well-controlled pregnant diabetic. J Reprod Med 34:274–276, 1989.

56. Santolaya J, Font G, Nobles G, Ramakrishnan V, Warsof L: Fetal hemodynamic evaluation by pulse Doppler in obese women. Ultrasound Obstet Gynecol 1:S60, 1991.

57. Stoz F, Schuhmann RA, Schmid A: Morphometric investigations of terminal villi of diabetic placentas in relation to the white classification of diabetes mellitus. J Perinat Med 15:193–198, 1987.

58. Teasdale F: Hystomorphometry of the human placenta in class B diabetes mellitus. Placenta 4:1–12, 1983.
59. Santolaya J, Seltman H, Meyer W, Warsof SL: Maternal characteristics can influence umbilical artery blood velocity waveforms in IUGR fetuses. Society for Gynecological Investigation, Annual meeting, San Antonio, Tex., March 1991. Abstract 109.
60. Trudinger BJ, Cook CM: Umbilical and uterine artery flow velocity waveforms in pregnancy associated with major fetal abnormality. Br J Obstet Gynecol 92:666–670, 1985.
61. Meizner I, Katz M, Lunenfield E, Insler V: Umbilical and uterine flow velocity waveforms in pregnancies complicated by major fetal anomalies. Prenat Diag 7:491–496, 1987.
62. Gaziano EP, Knox GF, Wager GP, Bendel RP, Olson JD: Pulsed Doppler umbilical artery waveform. Significance of an elevated umbilical artery systolic/diastolic ratios in the normally grown fetus. Obstet Gynecol 75:189–193, 1990.
63. Al-Gazali W, Chapman MG, Chita SK, Crawford DC, Allan LD: Doppler assessment of umbilical artery blood flow for the prediction of outcome in fetal cardiac abnormality. Br J Obstet Gynaecol 94:742–745, 1987.
64. Hsieh F, Chang F, Ko T, Chen H, Chen Y: Umbilical artery flow velocity waveforms in fetus dying with congenital anomalies. Br J Obstet Gynaecol 95:478–482, 1988.
65. Hata K, Hata T, Senoh D, Aoki S, Takamiya O, Kitao M: Umbilical artery blood flow velocity waveforms and associations with fetal abnormality. Gynecol Obstet Invest 27:179–182, 1989.
66. Giles WB, Trudinger BJ, Cook CM: Fetal umbilical artery flow velocity-time waveforms in twin pregnancies. Br J Obstet Gynaecol 92:490–497, 1985.
67. Gaziano EP, Knox E, Bendel RP, Calvin S, Brandt D: Is pulsed Doppler velocimetry useful in the management of multiple-gestation pregnancies? Am J Obstet Gynecol 164:1426–1433, 1991.
68. Santolaya J, Sampson M, Nobles G, Font G, Ramakrishnan V, Warsof S: Doppler evaluation of the fetoplacental circulation in the latent phase of preterm premature rupture of membranes. J Ultrasound Med 10:327–330, 1991.
69. Pearce JM, McParland PJ: A comparison of Doppler flow velocity waveforms, amniotic fluid columns, and the nonstress test as a means of monitoring post-dates pregnancies. Obstet Gynecol 77:204–208, 1991.
70. Nicolini U, Santolaya J, Ojo OE, Fisk NM, Hubinont C, Tonge M, Rodeck CH: Fetal blood sampling from the intrahepatic vein: an alternative to cord needling for prenatal diagnosis and therapy. Prenat Diag 8:665–671, 1988.
71. Nicolini U, Tonge HM, Santolaya J, Fisk NM, Rodeck CH: Transitory changes in umbilical artery blood velocity waveforms in association with fetal acidemia during intrauterine intravascular transfusion, 1991. Submitted for publication.
72. Defoort P, Thiery M, Vahasebrouk P: Uteroplacental and umbilical artery blood velocity waveforms in placental abruption assessed by Doppler ultrasound (letter, comment). Br J Obstet Gynaecol 29:254–255, 1989.
73. Farine D, Fox HE, Jakobson S, Timor-Tritsch IE: Vaginal ultrasound for diagnosis of placenta previa. Am J Obstet Gynecol 159:566–569, 1988.
74. Guy GP, Peisner DB, Timor-Tritsch IE: Ultrasonographic evaluation of uteroplacental blood flow patterns of abnormally located and adherent placentas. Am J Obstet Gynecol 163:723–727, 1990.
75. Jauniaux E, Campbell S, Vyas S: The use of color Doppler imaging for prenatal diagnosis of umbilical cord anomalies: report of three cases. Am J Obstet Gynecol 161:1195–1197, 1989.
76. Nelson LH, Melone PJ, King M: Diagnosis of vasa previa with transvaginal and color flow Doppler ultrasound. Obstet Gynecol 76:506–509, 1990.
77. Harding JA, Lewis DF, Major CA, Grade M, Patel J, Nageotte MP: Color flow Doppler—A useful instrument in the diagnosis of vasa previa. Am J Obstet Gynecol 163:1566–1568, 1990.

THE USE OF COLOR DOPPLER IMAGING TO EXAMINE THE FETAL HEART. NORMAL AND PATHOLOGIC ANATOMY

GREGGORY R. DeVORE

In the mid 1980s color Doppler imaging (CDI) was introduced to diagnostic ultrasound for use in evaluation of the cardiovascular system in pediatric and adult patients. In 1987 DeVore et al. published the first reports using CDI to diagnose congenital heart disease in the fetus.[1,2] Since 1987 a number of investigators have reported their experiences using CDI to diagnose abnormalities of the fetal heart which include (1) tricuspid and mitral insufficiency, (2) stenosis of the aortic and pulmonic valves, (3) reversed flow in the ascending aorta and main pulmonary artery, (4) abnormal communications, (5) abnormal ventricular anatomy such as Ebstein's anomaly, hypoplastic left and right ventricles, single ventricle, atrioventricular canal defect, and (6) ventricular and atrial septal defects.[1–14]

With the development of CDI for fetal applications, it is important for the physician evaluating the fetal heart to understand the principles of CDI and its use in examination of the cardiovascular system. The purpose of this chapter is to (1) review CDI imaging principles and potential pitfalls as they relate to the fetal heart, (2) review normal fetal cardiovascular anatomy, (3) illustrate examples of pathology, and (4) present case studies.

DOPPLER COLOR FLOW IMAGING PRINCIPLES AND POTENTIAL PITFALLS

From our experience there are three common problems that the imager should be familiar with which could influence the interpretation of CDI in the fetal heart:

assignment of maximal velocity, CDI sample rate, and orientation of the heart to the CDI ultrasound transducer beam.

Assignment of Maximal Velocity

Because of the need for imaging of the Doppler shift at both low as well as high flow states, manufacturers provide the user a selection of maximal velocity settings that are user-defined. When the blood velocity exceeds the maximal velocity setting aliasing, as manifest by reversal of the color map, occurs. This is often observed when the maximal velocity is not set appropriately for the structure being examined. However, when the setting is correct, then one must consider pathology due to increased or disturbed flow. Figure 8-1 illustrates aliasing which occurs as blood flows into the ventricles from the atria during ventricular diastole.

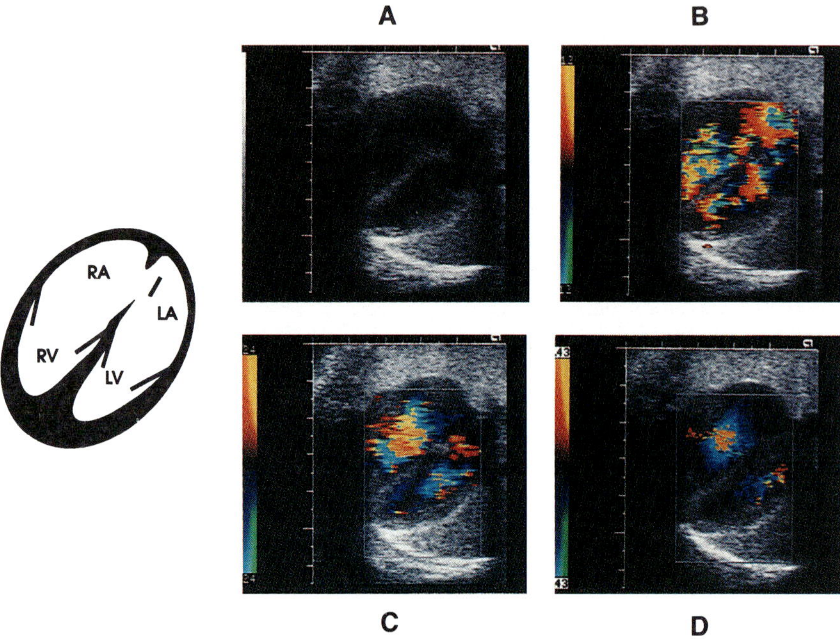

Figure 8-1 *Aliasing observed in the four-chamber view during ventricular diastole.* *A*. Real-time four-chamber view. *B*. Aliasing at a velocity setting of 0.12 m/s as manifest by multiple colors within the ventricular and atrial chambers. At this velocity setting blood flow is observed in the right and left atrial chambers. *C*. As the velocity setting is increased to 0.24 m/s, the aliasing is decreased in the left ventricle, but still present in the right ventricle. Identification of flow within the right and left atrial chambers is minimal at this velocity setting. *D*. Maximal velocity of 0.43 m/s demonstrates ventricular flow with aliasing at the inflow portion of the right ventricle. This is pathologic and due to early volume overload of the right ventricle. The schematic identifies the atrial and ventricular chambers. RA = right atrium; LA = left atrium; RV = right ventricle; LV = left ventricle.

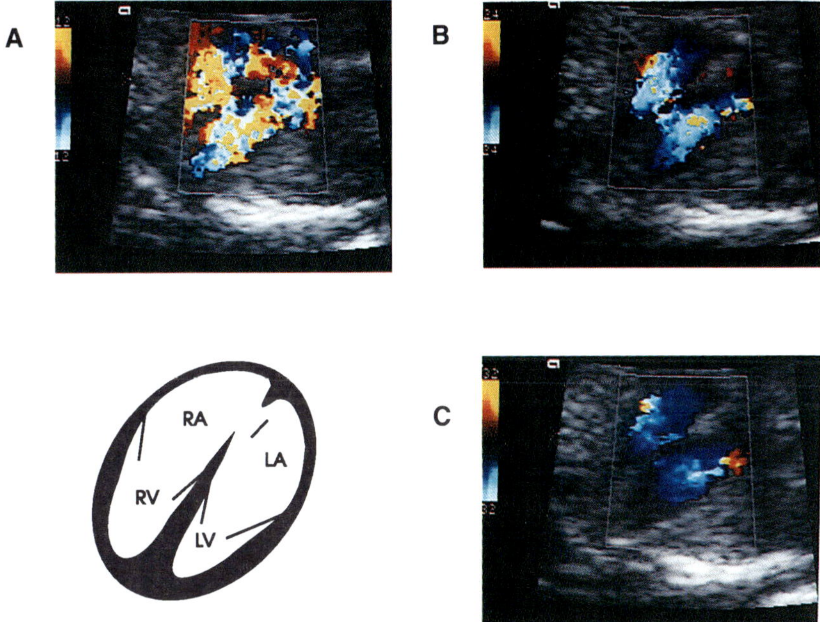

Figure 8-2   *CDI of the four-chamber view during diastole with aliasing and a ventricular septal defect. A.* Real-time four-chamber view with aliasing at a velocity setting of 0.12 m/s. CDI is observed to cross the ventricular septum suggesting a ventricular septal defect. *B.* As the velocity setting is increased to 0.24 m/s, the aliasing is decreased in the left ventricle, but flow across the ventricular septum is still present, again suggesting a ventricular septal defect. *C.* At a velocity of 0.32 m/s the ventricular septal defect is not present. The schematic identifies the atrial and ventricular chambers. RA = right atrium; LA = left atrium; RV = right ventricle; LV = left ventricle.

If the maximal velocity setting is too low, CDI will demonstrate aliasing within the chambers of the heart. Evaluation of flow when aliasing is present may be useful in situations when the flow of blood through a septal defect is identified at low velocity settings in which aliasing occurs, but not higher velocity settings (Fig. 8-2).

CDI Sample Rate

If the sample rate of CDI is too slow to discriminate independent events within the cardiac cycle, then the information may be misinterpreted. The CDI sample rate is dependent on (1) the size of the CDI area being interrogated, (2) the distance the heart is from the transducer, and (3) the user-selected variables unique to each imaging device. Figure 8-3 illustrates this problem in which a sampling rate of 16 Hz records both diastolic and systolic events, while a sampling rate of 22 Hz discriminates between systole and diastole. If one considers a fetal heart rate of 150 beats per minute, this would equate to 2.5 cardiac cycles per

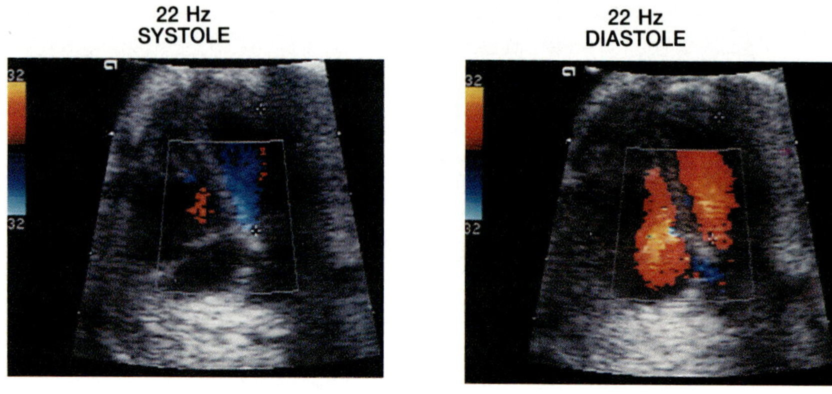

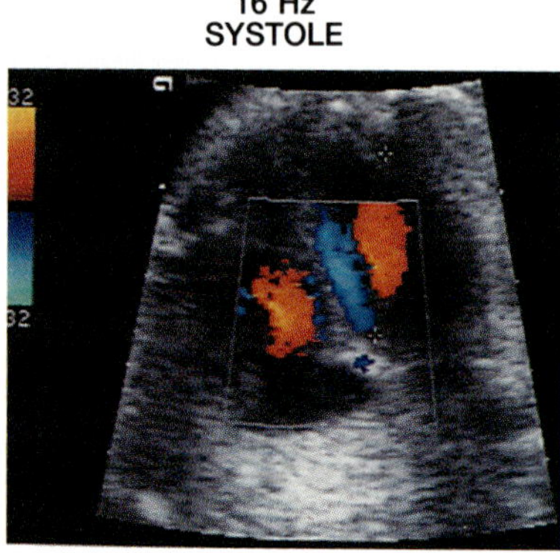

Figure 8-3 *Four-chamber CDI at two sampling rates.* At 22 Hz systole (blue observed along the ventricular septum) is separate from diastole (orange filling both ventricular chambers). However, at a lower sampling rate of 16 Hz, CDI does not discriminate between systole (blue) and diastole (orange).

second. If CDI were sampling at 16 Hz, then 6.4 frames per cardiac cycle would be recorded, while at 22 Hz 8.6 frames per cardiac cycle would be recorded.

Orientation of the Heart to the CDI Ultrasound Transducer Beam

Unlike real-time ultrasound in which maximal resolution occurs, when the ultrasound beam is perpendicular to the object to be imaged, CDI is optimal when the vascular structures (chambers of the heart, vessels) to be imaged are parallel to the ultrasound beam. Therefore, if one were to image the four-chamber view of the fetal heart in real-time, maximal information is obtained when the interventricular septum of the four-chamber view is perpendicular to the ultrasound beam. While CDI may be obtained when the interventricular septum is perpendicular to the ultrasound beam at low velocity settings, aliasing occurs within the ventricles and atria. When the velocity setting is set for ventricular flow, blood flowing into the ventricles from the atria is poorly imaged. As the interventricular septum approaches a plane parallel to the ultrasound beam, the CDI image fills more of the ventricular chambers (Figs. 8-4 and 8-5).

NORMAL CDI CARDIAC ANATOMY

The Four-Chamber View

The fetal heart may be identified with CDI as early as 6 to 7 weeks of gestation by last menstrual period (4 to 5 weeks conceptional age) (Fig. 8-6). CDI demonstrates two separate ventricles in the early second trimester (Fig. 8-7) which may be identified by transvaginal or transabdominal approaches to image ac-

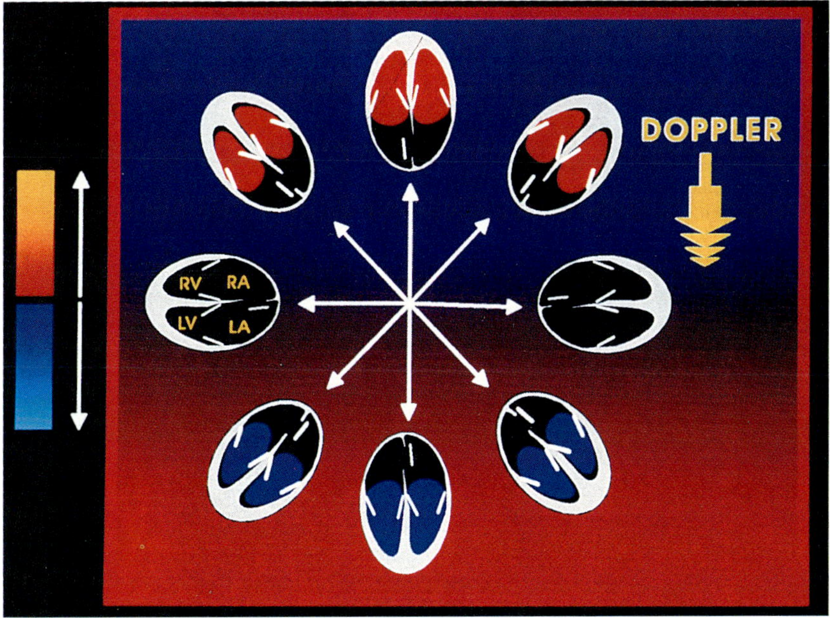

Figure 8-4   *Color schematic of the effect of the position of the heart as it relates to optimal CDI imaging.* When the four-chamber view is perpendicular to the ultrasound beam (*yellow arrow*), minimal to no CDI is observed at velocity settings appropriate for ventricular flow. However, as the heart approaches a parallel orientation to the ultrasound beam, CDI is displayed optimally. The schematic demonstrates CDI with the flow of blood toward the transducer (red) or away from the transducer (blue). RA = right atrium; LA = left atrium; RV = right ventricle; LV = left ventricle.

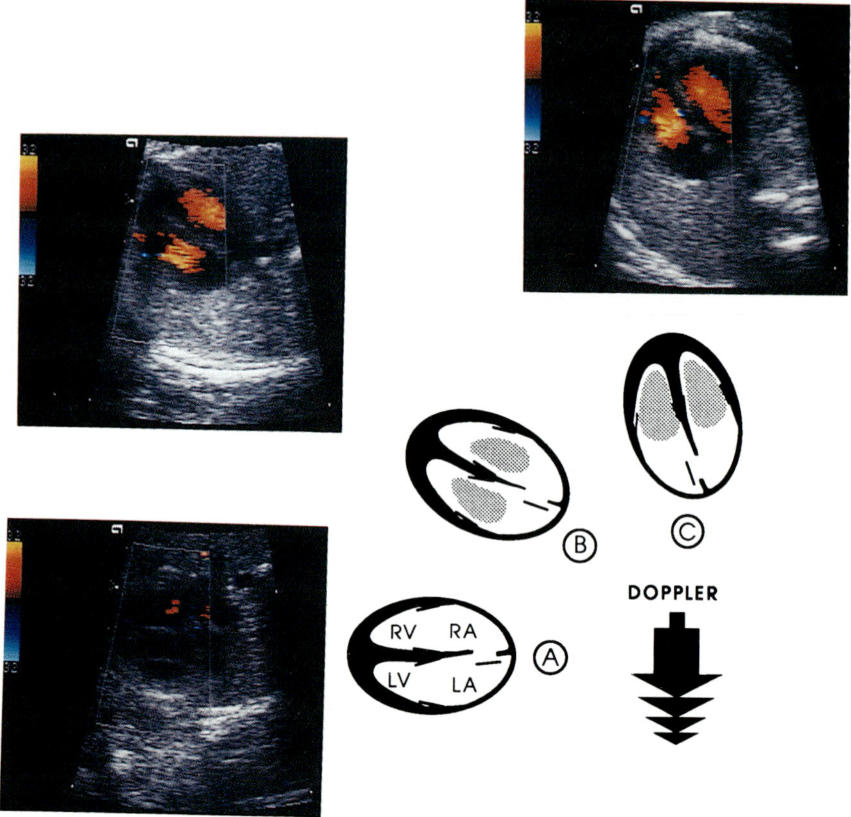

Figure 8-5 *The effect of the position of the heart as it relates to optimal CDI imaging during ventricular diastole. A.* The four-chamber view is perpendicular to the ultrasound beam (*black arrow*) demonstrating absent CDI of the ventricular or atrial chambers. *B.* As the heart approaches a 45° angle, CDI begins to fill the ventricles during diastole. *C.* As the four-chamber view approaches a plane parallel to the ultrasound beam, optimal CDI occurs. The color bars represent flow of blood toward the transducer (red) or away from the transducer (blue). RA = right atrium; LA = left atrium; RV = right ventricle; LV = left ventricle.

quisition.[15] After 16 weeks menstrual age, the four-chamber view of the heart enables one to evaluate flow of blood into the atrial chambers from the vena cava and pulmonary veins, across the foramen ovale, into the ventricles, and out the left ventricle. To evaluate intracardiac flow, the heart must be in an optimal position in relation to the transducer beam.

Pulmonary venous return. Because of the low velocity of blood flow in the pulmonary veins, the maximum velocity setting is lower (0.08 to 0.16 m/s) than that used to record ventricular flow. The pulmonary veins may be imaged when

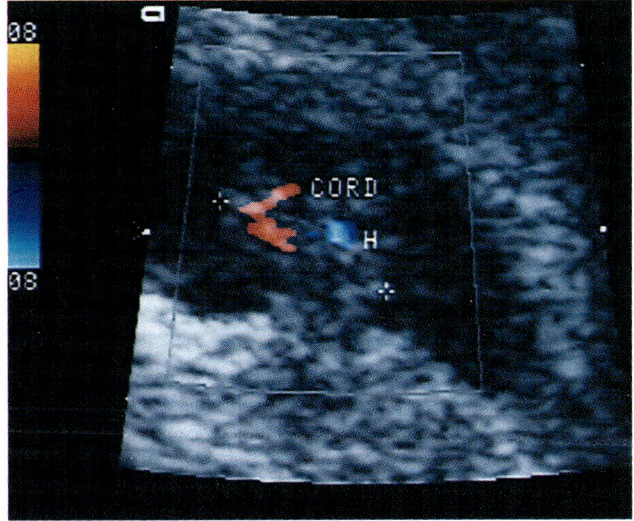

Figure 8-6 *Transvaginal CDI of an embryo at 7.1 weeks menstrual age (5.1 weeks conceptual age)*. The asterisk (*) represents the crown rump length and the blue in the center of the embryo is the heart (H). Because of the low flow velocity of the embryo, the velocity setting is 0.08 m/s. The color bars represent flow of blood toward the transducer (red) or away from the transducer (blue).

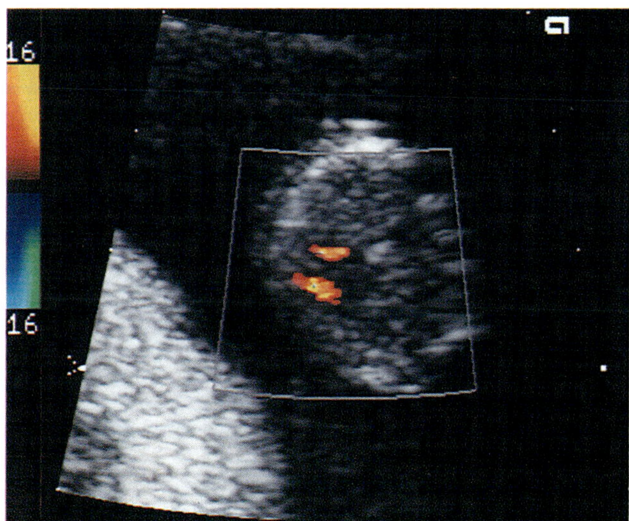

Figure 8-7 *Transabdominal evaluation of the four-chamber view of a 14-week fetus*. CDI demonstrates two separate ventricular chambers (orange represents flow and is divided by an interventricular septum). Because of the size of the fetus, the velocity setting is 0.16 m/s, which is twice that of Fig. 8-6 but less than a fetus in the late second and third trimesters of pregnancy. The color bars represent flow of blood toward the transducer (red) or away from the transducer (blue).

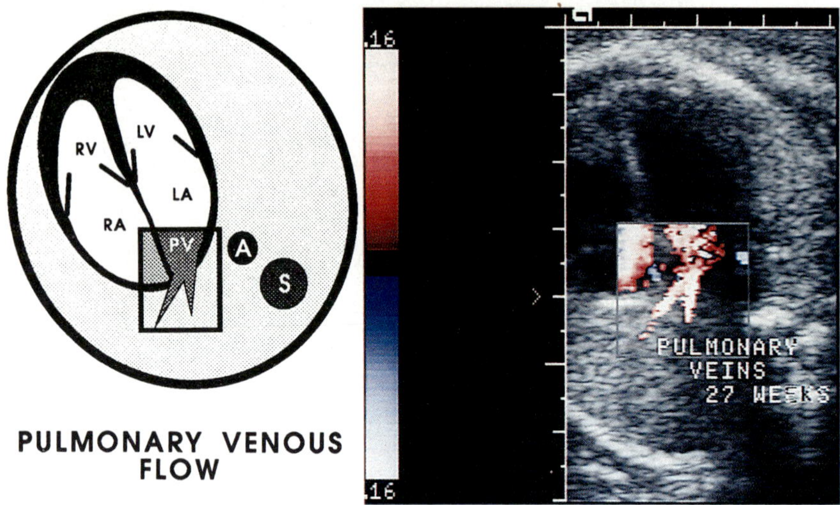

Figure 8-8 *CDI pulmonary venous return.* The four-chamber view is oriented with the interventricular septum parallel to the ultrasound beam. Because of the low flow of the pulmonary veins, the velocity setting is 0.16 m/s for a 27-week fetus. To avoid confusion, the CDI box is placed over the posterior aspect of the left and right atrial chambers. This minimizes aliasing and confusion with the interpretation of the image. The color bars represent flow of blood toward the transducer (red) or away from the transducer (blue). RA = right atrium; LA = left atrium; RV = right ventricle; LV = left ventricle; PV = pulmonary vein; A = descending aorta; S = spine.

the interventricular septum is tangential (Fig. 8-8) or perpendicular to the ultrasound beam (Fig. 8-9).

Flow into the right atrium from the vena cava. While the superior and inferior vena cava are not imaged with real time in the four-chamber view, blood flow entering the right atrium from the vena cava may be imaged with CDI. At the velocity setting used to image the pulmonary veins (0.08 to 0.16 m/s) blood flow within the atrial chambers can be recorded but may demonstrate aliasing, while at higher settings (0.17 to 0.33 m/s) flow appears normal (Fig. 8-9). When the interatrial septum is perpendicular to the ultrasound beam, minimal to no flow is observed when the velocity setting used to evaluate flow within the ventricles is used (> 0.32 m/s) except when there is an increased flow from the inferior vena cava associated with a dilated right atrium (Figs. 8-4, 8-5, and 8-10).

Flow across the foramen ovale. CDI may be observed from the right atrium to the left atrium across the foramen ovale, which is unidirectional (Fig. 8-11).

Intraventricular flow. The velocity setting for flow within the ventricles is the highest when imaging the four-chamber view. During ventricular diastole CDI may be observed with blood entering and filling the ventricular chambers.

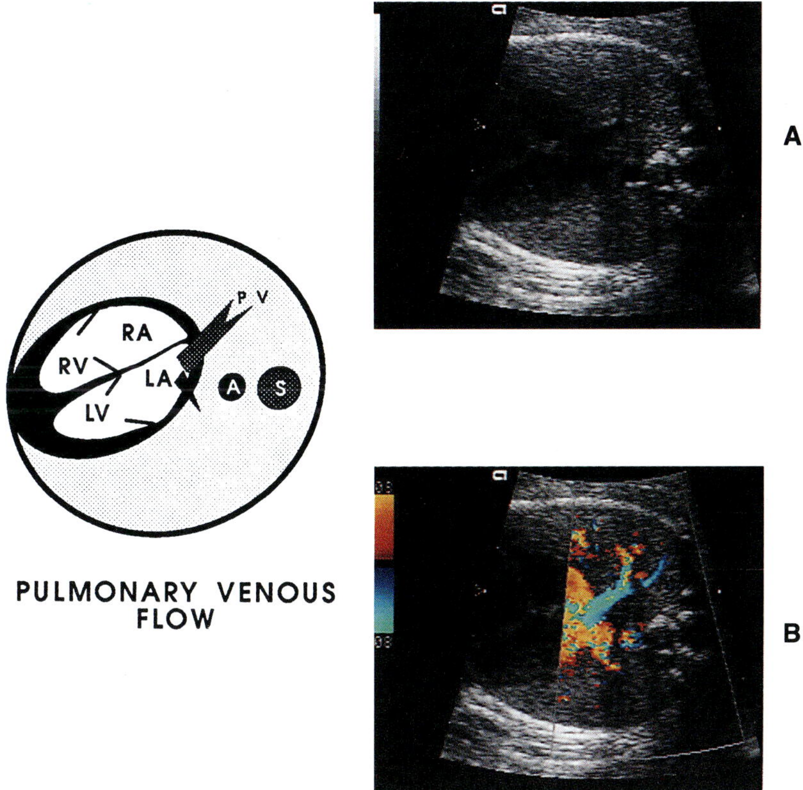

Figure 8-9   *Pulmonary venous return. A.* Real-time image of the four-chamber view with the interventricular septum tangential to the ultrasound beam. The pulmonary vein is present but may be difficult to identify from the real-time image. *B.* CDI of the same image in which the pulmonary vein (blue) and its branches are readily identified. Venous blood is observed entering the left atrial chamber. The yellow-orange represents blood flow within the atrial chambers with minimal aliasing in the left atrium. The color bars represent flow of blood toward the transducer (red) or away from the transducer (blue). RA = right atrium; LA = left atrium; RV = right ventricle; LV = left ventricle; PV = pulmonary vein; A = descending aorta; S = spine.

In the normal, nondilated fetal heart, the CDI is unidirectional during diastole. When the velocity setting is optimal, aliasing should not be observed (Fig. 8-3). However, when volume overload occurs in the right atrium, aliasing due to increased velocity may be observed during ventricular diastole (Fig. 8-1). During ventricular systole CDI is observed to occur adjacent to the interventricular septum of the left ventricle (Fig. 8-3). Minimal to no flow is observed within the right ventricle during systole. In approximately 2 percent of fetuses an echodensity may be observed within the left ventricle. The echodensity is a single structure which has minimal movement during systole or diastole and is within the ventricular chamber (Fig. 8-12).

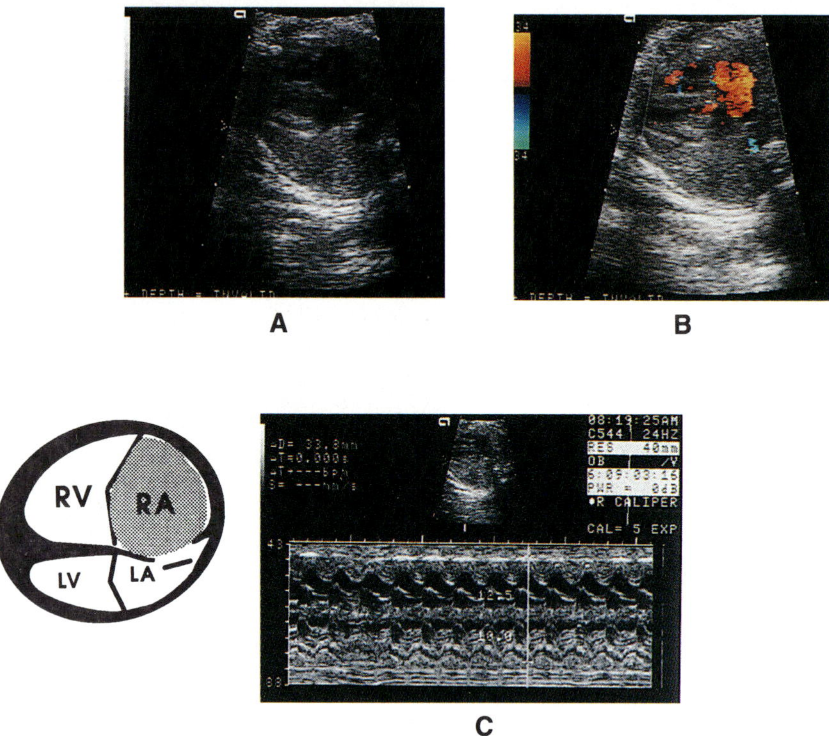

Figure 8-10 *Right atrial and ventricular volume overload. A.* Real-time four-chamber view illustrating right/left atrial and ventricular disproportion. *B.* CDI illustrates increased flow within the right atrial chamber (orange). *C.* M-mode measurements from the four-chamber view in which the M-mode cursor is perpendicular to the mitral and tricuspid valves demonstrating the right ventricle (12.5 mm) to be larger than the left ventricle (10.0 mm).

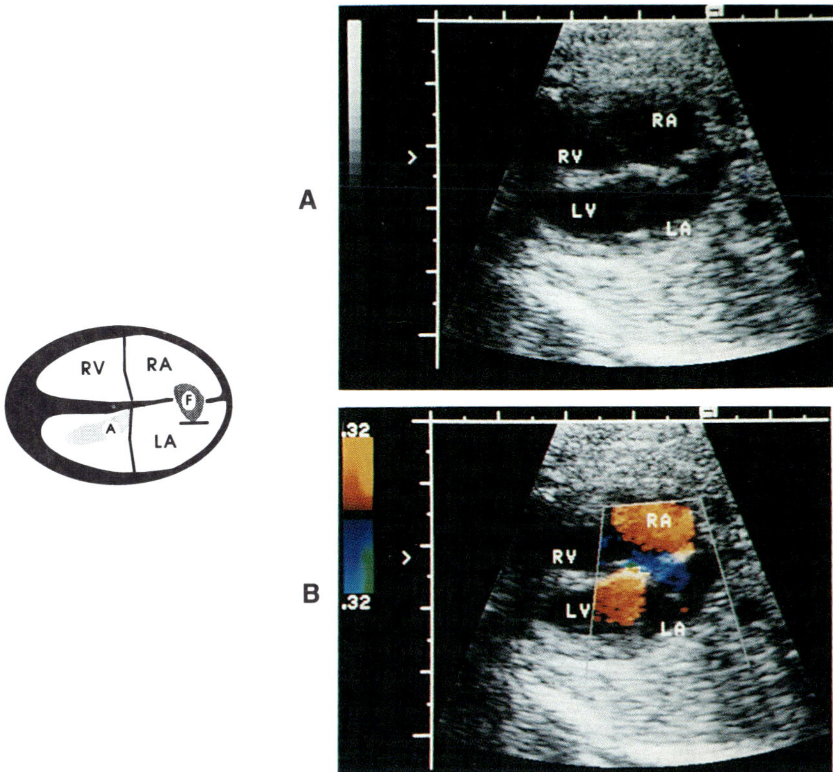

Figure 8-11   *Four-chamber view of flow across the foramen ovale.* A. Real-time four-chamber view illustrating the interruption of the interatrial septum which represents the foramen ovale. *B.* CDI demonstrating flow across the foramen ovale (blue) from the right atrium to the left atrium. The orange in the left ventricle represents flow along the interventricular septum during ventricular systole as blood leaves the left ventricle. The orange in the right atrium represents interatrial flow. The color bars represent flow of blood toward the transducer (red) or away from the transducer (blue). RA = right atrium; LA = left atrium; RV = right ventricle; LV = left ventricle; A = aortic flow; F = flow across the foramen ovale.

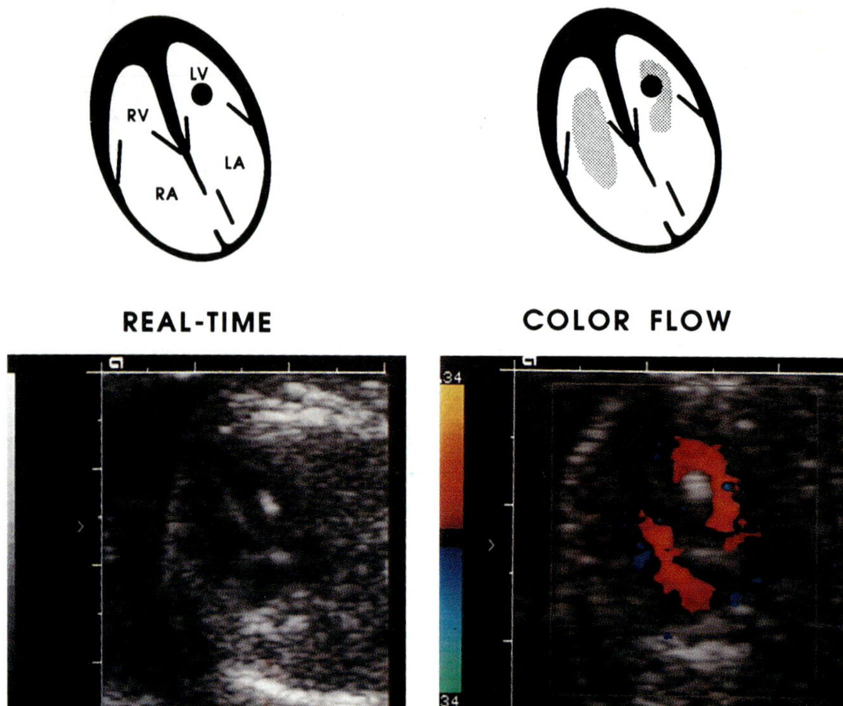

Figure 8-12 *Ventricular echodensity*. The real-time image (*left panel*) illustrates a bright echodensity within the left ventricle. CDI (*right panel*) demonstrates flow of blood to be displaced around the echodensity, thus illustrating the echodensity to be within the left ventricular chamber. The echodensity most likely represents an aberrant papillary muscle. The color bars represent flow of blood toward the transducer (red) or away from the transducer (blue). RA = right atrium; LA = left atrium; RV = right ventricle; LV = left ventricle.

THE AORTIC AND PULMONARY OUTFLOW TRACTS

Five-Chamber View

With the fetus supine, the five-chamber view is obtained by angling the transducer cephlad from the four-chamber view until the aortic outflow tract is identified. CDI demonstrates flow along the interventricular septum (Fig. 8-13). This view is useful for identification of septal overriding as observed with tetralogy of Fallot and obtaining pulsed Doppler information from the aorta.

Short-Axis View

The short-axis view of the heart is imaged as previously described with the fetus lying in the supine position with the interventricular septum parallel or tangential to the ultrasound beam (Fig. 8-11).[16] The velocity setting for CDI should be maximal because of the increased velocity through the aortic and pulmonary outflow tracts. With the velocity setting appropriately selected, CDI demonstrates blood entering the right ventricle during ventricular diastole and exiting

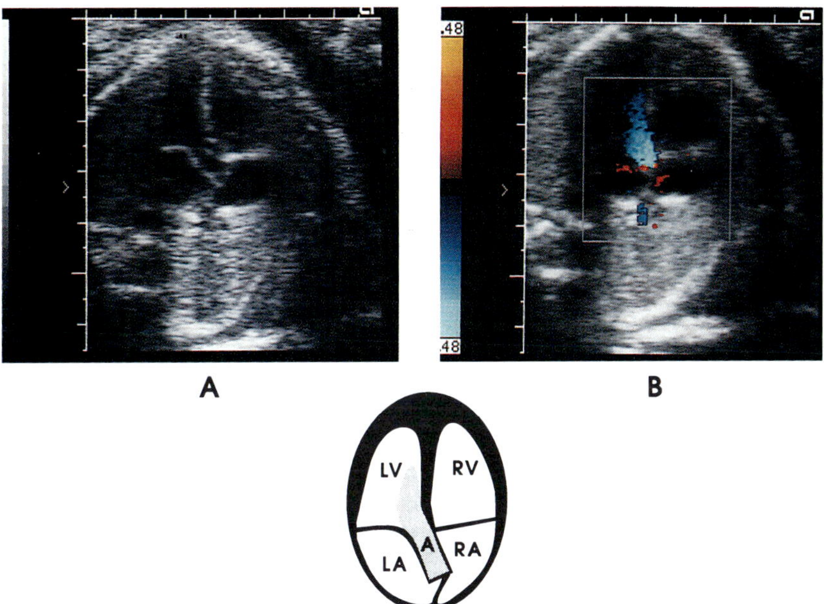

Figure 8-13   *The five-chamber view. A.* Real-time image of the five-chamber view in which the aortic outflow tract is identified as it exits the left ventricle. *B.* CDI of the five-chamber view in which there is no blood flowing across the interventricular septum into the right ventricle. The color bars represent flow of blood toward the transducer (red) or away from the transducer (blue). RA = right atrium; LA = left atrium; RV = right ventricle; LV = left ventricle.

the pulmonary outflow tract during systole. In the normal fetus CDI distal to the level of the pulmonary valve should not demonstrate aliasing. However, as the main pulmonary artery divides into the right pulmonary artery and the ductus arteriosus, aliasing may be observed at the level of the ductus arteriosus just as it enters the descending aorta (Fig. 8-14). The aorta, which is circular and perpendicular to the main pulmonary artery, demonstrates CDI which is dependent on the angle of insonation.

Long-Axis View

When the fetus is lying on its side, the interventricular septum imaged in the four-chamber view is perpendicular to the ultrasound beam (Figs. 8-15 and

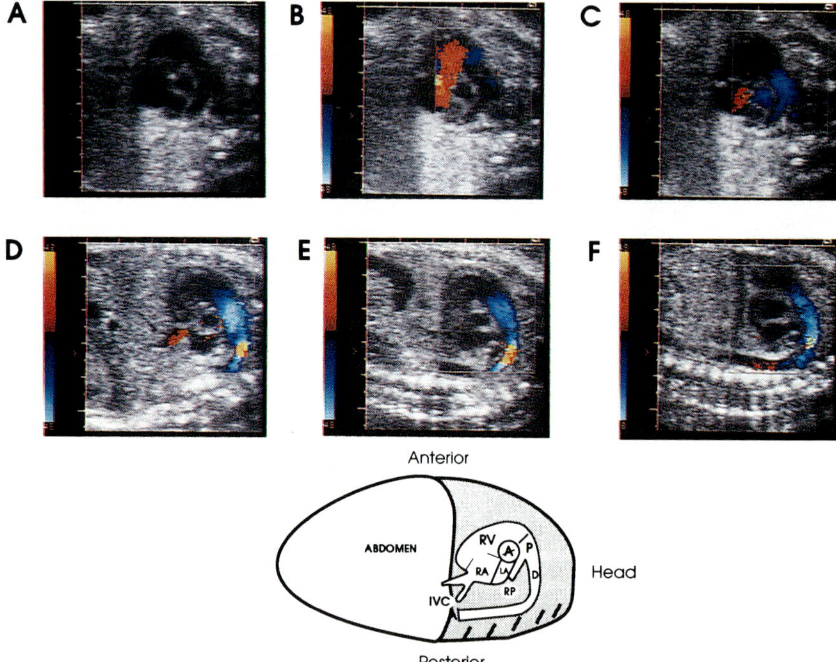

Figure 8-14 *The short axis of the aortic and pulmonic outflow tracts. A.* Real-time short-axis view of the outflow tracts. *B.* Early diastole in which CDI demonstrates blood entering the right ventricle from the right atrial chamber. *C.* Systole in which blood is leaving the pulmonary outflow tract. Blood is also observed in the aorta. *D* to *F.* Systole in which blood is observed in the ductus arteriosus entering the descending aorta. The yellow represents aliasing at the point of maximal velocity in the ductus. The color bars represent flow of blood toward the transducer (red) or away from the transducer (blue). RA = right atrium; LA = left atrium; RV = right ventricle; LV = left ventricle; IVC = inferior vena cava; RP = right pulmonary artery; A = aorta; P = main pulmonary artery; D = ductus arteriosus.

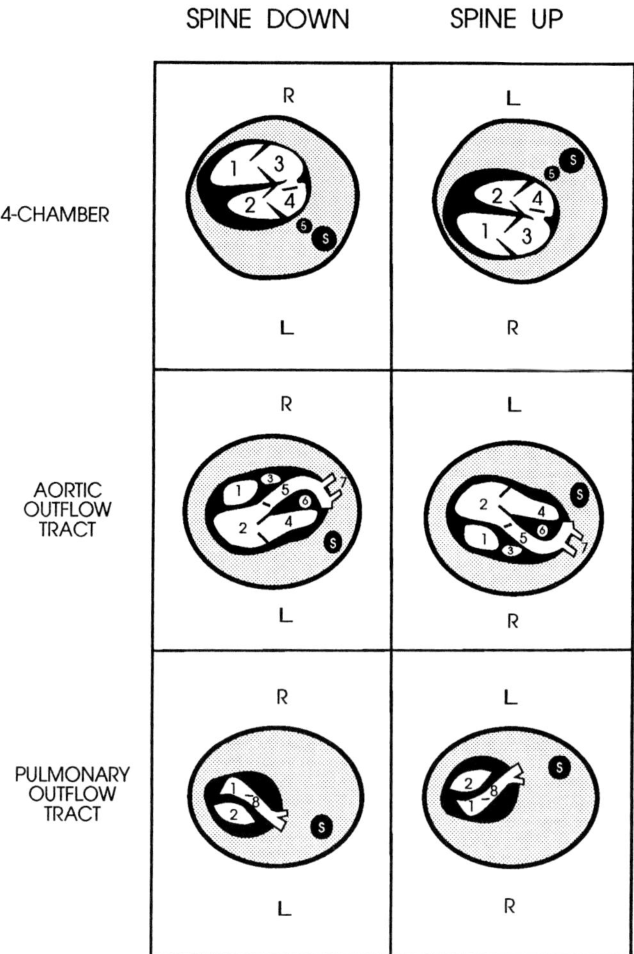

Figure 8-15 *Schematic of examination of the outflow tracts.* The schematic illustrates examination of the aortic and pulmonary outflow tracts when the interventricular septum is perpendicular to the ultrasound beam. The aortic outflow tract is identified by rotating the transducer from the four-chamber view until the aortic arch is identified. Once the arch is identified, the transducer is rocked demonstrating the pulmonary outflow tract perpendicular to the ascending aorta. R = right; L = left; 1 = right ventricle; 2 = left ventricle; 3 = right atrium; 4 = left atrium; 5 = aorta; 6 = right pulmonary artery; 7 = brachiocephalic arteries; 8 = pulmonary artery; S = spine.

8-16). Once this view is obtained, the transducer can be rotated to image the aorta and pulmonary outflow tracts (Figs. 8-15 and 8-16). In this view CDI demonstrates blood in the ascending and descending aorta (Figs. 8-16 and 8-17). Once this view is obtained, rocking the transducer will demonstrate CDI from the pulmonary outflow tract as it exits the right ventricle (Fig. 8-18).

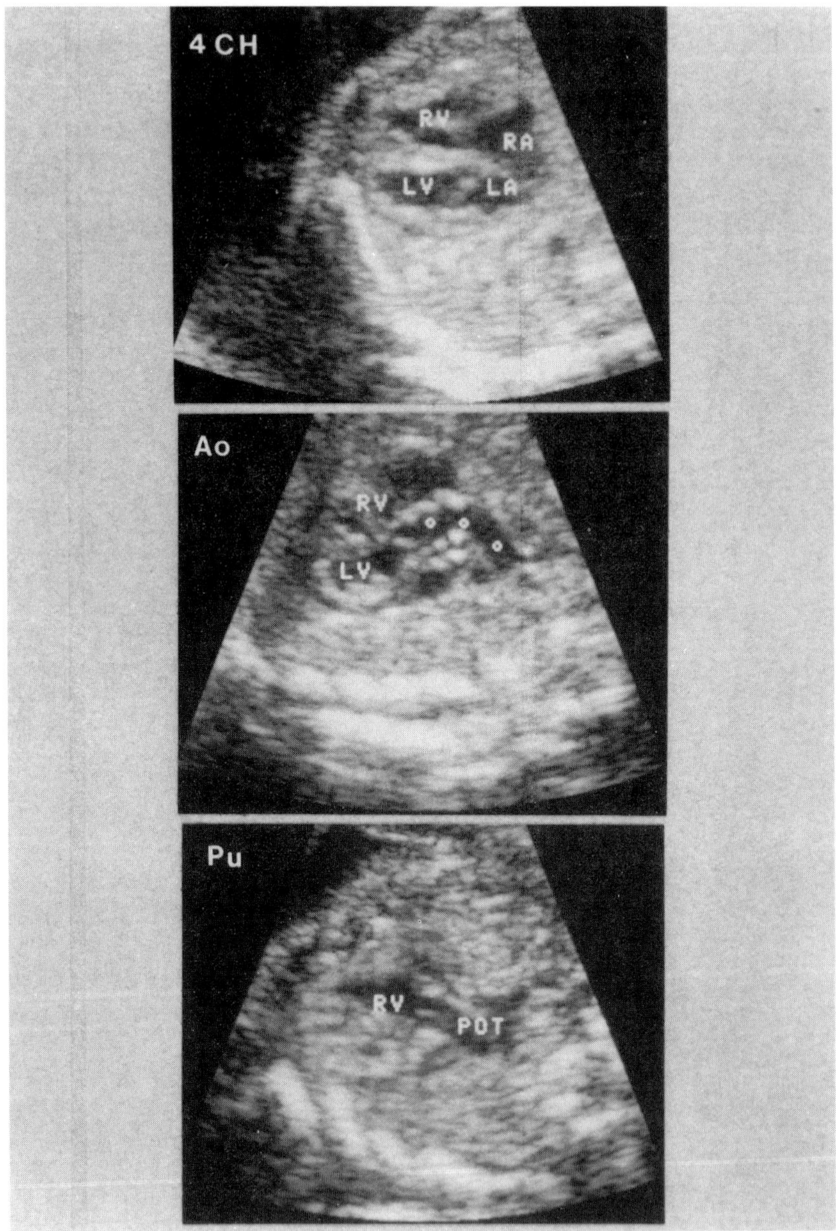

Figure 8-16 *Real-time examination of the outflow tracts.* The images correspond to the schematic of Fig. 8-15. 4-CH = four-chamber view; RV = right ventricle; LV = left ventricle; RA = right atrium; LA = left atrium; Ao = Aortic outflow tract; Pu = pulmonary artery; POT = pulmonary outflow tract.

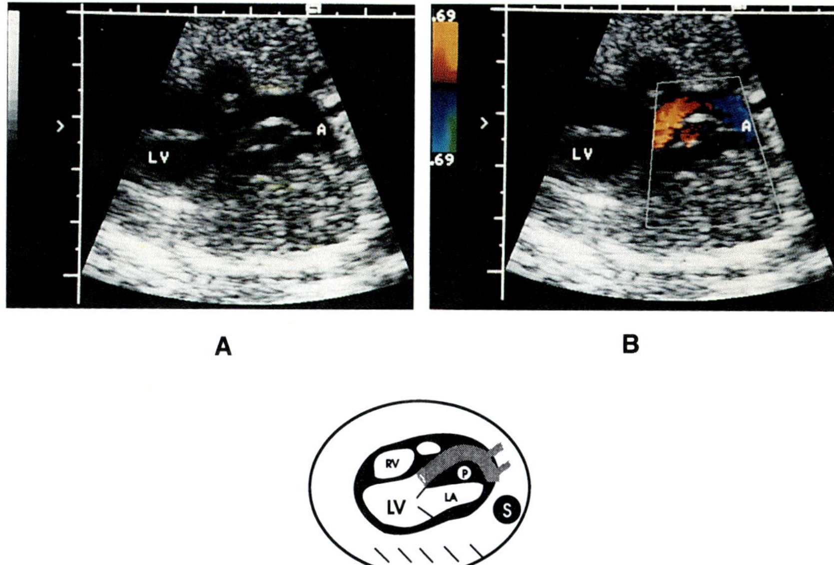

Figure 8-17 *The aortic outflow tract. A.* Real-time image of the arch of the aorta as it leaves the left ventricle. This view corresponds to the views identified in Figs. 8-15 and 8-16. *B.* CDI of the real-time image demonstrating flow of blood in the aortic arch. As blood leaves the left ventricle, it is flowing toward the transducer (orange). As it is perpendicular to the transducer, no CDI is recorded (black). As it flows along the descending aortic arch, it is depicted in blue. The color bars represent flow of blood towards the transducer (red) or away from the transducer (blue). RA = right atrium; LA = left atrium; RV = right ventricle; LV = left ventricle; A = aorta.

Aortic Arch

This may be imaged with CDI when the fetus is supine or when the spine is up. It is not unusual to observe aliasing or disturbed flow at the junction of the aorta and ductus arteriosus (Fig. 8-19).

VENA CAVA

Inferior and Superior Vena Cava

This is imaged with the fetus in supine position. CDI identifies blood entering the right atrium from the vena cava and the liver (Fig. 8-20).

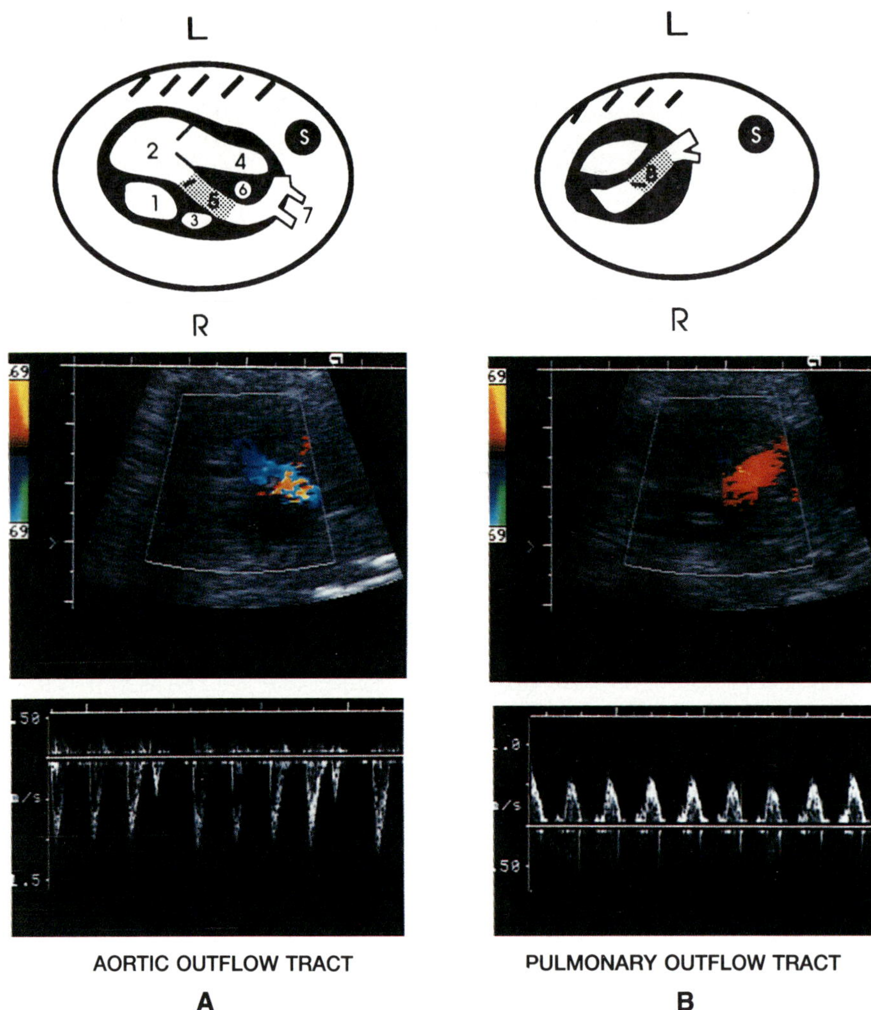

Figure 8-18 *The aortic and pulmonary outflow tracts.* *A.* CDI and pulsed Doppler of the aorta. This fetus demonstrated premature atrial contractions and increased flow across the aortic valve as manifest by aliasing (red-orange) at a velocity setting of 0.69 m/s. *B.* CDI and pulsed Doppler of blood leaving the pulmonary artery (orange), which is perpendicular to the aorta. No aliasing is noted. The color bars represent flow of blood toward the transducer (red) or away from the transducer (blue). 1 = right ventricle; 2 = left ventricle; 3 = right atrium; 4 = left atrium; 5 = aorta; 6 = right pulmonary artery; 7 = brachiocephalic vessels; 8 = pulmonary artery; S = spine.

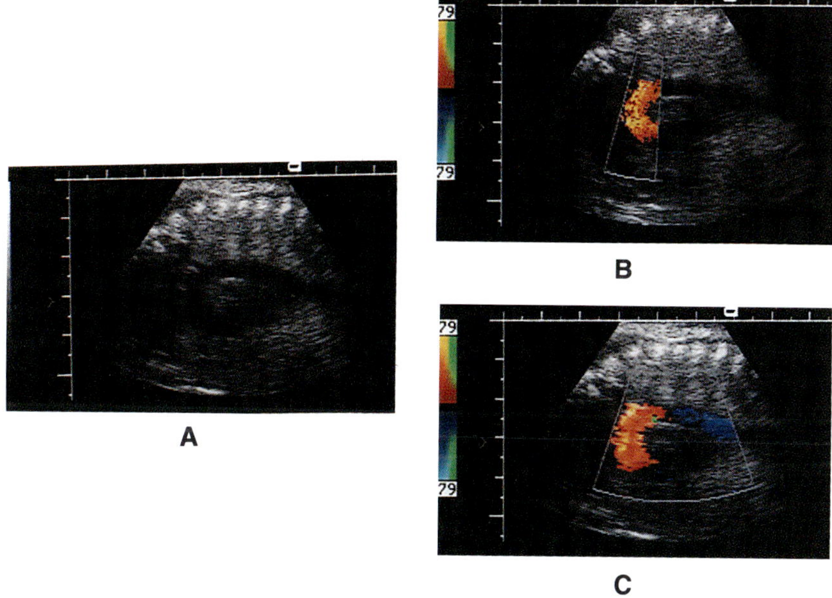

Figure 8-19 *The aortic arch. A.* Real-time image of the aortic arch with the spine in the up position. The aortic arch has the appearance of a candy cane. *B.* CDI demonstrating blood leaving the left ventricle (orange). *C.* CDI of blood leaving the left ventricle (orange) and flowing down the descending aorta (blue). The color bars represent flow of blood toward the transducer (red) or away from the transducer (blue).

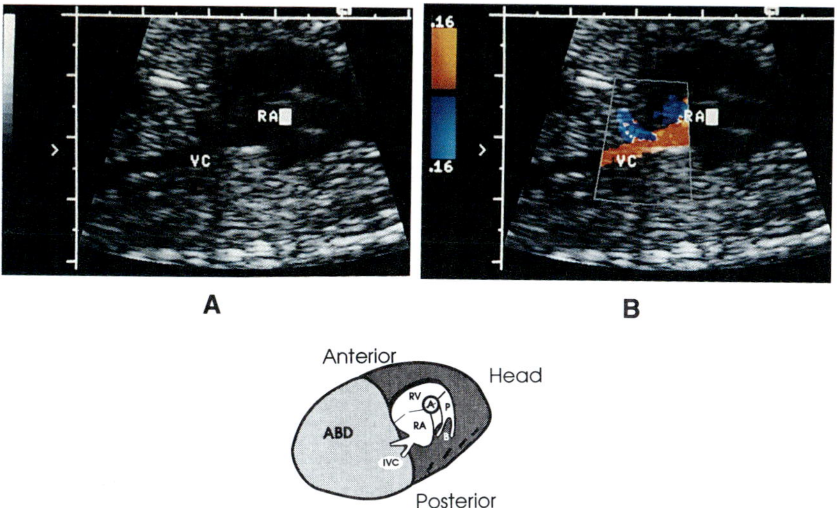

Figure 8-20 *The inferior vena cava. A.* Real-time of the inferior vena cava as it enters the right atrium. *B.* CDI illustrating blood entering the vena cava from the liver (blue) and the inferior vena cava (orange) entering the right atrium. The color bars represent flow of blood toward the transducer (red) or away from the transducer (blue). RA = right atrium; VC, IVC = inferior vena cava; RV = right ventricle; A = aorta; P = pulmonary artery; B = bifurcation.

ABNORMAL ANATOMY

Abnormal Intraventricular Flow

In the normal fetus CDI fills both ventricles during diastole (Figs. 8-2 and 8-3). If there is a marked difference in atrial or ventricular size due to abnormal anatomy, then the CDI may not be symmetric as is observed in the normal fetus (Fig. 8-1). Figure 8-21 illustrates an example of a fetus with endocardial fibroelastosis due to critical aortic stenosis. The real-time image of the four-chamber view demonstrated the left ventricle to be smaller than the right ventricle, but the difference was not as striking as one might observe with a hypoplastic left ventricle. CDI demonstrated filling of the right ventricle, but no filling of the left ventricle at the velocity setting chosen for ventricular flow. Because the aortic

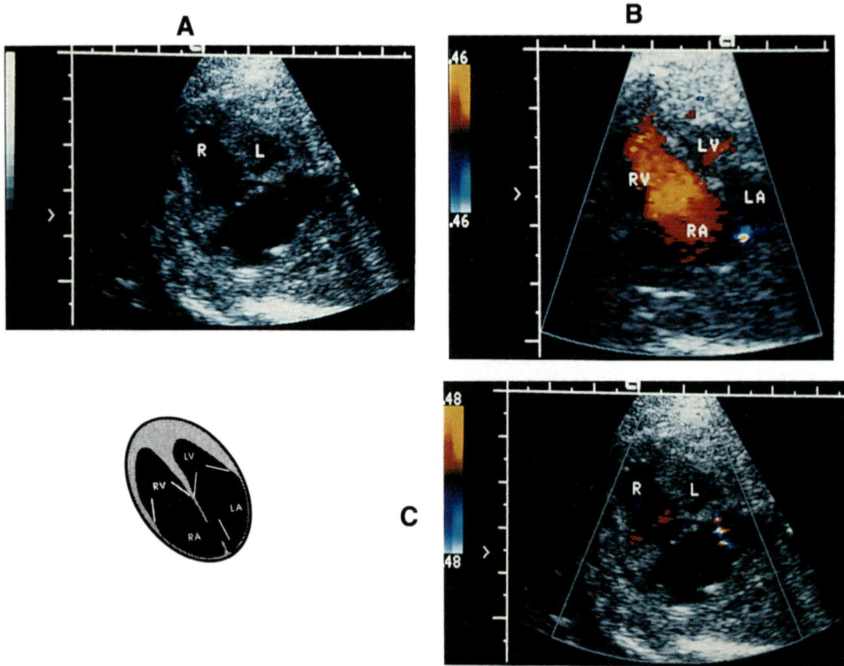

Figure 8-21 *Ventricular disproportion. A.* Real-time four-chamber view illustrating ventricular disproportion with the right ventricle larger than the left ventricle. *B.* CDI during ventricular diastole demonstrating flow into the right ventricle with minimal flow into the left ventricle. *C.* CDI during systole demonstrating absence of flow along the interventricular septum of the left ventricle and mitral regurgitation. The fetus had critical aortic stenosis with endocardial fibroelastosis. The color bars represent flow of blood toward the transducer (red) or away from the transducer (blue). R, RV = right ventricle; L, LV = left ventricle; RA = right atrium; LA = left atrium.

valve was completely stenotic with absent flow, the only exit for blood which entered the left ventricle was retrograde into the left atrium during ventricular systole. Figure 8-22 illustrates a fetus with a common ventricle in which the color flow image is not divided by the interventricular septum.

Ventricular Septal Defect

Unlike the pediatric and adult patient in whom there is a pressure gradient between the right and left ventricles which results in shunting across a *ventricular septal defect,* the pressure within the right and left ventricles in the fetus is almost identical. This is important because in many fetuses with a ventricular septal defect CDI does not demonstrate disturbed flow across the septum. Therefore, the CDI appears as a filling defect during diastole (Figs. 8-21, 8-23, and 8-24). During systole, however, one may observe shunting across the septum, with or without disturbed flow, especially when there is an associated abnormality of the outflow tract in which there is an increased resistance to the flow of blood leaving the ventricle (Figs. 8-25 and 8-26).

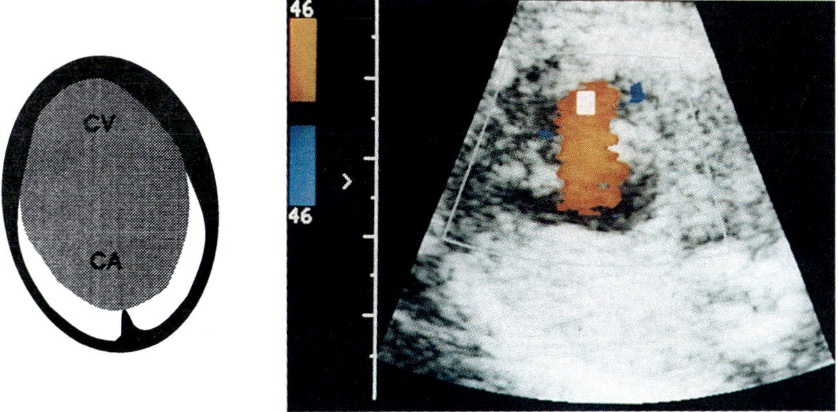

Figure 8-22 *Common atrium and ventricle.* CDI during ventricular diastole demonstrates a common ventricle and common atrium. The color bars represent flow of blood toward the transducer (red) or away from the transducer (blue). CV — common ventricle; CA — common atrium.

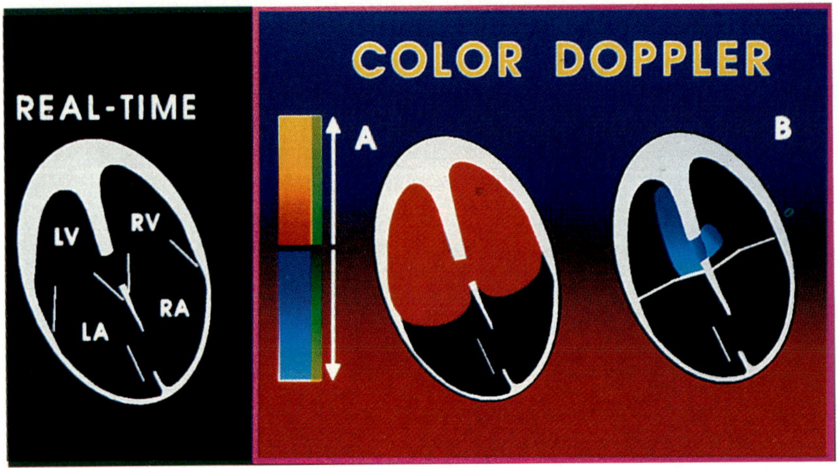

Figure 8-23 *Schematic of CDI illustrating a ventricular septal defect.* *A.* Four-chamber view of a ventricular septal defect in diastole with the color filling the defect. *B.* The same view during systole in which blood crosses the septum. The color bars represent flow of blood toward the transducer (red) or away from the transducer (blue).

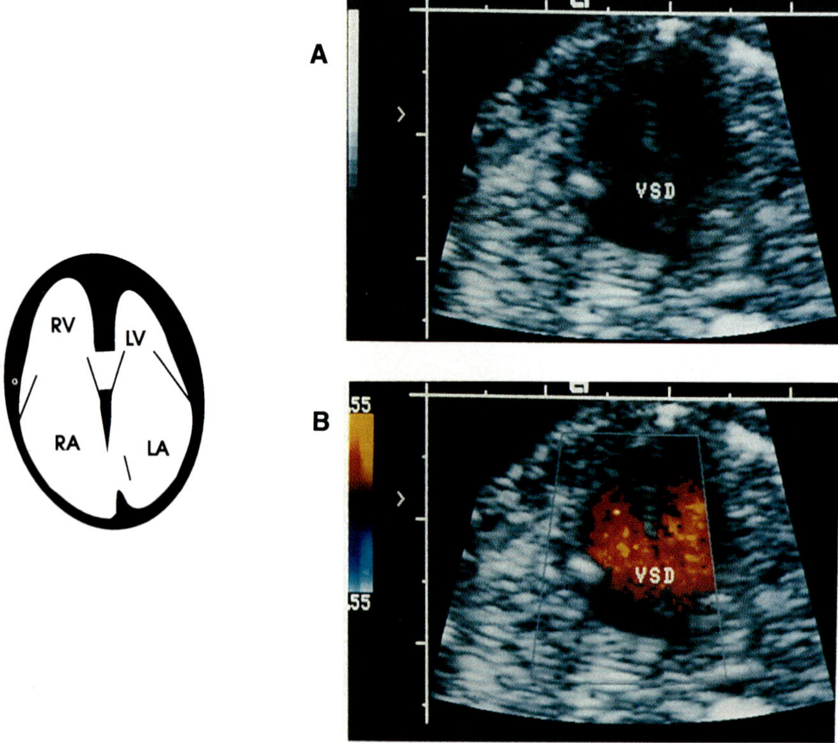

Figure 8-24 *Four-chamber ventricular septal defect.* *A.* Real-time four-chamber view in which a ventricular septal defect appears to be present. *B.* CDI of the same view confirming the ventricular septal defect during diastole. The color bars represent flow of blood toward the transducer (red) or away from the transducer (blue). RV = right ventricle; RA = right atrium; LV = left ventricle; LA = left atrium; VSD = ventricular septal defect.

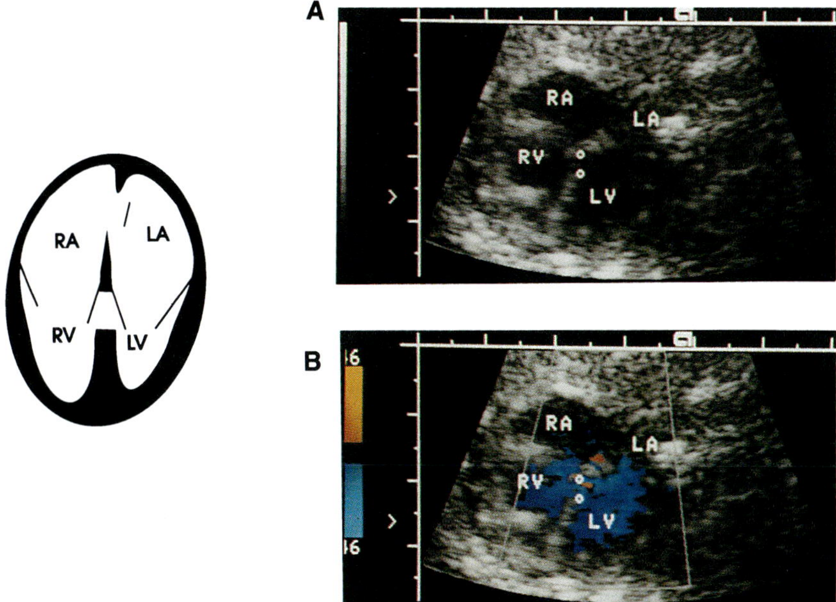

Figure 8-25 *Four-chamber ventricular septal defect. A.* Real-time four-chamber view in which a ventricular septal defect appears to be present as identified by the two circles. *B.* CDI of the same view confirming the ventricular septal defect during diastole in which the color does not demonstrate preferential shunting from one ventricle to another. The color bars represent flow of blood toward the transducer (red) or away from the transducer (blue). RV = right ventricle; RA = right atrium; LV = left ventricle; LA = left atrium.

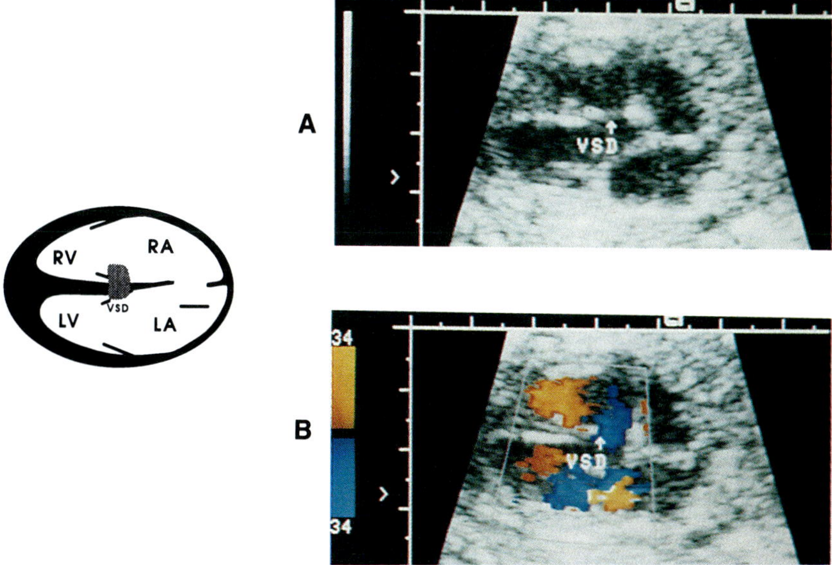

Figure 8-26 *Four-chamber ventricular septal defect. A.* Real-time four-chamber view of the heart in which a ventricular septal defect is suspected. *B.* CDI confirming the ventricular septal defect. However flow of blood is observed from the right ventricle to the left ventricle. The color bars represent flow of blood toward the transducer (red) or away from the transducer (blue). RV = right ventricle; RA = right atrium; LV = left ventricle; LA = left atrium; VSD = ventricular septal defect.

Atrioventricular Canal Defect

While this malformation is easily diagnosed with real time and M-mode echocardiography because of the large atrial and ventricular septal defects and the appearance of a common atrioventricular valve, CDI provides additional hemodynamic information (Fig. 8-27). In 1991 Gembruch et al. reported 14 cases of atrioventricular canal defect (ACD), in which they stated that CDI combined with pulsed Doppler provided information regarding prognosis.[6] They identified atrioventricular valve regurgitation in 10 of 14 cases and noted that the proportion of systolic time during which regurgitation occurred correlated with nonimmune hydrops fetalis. Five fetuses with hydrops had pansystolic regurgitation. In the fetuses with hydrops, CDI filled a large portion of the atrial chamber.

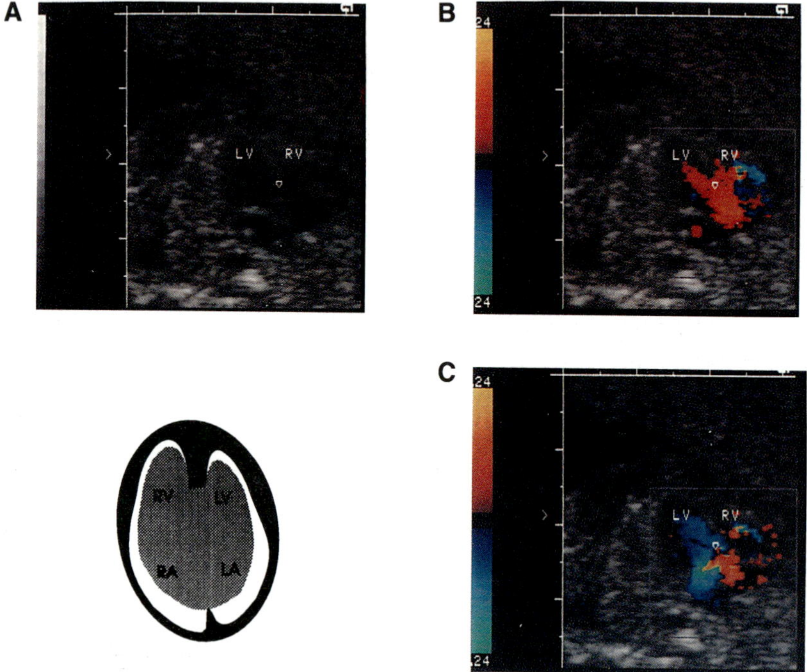

Figure 8-27 *Atrioventricular canal defect. A.* Real-time four-chamber view in which a large ventricular septal defect is suspected (triangle). *B.* CDI illustrates diastolic flow from the atrium, which also has a large septal defect (orange), into the right and left ventricles where bifurcation of flow occurs (orange) around the ventricular septum. *C.* CDI during systole demonstrating flow along the left side of the interventricular septum, crossing the septal defect into the right ventricle. There was no evidence of atrioventricular valve insufficiency in this fetus. The color bars represent flow of blood toward the transducer (red) or away from the transducer (blue). RV = right ventricle; RA = right atrium; LV = left ventricle; LA = left atrium.

Atrial Septal Defect

The most common manifestation of an ostium primum defect is when it is associated with large ventricular septal defect and abnormal atrioventricular valves (Fig. 8-27). An *atrial septal defect* (ASD) involving other areas of the interatrial septum may manifest itself as disproportion between the atrial chambers (right larger than left) as well as dilatation of the right ventricle. CDI demonstrates flow from the right atrium to the left atrium through the foramen ovale as well as reversal of flow back across the atrial septal defect (Fig. 8-28). The volume overload of the right atrium is subsequentially manifest by dilatation of the right ventricle.

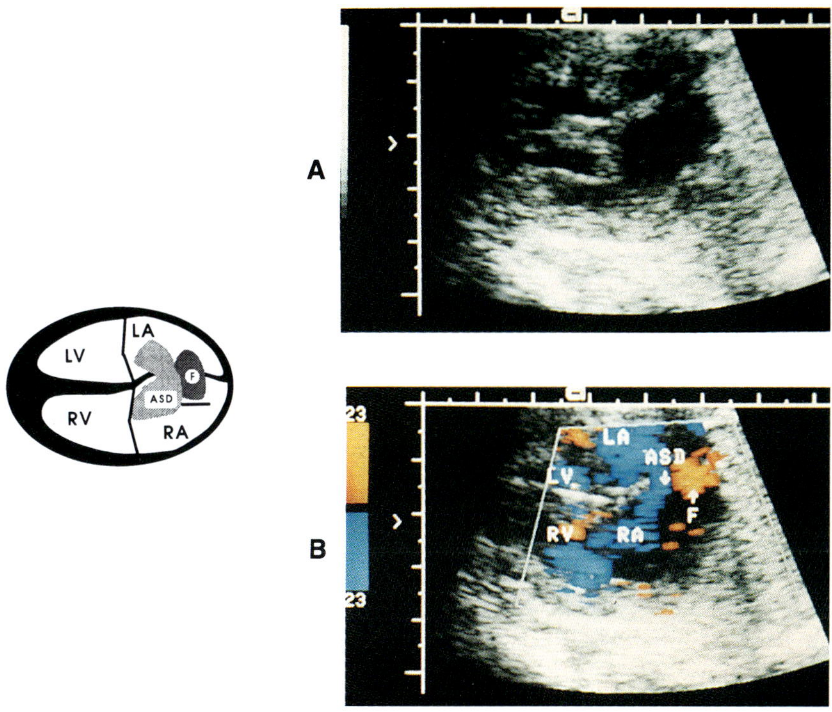

Figure 8-28   *Four-chamber atrial septal defect. A.* Four-chamber view in which dilatation of the right atrium is apparent with the interatrial septum deviated toward the left atrial chamber. *B.* CDI demonstrating flow (orange) from the right atrium into the left atrium, with return flow (blue) from the left atrium into the right atrium. This was the reason for the dilated right atrium. Following birth, the foramen ovale did not completely close. Thus an ostium secundum atrial septal defect was present. The color bars represent flow of blood toward the transducer (red) or away from the transducer (blue). RV = right ventricle; RA = right atrium; LV = left ventricle; LA = left atrium; ASD = atrial septal defect; F = foramen ovale.

Tricuspid Regurgitation

Tricuspid regurgitation (TR) is observed more frequently than mitral valve regurgitation in the fetus. From our experience TR observed with CDI is not physiologic in that there usually is an underlying etiology. TR may be present in one of three locations in relation to the interatrial septum and the right atrial chamber (Fig. 8-29). In fetuses with anemia, it is not uncommon to observe the TR jet adjacent to the interatrial septum, which, without CDI, might be unrecognized if one were using only pulsed Doppler. In the fetus with right ventricular volume overload, the TR jet is usually observed in the center of the right atrial chamber just above the closed tricuspid valve. When the fetus has ductal constriction (maternal ingestion of indomethacin), pulmonary hypertension (term or postterm fetuses), or congenital heart disease (Ebstein's malformation, pulmonary stenosis), the TR jet is observed in the midline and may fill the entire

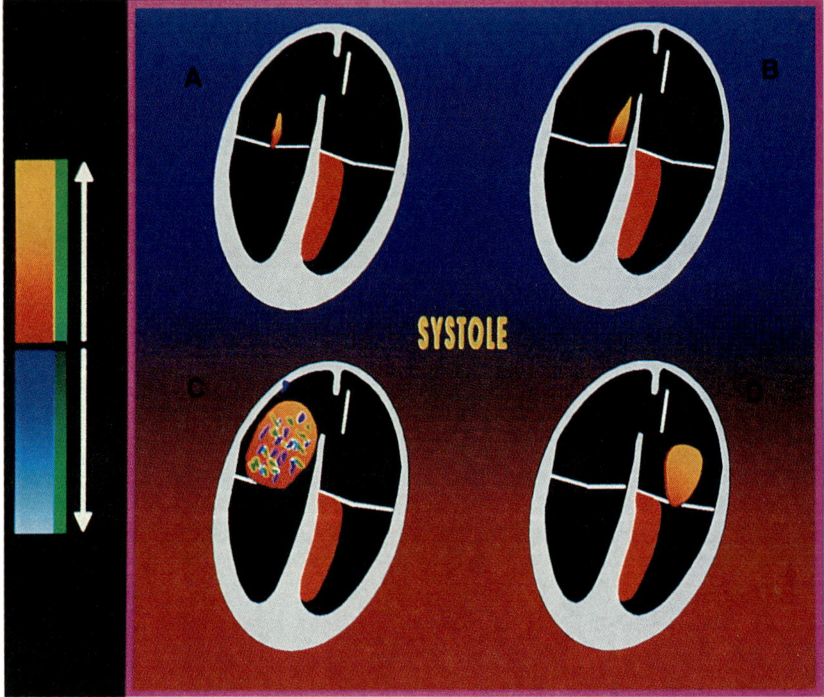

Figure 8-29 *CDI schematic illustrating tricuspid and mitral valve regurgitation during ventricular systole.* The red CDI demonstrates flow along the interventricular septum of the left ventricle during systole. *A.* Minimal tricuspid regurgitation (orange) located in the center of the right atrial chamber. *B.* Tricuspid regurgitation (orange) located adjacent to the interatrial septum. *C.* Severe tricuspid regurgitation in which aliasing (orange, blue, green, yellow) and disturbed flow is observed filling a major portion of the right atrial chamber. *D.* Mitral regurgitation (orange). The color bars represent flow of blood toward the transducer (red) or away from the transducer (blue).

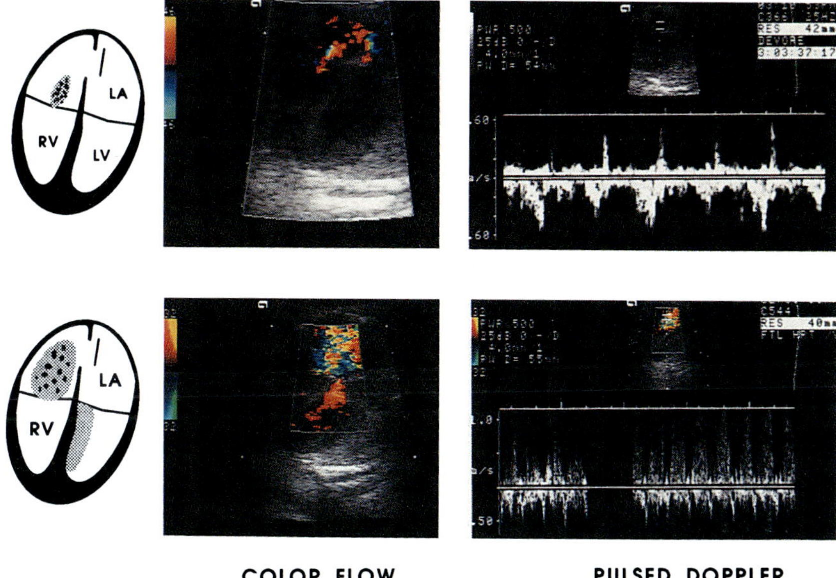

COLOR FLOW   PULSED DOPPLER

Figure 8-30   *Tricuspid regurgitation. Upper panel.* Tricuspid regurgitation which is adjacent to the interventricular septum (orange). Pulsed Doppler demonstrates the regurgitant jet, which occurs during the first quarter of systole. *Lower panel.* Severe tricuspid regurgitation with aliasing (orange, blue, yellow) which fills the right atrial chamber. Blood leaving the left ventricle is present (orange) as it is identified along the left interventricular septum. Pulsed Doppler demonstrates the regurgitant jet to be holosystolic. The color bars represent flow of blood toward the transducer (red) or away from the transducer (blue).

right atrial chamber (Fig. 8-30). The benefit of CDI in the assessment of TR is that it readily identifies the regurgitant jet and allows for easy placement of the pulsed Doppler sample gait to evaluate the maximal velocity and duration of systole the TR persists.

Mitral Regurgitation

Mitral regurgitation (MR) has been observed in fetuses with severe left ventricular function as well as congenital heart disease affecting the aortic valve in which the resistance to blood flow exiting the left ventricle is increased resulting in regurgitant flow from the left ventricle into the left atrium (Fig. 8-21). Fetuses in which there is placental dysfunction most often present with TR but rarely with MR, except in severe cases of myocardial dysfunction.

Pulmonary Stenosis

Pulmonary stenosis (PS) may be an isolated finding, if minimal, or may be associated with abnormal changes of the right ventricle or atrium depending on

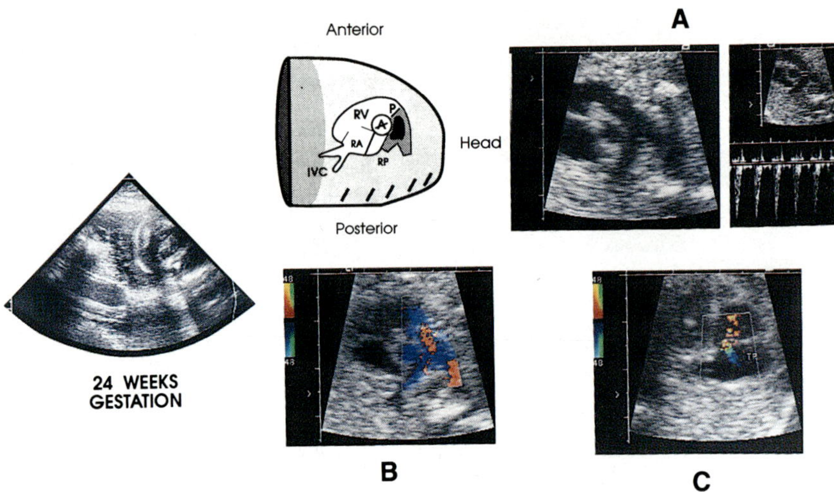

Figure 8-31 *Evolving pulmonary stenosis.* The sector scan demonstrates a thickened nuchal fold in a 24-week fetus with normal male chromosomes. *A.* Real time examination of the short axis of the aortic and pulmonic outflow tracts. The main pulmonary artery does not appear to be distended or dilated. The pulsed Doppler demonstrates a sharp peak with increased velocity. *B.* CDI illustrating aliasing (red) within the main pulmonary artery (blue) which should not be present in the normal fetus at this position in the pulmonary artery. This corresponds to the increased velocity identified with the pulsed Doppler. *C.* Four-chamber view illustrating tricuspid regurgitation (blue-green) which is observed with pulmonary stenosis. RV = right ventricle; P = pulmonary artery; RA = right atrium; A = aorta; RP = right pulmonary artery; IVC = inferior vena cava; TR = tricuspid regurgitation. The color bars represent flow of blood toward the transducer (red) or away from the transducer (blue).

the severity and duration of the lesion. In fetuses with evolving PS, we have observed the stenotic jet to decrease in velocity as the valve progresses to complete stenosis (Fig. 8-31). When PS is present, tricuspid regurgitation is usually present as well.

Aortic Stenosis

In fetuses with *aortic stenosis* (AS), one may observe findings similar to pulmonary stenosis which may or may not be associated with poststenotic dilatation of the aortic outflow tract. In cases of complete aortic stenosis or atresia (no flow through the valve), one may observe retrograde flow from the ductus arteriosus filling the ascending aorta (Fig. 8-32).

Aortic Regurgitation

We have observed one case of *aortic regurgitation* (AR) which occurred in a fetus with severe left ventricular dysfunction associated with a markedly dilated left ventricle (Fig. 8-33).

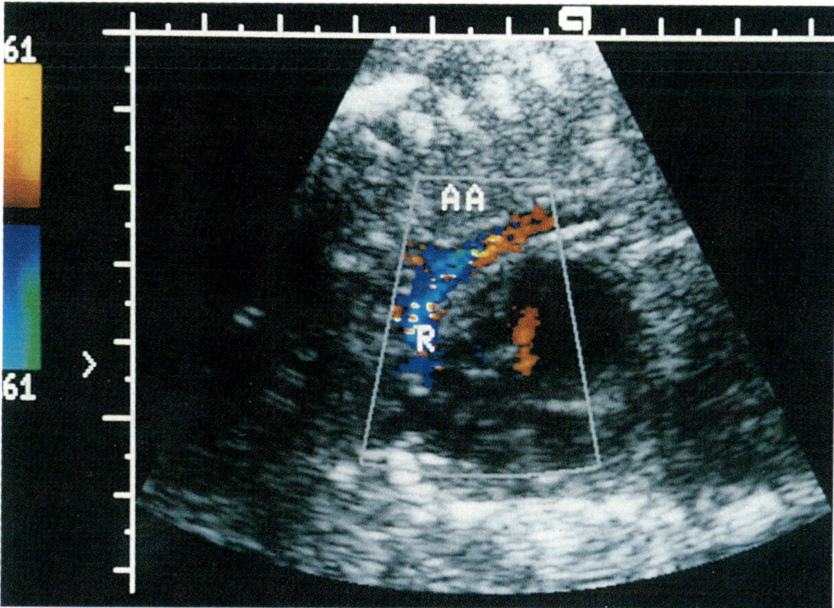

Figure 8-32 *Reversal of flow within the aortic arch.* Unlike Fig. 8-19, in which blood leaving the aorta in the ascending aorta (fetal spine up) is red, the CDI of the ascending aorta is blue owing to reversal of flow as blood flows back into the ascending aorta from the ductus arteriosus. Blood flowing in the descending aorta is depicted as red. The color bars represent flow of blood toward the transducer (red) or away from the transducer (blue).

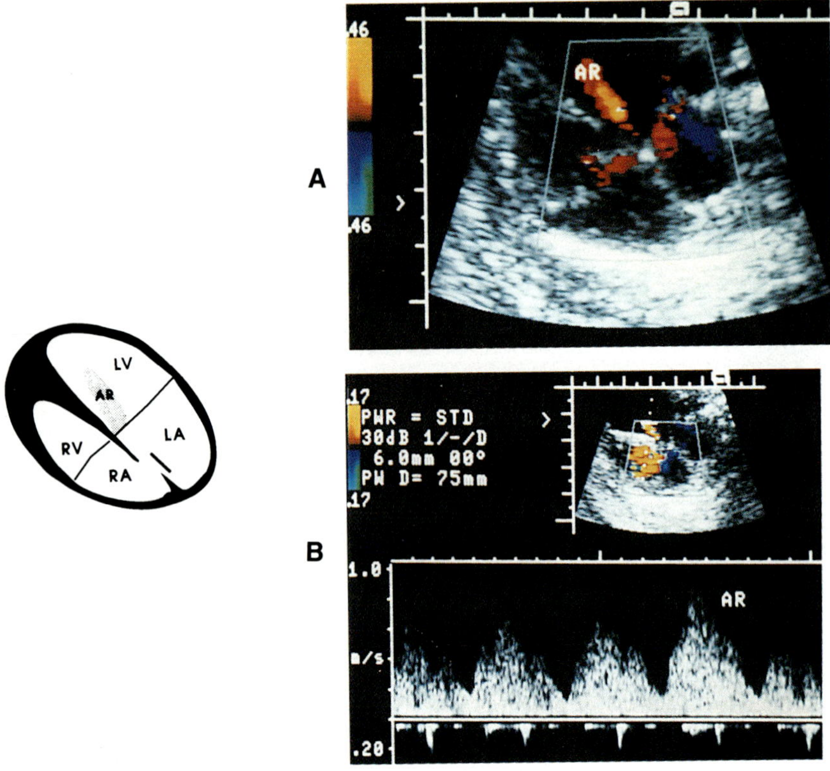

Figure 8-33 Aortic Regurgitation. *A.* CDI demonstrating regurgitant blood along the interventricular septum from the aortic valve. *B.* Pulsed Doppler demonstrates the regurgitant waveform. The color bars represent flow of blood toward the transducer (red) or away from the transducer (blue).

CASE REPORTS

Case 1

The patient was 42 years of age. She was informed by her obstetrician of the increased risk for fetal trisomy associated with her age (4 percent) and the risk of fetal loss from amniocentesis (0.5 percent). Although the patient understood the risks and benefits of amniocenteses, she did not desire an amniocentesis because she felt that her fetus had a 96 percent chance of being normal. However, she inquired of her obstetrician as to whether ultrasound would be helpful for decreasing or increasing her risk for a fetus with abnormal chromosomes. She was referred for fetal echocardiography because of the association between chromosomal aneuploidy and congenital heart disease. Ultrasound examination demonstrated measurements of the head, abdomen, and femur to be consistent with 16.8 weeks of gestation. The fetal heart demonstrated abnormal flow within the

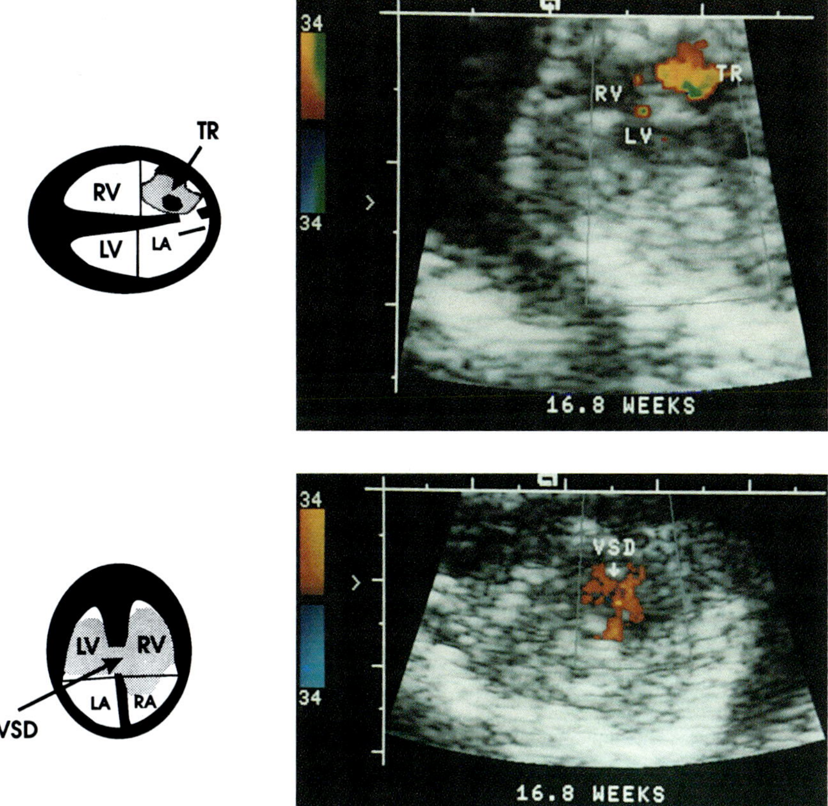

Figure 8-34 *Case 1 trisomy 13. Top panel.* The four-chamber view at 16.8 weeks of gestation. The orange-yellow-green demonstrates CDI of tricuspid regurgitation. Prior to activating CDI, the real-time image did not suggest a dilated right atrial chamber. *Bottom panel.* An image obtained cephalid to the inflow four-chamber view demonstrating a ventricular septal defect (orange). RV = right ventricle; LV = left ventricle; TR = tricuspid regurgitation; LA = left atrium; RA = right atrium; VSD = ventricular septal defect. The color bars represent flow of blood toward the transducer (red) or away from the transducer (blue).

right atrial chamber which was identified with pulsed Doppler to be consistent with tricuspid regurgitation (Fig. 8-34). A ventricular septal defect was also present. Following the examination the patient was encouraged to undergo genetic amniocentesis which demonstrated trisomy 13.

Case 2

A 29 year old was referred because of fetal ascites. Ultrasound examination demonstrated fetal ascites, a pericardial effusion, and right-to-left ventricular

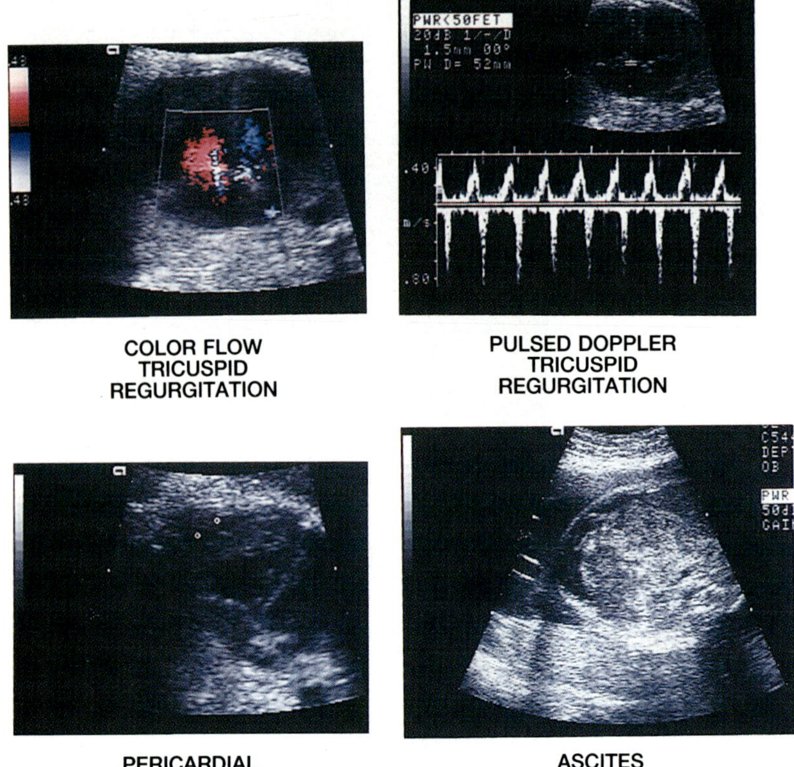

Figure 8-35 *Case 2 fetal cytomegalovirus infection. Top panel.* CDI demonstrating tricuspid regurgitation (blue line within the red) and blood leaving the left ventricle along the interventricular septum (blue). The blue and red are mixed because the sample rate in the last part of diastole is recorded with ventricular systole. Pulsed Doppler demonstrates the regurgitant jet. *Bottom panel.* The pericardial effusion (*circles*) along the right ventricle and ascites. The color bars represent flow of blood toward the transducer (red) or away from the transducer (blue).

disproportion with right ventricular dilatation. The differential diagnosis consisted of fetal anemia, congenital heart disease involving the right heart (tricuspid or pulmonary valves), fetal arrhythmia, abnormal chromosomes, and fetal infection. CDI demonstrated the following (Fig. 8-35):

1. Tricuspid regurgitation which was present in the center of the right atrial chamber
2. Right atrial volume overload
3. Absence of pulmonary stenosis or premature closure of the ductus arteriosus
4. Normal mitral and aortic valves
5. No evidence of coarctation of the aorta

Because of the above findings, fetal anemia was less likely as well as congenital heart disease. The most likely diagnosis was a right atrial and ventricular volume overload. A number of tests were obtained which demonstrated that the etiology of the fetal condition was a recent maternal infection with cytomegalovirus.

Case 3

A 24 year old presented for diagnostic ultrasound in the third trimester to exclude intrauterine growth retardation. Examination of the fetal heart demonstrated dilated right atrial and ventricular chambers. The differential diagnosis was similar to that in case 2. When the heart was examined with CDI, it was apparent that the reason for the volume overload was an atrial septal defect with shunting of blood from the left atrium into the right atrium (Fig. 8-36).

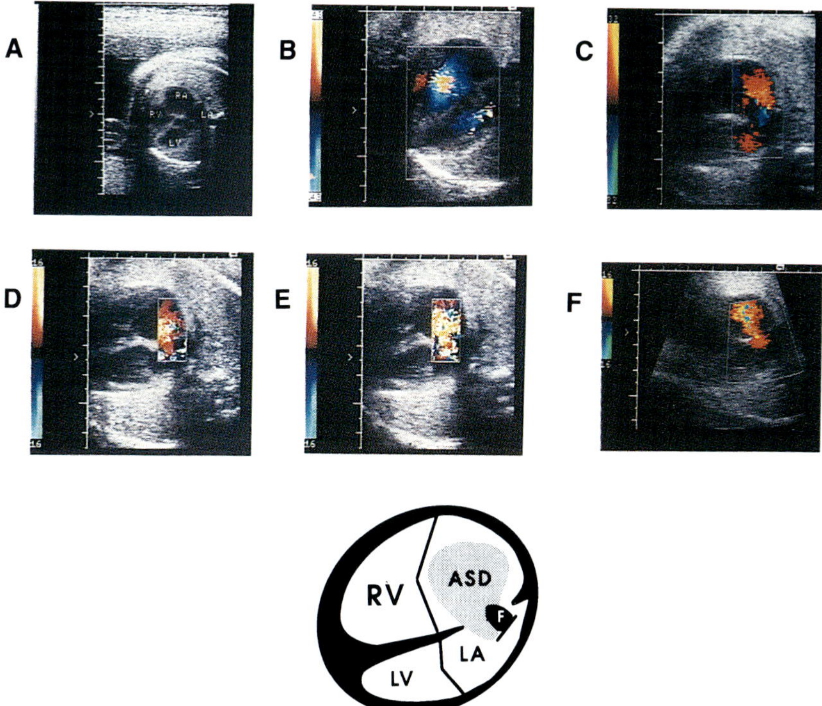

Figure 8-36 *Case 3 atrial septal defect. A.* Real-time four-chamber view illustrating right-left atrial disproportion. *B.* Increased blood flow through the right ventricle. *C.* Flow across the foramen ovale (blue) with increased flow within the right atrium. *D* to *F.* Flow from the left atrium to the right atrium (orange, yellow). RV = right ventricle; LV = left ventricle; ASD = atrial septal defect; F = foramen ovale. The color bars represent flow of blood toward the transducer (red) or away from the transducer (blue).

REFERENCES

1. DeVore GR, Brar HS, Platt LD: Doppler ultrasound in the fetus: a review of current applications. J Clin Ultrasound 15:687–703, 1987.
2. DeVore GR, Horenstein J, Siassi B, Platt LD: Fetal echocardiography. VII. Doppler color flow mapping: a new technique for the diagnosis of congenital heart disease. Am J Obstet Gynecol 156:1054–1064, 1987.
3. Jacobson RL, Perez A, Meyer RA, Miodovnik M, Siddiqi TA: Prenatal diagnosis of fetal left ventricular aneurysm: a case report and review. Obstet Gynecol 78:525–528, 1991.
4. Gembruch U, Chatterjee MS, Bald R, Redel DA, Hansmann M: Color Doppler flow mapping of fetal heart. J Perinat Med 19:27–32, 1991.
5. Copel JA, Morotti R, Hobbins JC, Kleinman CS: The antenatal diagnosis of congenital heart disease using fetal echocardiography: is color flow mapping necessary? Obstet Gynecol 78:1–8, 1991.
6. Gembruch U, Knopfle G, Chatterjee M, Bald R, Redel DA, Fodisch HJ, Hansmann M: Prenatal diagnosis of atrioventricular canal malformations with up-to-date echocardiographic technology: report of 14 cases. Am Heart J 121:1489–1497, 1991.
7. Sharland GK, Chita SK, Allan LD: The use of colour Doppler in fetal echocardiography. Int J Cardiol 28:229–236, 1990.
8. Gentile R, Pearlman AS, Lagana B, Marsocci A: Development of echocardiographic diagnosis of congenital cardiopathies: from M-mode to color Doppler. Medicina (Firenze), 9:147–154, 1989.
9. Chiba Y, Kanzaki T, Kobayashi H, Murakami M, Yutani C: Evaluation of fetal structural heart disease using color flow mapping. Ultrasound Med Biol 16:221–229, 1990.
10. Matsuura T: Study on intracardiac blood flow with color flow mapping in human fetus—the reverse flow at tricuspid valve in human fetus during labor. Nippon Sanka Fujinka Gakkai Zasshi 41:1373–1379, 1989.
11. Gembruch U, Hansmann M, Redel DA, Bald R: Fetal two-dimensional Doppler echocardiography (colour flow mapping) and its place in prenatal diagnosis. Prenat Diagn 9:535–547, 1989.
12. Huhta JC: Future directions in noninvasive Doppler evaluation of the fetal circulation. Cardiol Clin 7:239–253, 1989.
13. Gembruch U, Hansmann M, Redel DA, Bald R: Two-dimensional color-coded fetal Doppler echocardiography—its value in prenatal diagnosis. Geburtshilfe Frauenheilkd 48:381–388, 1988.
14. Kurjak A, Breyer B, Jurkovic D, Alfirevic Z, Miljan M: Color flow mapping in obstetrics. J Perinat Med 15:271–281, 1987.
15. DAmelio R, Giorlandino C, Masala L, Garofalo M, Martinelli M, Anelli G, Zichella L: Fetal echocardiography using transvaginal and transabdominal probes during the first period of pregnancy: a comparative study. Prenat Diagn 11:69–75, 1991.
16. DeVore GR: The prenatal diagnosis of congenital heart disease—a practical approach for the fetal sonographer. J Clin Ultrasound 13:229–245, 1985.

NORMAL FETAL ARTERIAL AND VENOUS FLOW-VELOCITY WAVEFORMS IN EARLY AND LATE GESTATION

JURIY W. WLADIMIROFF
TJEERD W. A. HUISMAN
PATRICIA A. STEWART

Doppler ultrasonography is well recognized as a valuable tool for the study of the fetal heart. With improved technology and the introduction of color Doppler imaging, we can now study the whole fetal circulation. The observed characteristics of flow in fetal peripheral vessels will provide us with important information on normal fetal physiology as well as a better understanding of the pathophysiology of complicated pregnancies. The normal development of flow characteristics in fetal peripheral vessels and the value of color Doppler in the study of these vessels are discussed in this chapter.

VENOUS BLOOD FLOW

The ductus venosus and inferior vena cava ensure optimal mixture of oxygen-rich umbilical venous blood and oxygen-poor systemic venous blood. The ductus venosus forms a shunt, which maintains a short circuit between the umbilical vein and the inferior vena cava, thus bypassing the hepatic microcirculation.[1] In fetal sheep it was shown that more than half of the blood flow entering the fetus via the umbilical vein is shifted through the ductus venosus and preferentially streams through the foramen ovale to favor left heart hemodynamics.[2] Moreover, umbilical cord compression decreases hepatic and pulmonary blood flow and increases the preferential distribution of blood through the ductus venosus as well as through the foramen ovale.[3]

Ductus Venosus

The fetal ductus venosus is localized in the liver, approximately between the right and left lobes. Its course is from caudal to cranial, from ventral to dorsal, and slightly oblique to the left side. It originates from the ventral side of the umbilical sinus and joins the inferior vena cava close to the right atrium (Fig. 9-1). The sample volume (2 to 4 mm) is placed under two-dimensional ultrasonic guidance immediately above the umbilical sinus, visualized in a transverse to oblique view. On a few occasions with excellent visualization it is also possible to place the sample volume immediately proximal to the connection with the inferior vena cava.

The ductus venosus flow-velocity waveform depicts a pulsatile pattern, which consists of two forward components (Fig. 9-2). During systole and early diastole

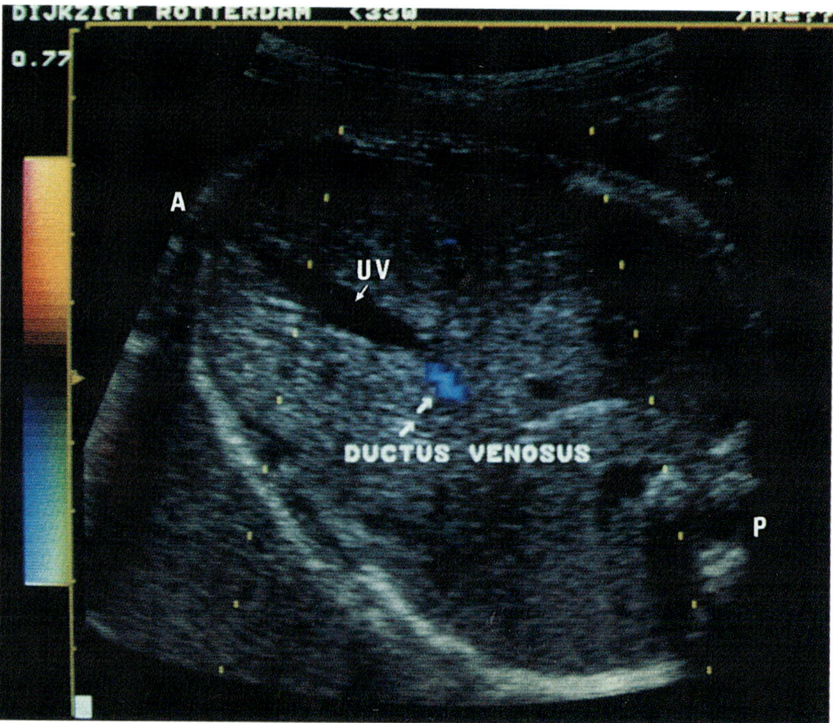

Figure 9-1 Two-dimensional real-time color Doppler image of an oblique section through the upper fetal abdomen demonstrating the umbilical vein (UV) and ductus venosus at 33 weeks of gestation.

both the ductus venosus and inferior vena cava waveforms exhibit forward flow. During late diastole, forward flow in the ductus venosus coincides with the reverse flow in the inferior vena cava. Time-averaged velocity depicts a nearly twofold increase between 11 and 40 weeks of gestation, which may be determined by the increased volume flow through the ductus venosus and reduced cardiac afterload. Of interest are the high time-averaged velocities (20 to 30 cm/s) established as early as 11 to 12 weeks of gestation, indicating that throughout pregnancy ductus venosus flow velocities appear to be highest in the fetal venous system.

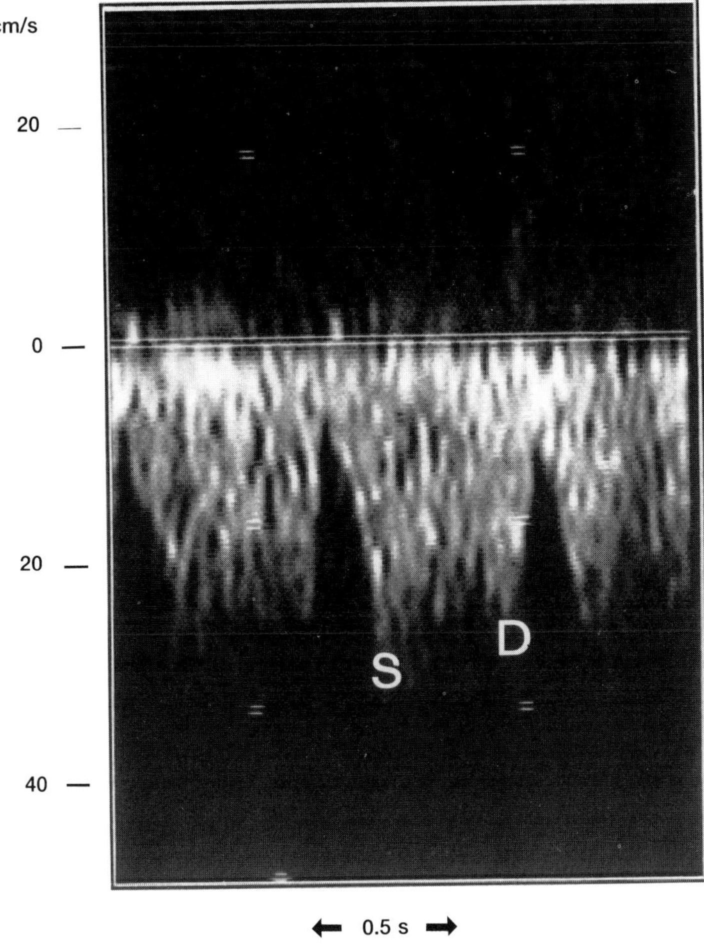

Figure 9-2 Flow-velocity waveform recordings from the ductus venosus at 11 weeks (*A*) and 30 weeks of gestation (*B*). S = systole; D = diastole.

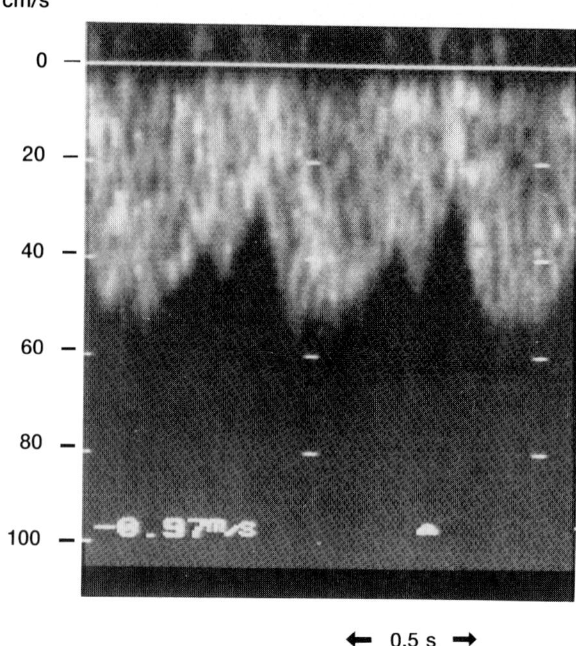

B

Figure 9-2 (*Continued*).

Inferior Vena Cava

The fetal inferior vena cava is localized in a sagittal view directly under the fetal spine, to the right and parallel with the descending aorta. Only those waveform recordings were accepted in which the interrogation angle between the Doppler beam and assumed direction of blood flow was less than 30°. The sample volume (2 to 4 mm) is placed under two-dimensional ultrasonic guidance immediately proximal to the right atrium. The inferior vena cava flow velocity waveform consists of three components[4]: the first and largest component represents forward flow during late diastole (atrial relaxation) and ventricular systole; the second component represents forward flow, which is coincident with early diastolic filling; the third component depicts reverse flow, reflecting atrial contraction (Fig. 9-3).

Time-averaged velocity (in centimeters per second) of forward flow and *time-velocity integral* (TVI, in centimeters) during reverse flow coincident with atrial contraction were measured. TVI of reverse flow was expressed as a percentage of combined forward flow during systole and early diastole. Time-averaged velocity displays a nearly threefold increase between 11 and 40 weeks of gestation, which may be determined by increased volume flow in this vessel, raised cardiac contractility, and reduced afterload with advancing gestational age. Percentage

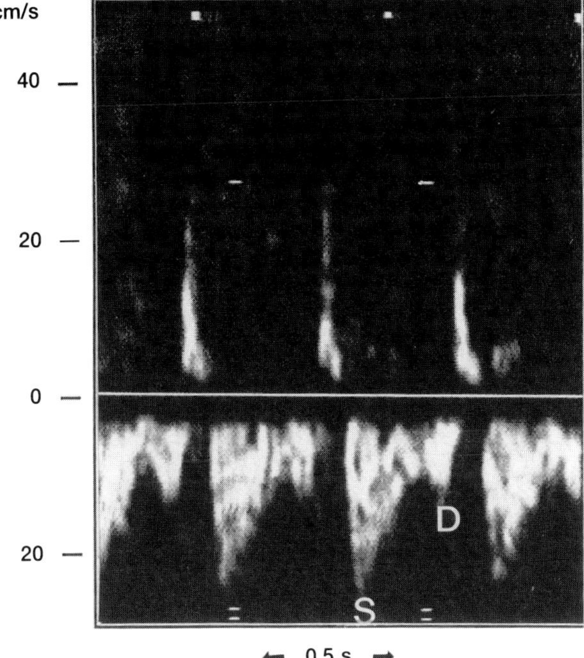

reverse flow at 11 to 12 weeks is a twofold increase over the values found at 16 weeks and a fourfold increase over the values established during late third trimester pregnancies. Also here, ventricular compliance and cardiac afterload may play a role.

Recently we studied the anatomic relationship between the fetal inferior vena cava and adjacent vessels, e.g., the ductus venosus and hepatic veins at the level of venous entrance into the right atrium in a postmortem specimen. It was found that at this level the inferior vena cava together with the ductus venosus and hepatic veins constitute a funnellike structure in which the distance between the individual vessels varies only between 2 and 5 mm, depending on gestational age. From these data it is suggested that inferior vena cava flow-velocity waveforms should be collected more distal to the venous entrance into the right atrium.

THE UMBILICAL CIRCULATION

The umbilical circulation has been studied extensively in the fetal lamb. Umbilical blood flow increases with advancing gestational age and represents 40 percent of the combined ventricular output in the fetal lamb at term.

Using transvaginal color-coded Doppler techniques, the umbilical circulation can be visualized as early as 8 weeks of gestation (Fig. 9-4). Because of the

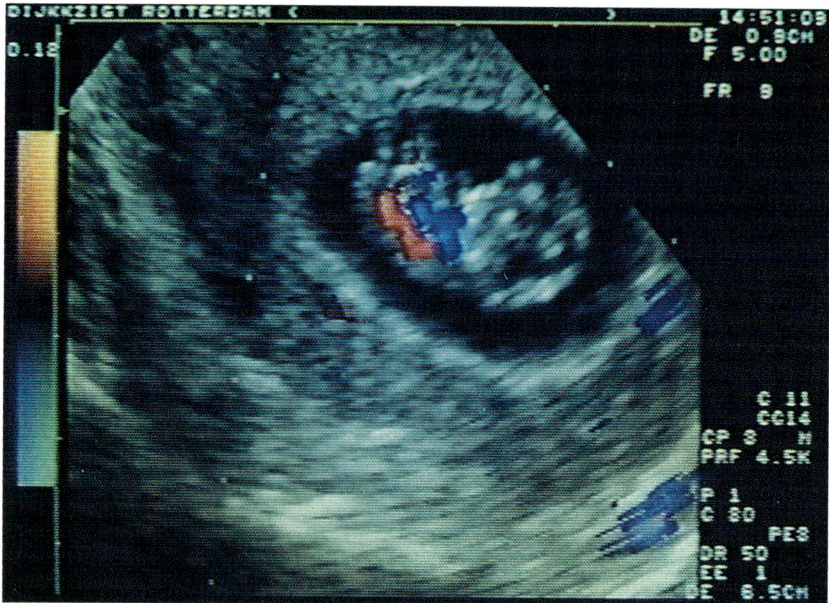

Figure 9-4   Color-coded transvaginal Doppler recording of the cardiac, extracardiac, and umbilical flow in the early embryo at 8 weeks of gestation.

coiling of the umbilical cord and its vessels, it is not possible to determine the exact interrogation angle between the Doppler beam and flow direction.[5] Instead, an angle-independent parameter, the *pulsatility index* (PI) is being used to determine the degree of umbilical placental vascular resistance in any particular pregnancy. The PI is defined as the *difference between the peak systolic and end-diastolic Doppler shift divided by the averaged Doppler shift.*[6]

End-diastolic flow velocities are absent in the umbilical artery between 8 and 12 weeks of gestation, with PI values ranging between 2.4 and 3.0, reflecting a high umbilical placental vascular resistance.[7] At 12 to 13 weeks, end-diastolic flow velocities gradually appear (cutoff level of high-pass filter: 100 Hz), and as a result PI will drop to values of 1.6 to 1.8 at 16 weeks of gestation (Figs. 9-5 and 9-6). This reduction in PI from the umbilical artery suggests a transition from a high-resistance to a low-resistance placenta. A further decrease in PI can be seen as a result of an increase in end-diastolic flow velocity relative to systolic peak velocity during the remainder of pregnancy (Fig. 9-7), reflecting a further reduction in placental vascular resistance. It is essential that the flow-velocity waveform recording is performed during fetal apnea, since breathing movements have a profound effect on the umbilical artery waveform. It should be realized that the PI is inversely related to fetal heart rate.[8]

BLOOD FLOW AT FETAL TRUNK AND LOWER EXTREMITY LEVEL

Flow-velocity waveforms are discussed at the descending aorta, external iliac artery, and renal artery level.

Descending Aorta

The fetal aortic flow pattern is very much dependent on the presence of the placenta as part of the systemic circulation. As in the umbilical artery, the flow-velocity waveform in the descending aorta during the first trimester of pregnancy is characterized by absent end-diastolic flow velocities (Fig. 9-8).

At 12 to 13 weeks, end-diastolic flow velocities gradually appear, suggesting a lowering of systemic vascular resistance (Fig. 9-8). PI in the descending aorta depicts a similar drop to that seen in the umbilical artery, from 2.5 to 3.0 and 1.8 to 2.0.

Particularly in later pregnancy, it is important to establish the site of Doppler recording. The most common place to measure is in the midthoracic part of the descending aorta, 1 to 2 cm above the aortic bifurcation. Of interest is that after 17 to 18 weeks of gestation there is no significant further decrease in aortic PI with advancing gestational age. Changes with time in the distribution of aortic blood flow may affect the total vascular impedance and as such the PI in the descending aorta.[9]

(Text continues on page 165.)

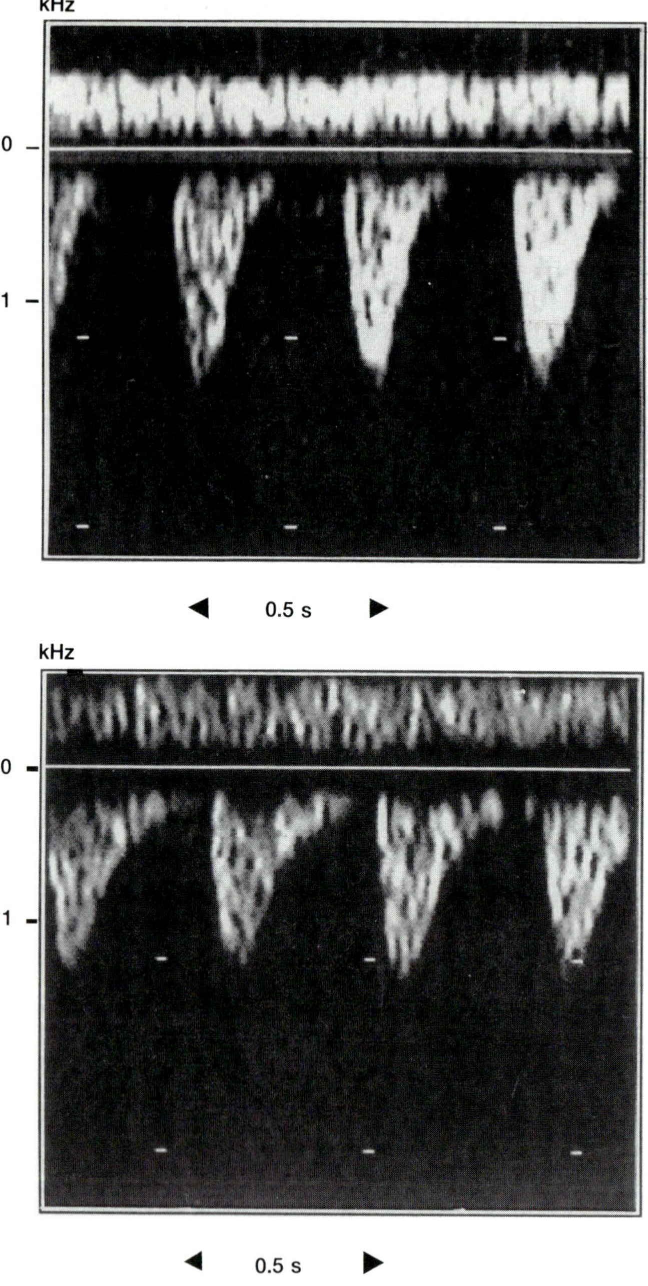

Figure 9-5 Venous and arterial umbilical artery flow-velocity waveforms at 11 weeks (*upper panel*) and 16 weeks (*lower panel*). Note the absence of end-diastolic flow at 11 weeks and the presence of end-diastolic flow at 16 weeks.

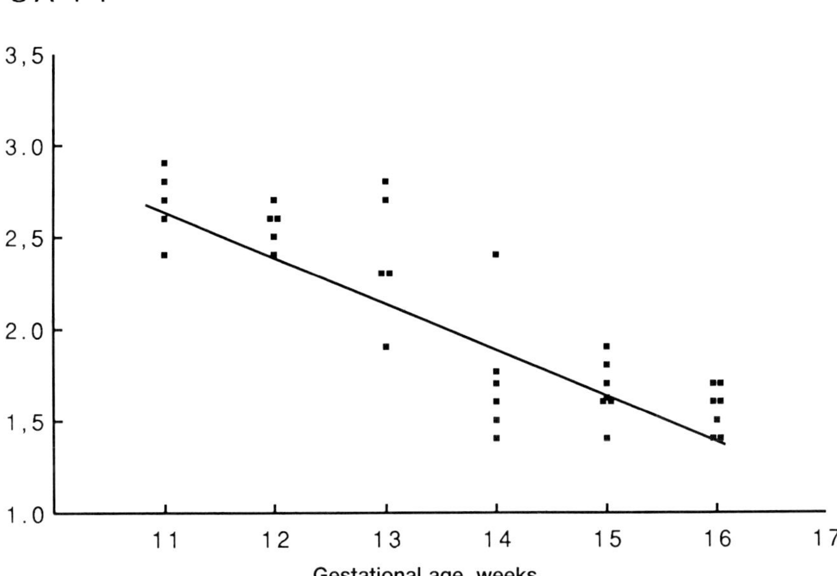

Figure 9-6   Normal pulsatility index (PI) values from the umbilical artery between 11 and 16 weeks of gestation.

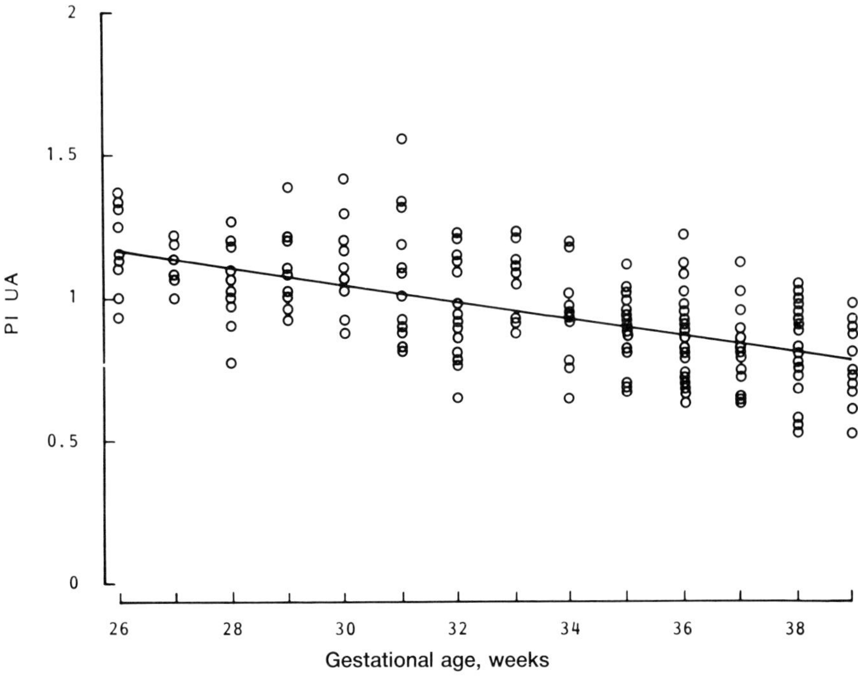

Figure 9-7   Normal pulsatility index (PI) values from the umbilical artery between 26 and 39 weeks of gestation. *(By permission of Pediatric Research.[21])*

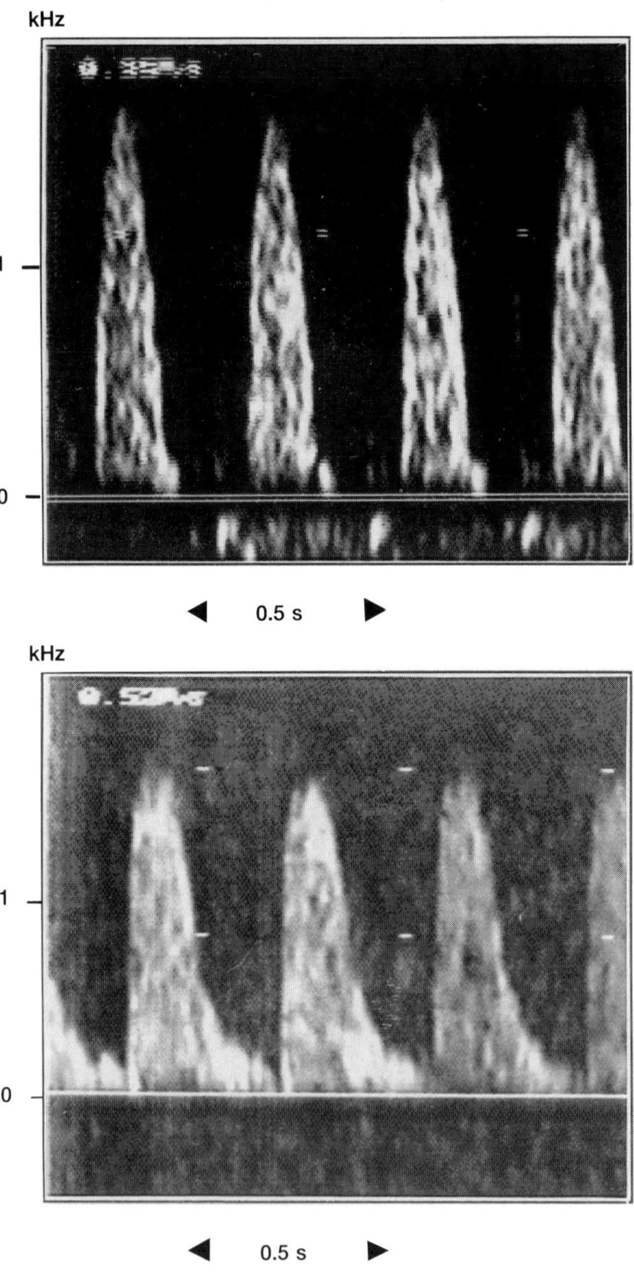

Figure 9-8 Flow-velocity waveforms from the fetal descending aorta at 11 weeks (*upper panel*) and 16 weeks (*lower panel*). Note the absence of end-diastolic flow velocities at 11 weeks and the presence of end-diastolic flow velocities at 16 weeks.

Fetal variables such as fetal heart rate, breathing movements, and behavioral states affect flow-velocity waveform patterns in the descending aorta.[10] After 32 to 34 weeks, active and quiet sleep states can be recognized in the fetus.[11] A significantly lower PI was observed in the fetal descending aorta during active sleep as compared to quiet sleep, suggesting a reduction in systemic resistance during the former sleep state (Fig. 9-9). Indeed, a higher blood supply is needed

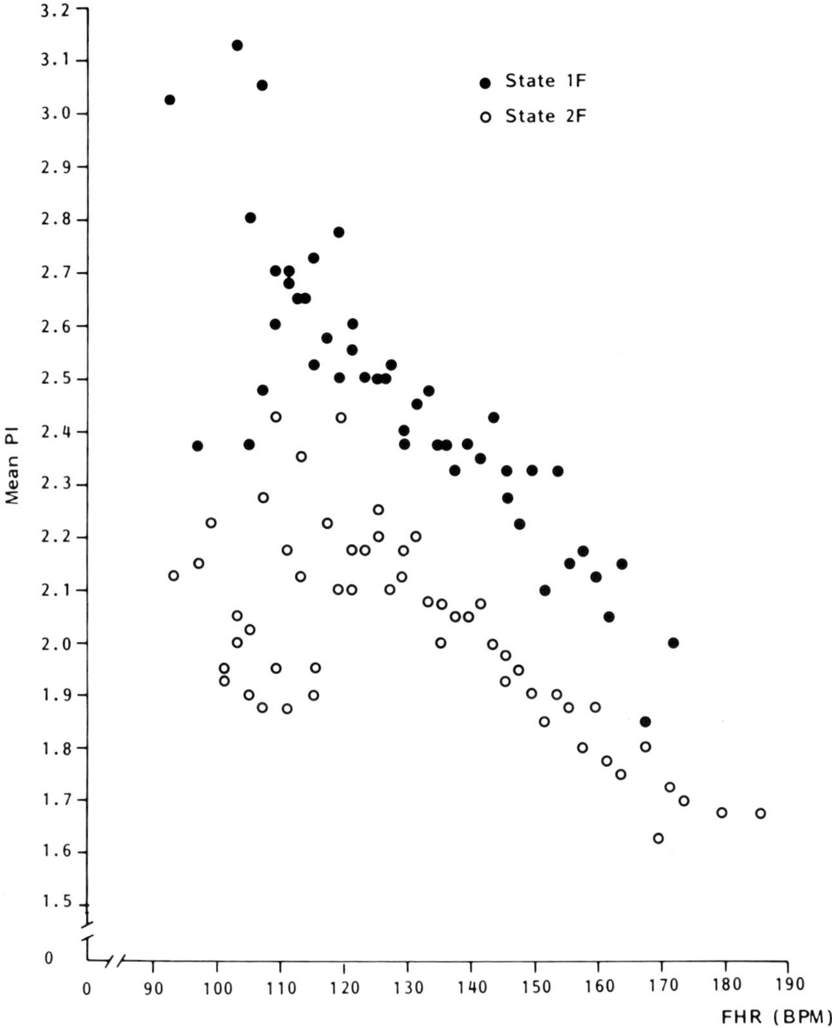

Figure 9-9   Normal pulsatility index (PI) values from the fetal descending aorta relative to fetal heart rate (BPM) during quiet sleep (stage 1F, *closed circles*) and active sleep (stage 2F, *open circles*) at 37 to 38 weeks of gestation.

to the skeletal musculature to meet the increased energy demand during active sleep, which is characterized by raised motor activity.

Volume flow measurements have been carried out in the fetal descending aorta.[12] Insonation of the aorta is always done at an angle of 45°. The aortic diameter is measured either in the frozen real-time image using electronic calipers or from on-line pulsatile diameter changes obtained with a time-distance recorder.[13] Volume flow measurement may display a percentage of error of 20 to 25 percent. Comparison of pulsatile flow velocity and pulsatile vessel diameter in cardiac cycles of equal R-R intervals as obtained by external fetal ECG may improve the accuracy of volume measurement.[14,15]

Renal Blood Flow

The flow-velocity waveforms in the fetal descending aorta represent the summation of flow to the kidneys, other abdominal organs, the femoral arteries, and the placenta. The fetal renal arteries are best visualized from a longitudinal view of the fetal kidneys using color-coded Doppler ultrasound (Fig. 9-10). Pulsatility index calculations have demonstrated that impedance to flow in the renal cir-

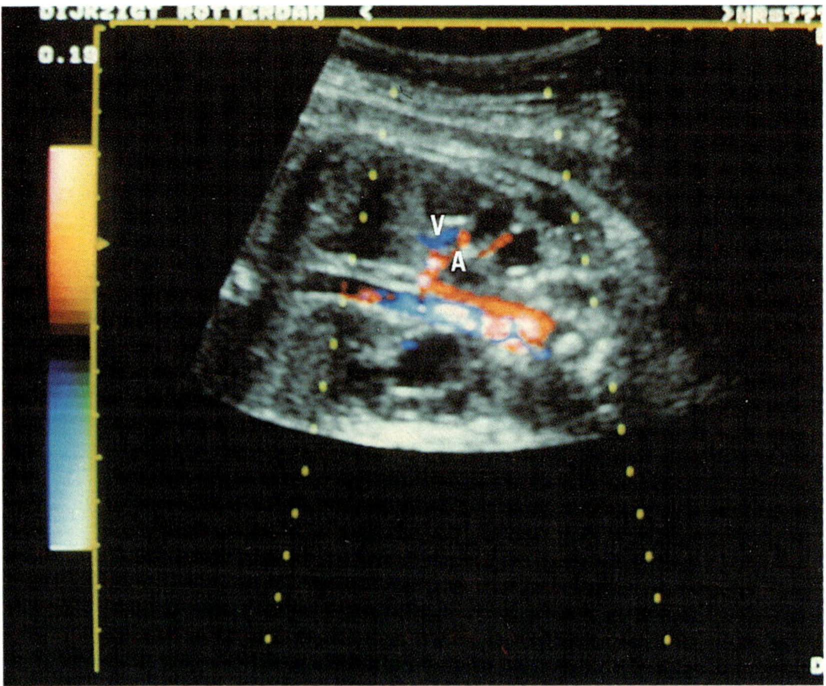

Figure 9-10   Two-dimensional color-coded Doppler recording of the renal artery (A) and vein (V) at 28 weeks of gestation.

culation decreases with advancing gestation.[16] If it is assumed that arterial pressure remains constant, then fetal renal perfusion increases. This may explain the increase in fetal urine production with advancing gestation.[17]

Lower Extremity Blood Flow

Flow-velocity waveforms can be successfully obtained from the fetal external iliac artery. The femoral artery would have been a more obvious choice for assessing lower extremity blood flow. However, despite color-coded Doppler, we only rarely succeeded in visualizing this particular vessel. The principal reason for this is the closely related course of the femoral artery and femur, thus often concealing the vessel from ultrasound visualization. The external iliac artery is easily identified using color-coded Doppler techniques.[18] In color-coded Doppler systems the Doppler shift is displayed in real time and color encoded, with red indicating flow toward the transducer and blue flow away from the transducer. Thus, regardless of fetal position, it is possible to identify direction of flow in specific vessels unequivocally. First, the fetal bladder was identified and the transducer placed in a longitudinal or slightly oblique axis. The most distal portion of the fetal bladder, just above the genitalia, was brought into view. Clearly

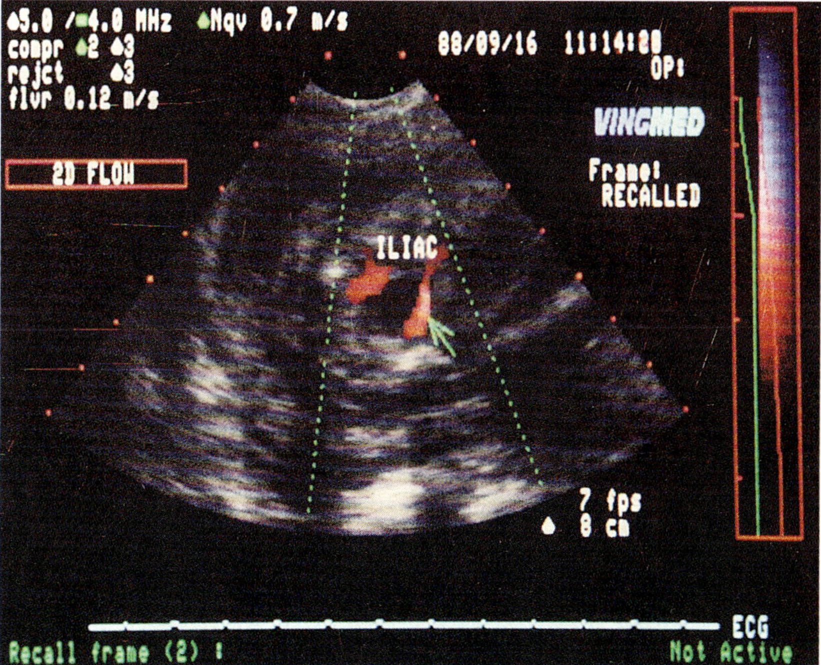

Figure 9-11   Two-dimensional color-coded Doppler recording of the external iliac arteries at 33 weeks of gestation.

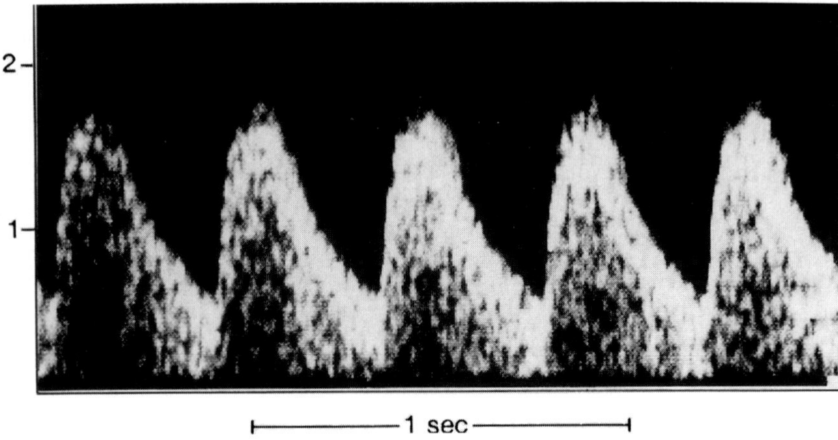

Figure 9-12 Normal flow-velocity waveform recording from the external iliac artery at 28 weeks of gestation. Note the presence of end-diastolic flow velocities.

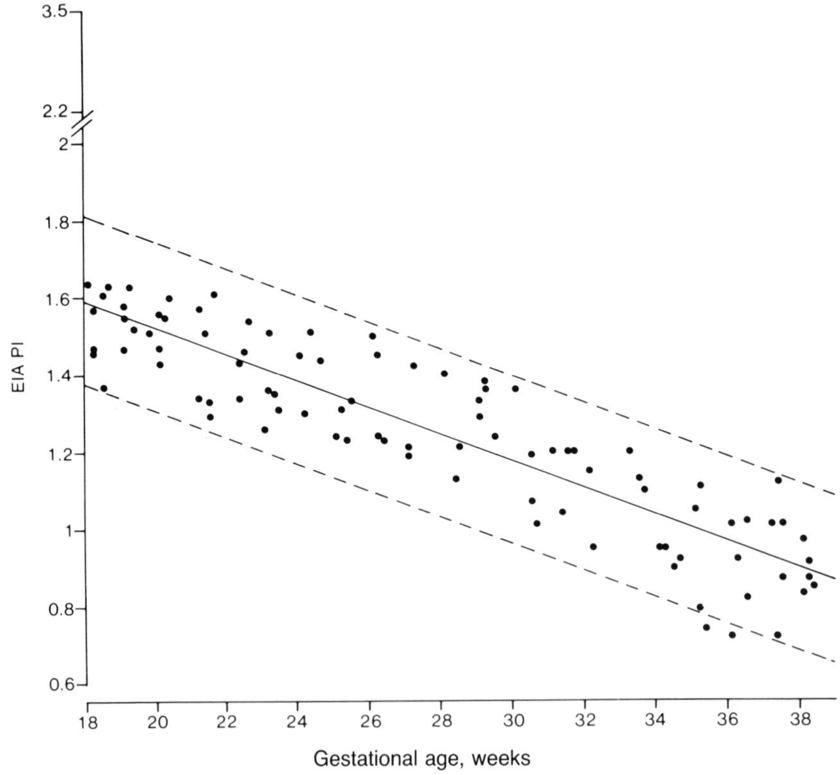

Figure 9-13 Normal pulsatility index values (PI) (mean ± 1 SD) from the external iliac artery between 18 and 38 weeks of gestation.

pulsating vessels were readily identified in this region. Precise placement of the sample volume was facilitated by switching to color mode, whereby a differentiation could be made between the external iliac artery and the intraabdominal umbilical artery. Although these vessels are very close to each other, color-coded flow mapping (Fig. 9-11) clearly identified flow direction toward the fetal legs (i.e., external iliac artery) and flow away from the legs (i.e., intrabdominal umbilical artery). Following identification of the external iliac artery, the maximum flow-velocity waveform was recorded (Fig. 9-12) on hard copy. All measurements were made under an angle of less than 20° between transducer and vessel.

The presence of forward flow in the external iliac artery throughout the cardiac cycle in normal pregnancy reflects low fetal vascular resistance as has also been established from other fetal vessels.[5,19–21] PI in the external iliac artery decreases with advancing gestational age, indicating a reduction in lower extremity vascular resistance during the second half of gestation (Fig. 9-13). The decline in external iliac artery PI/umbilical artery PI ratio with advancing gestational age suggests that in the lower extremities decrease in vascular resistance is more pronounced than in the umbilical artery. Of interest is that volume flow mea-

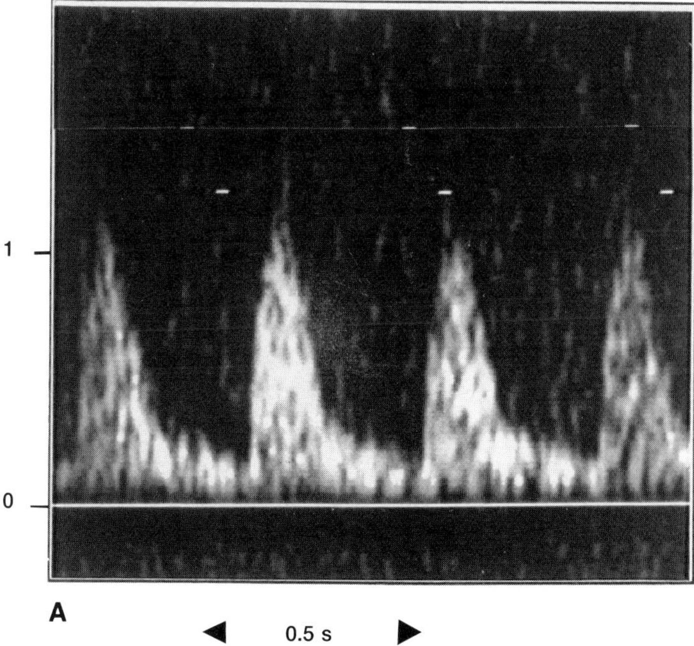

Figure 9-14   Flow-velocity waveform recordings from the intracerebral arteries at 12 weeks of gestation. Note the presence of end-diastolic flow velocities.

surements in the descending aorta and umbilical vein during the third trimester of pregnancy[9] suggest an increase in volume flow to the lower extremities relative to placental blood flow.

INTRACEREBRAL BLOOD FLOW

Intracerebral flow velocities were first described in the fetal internal carotid artery.[22] Since then, Doppler waveforms have also been collected in the anterior, middle, and posterior cerebral artery.[8,23–25] Color-coded Doppler allows detailed visualization of the cerebral circulation. The middle cerebral artery is probably the technically most accessible vessel for reproducible intracerebral arterial waveform recording. Intracerebral waveforms can now be collected as early as 10 to 11 weeks of gestation. Of interest is that in contrast to aortic and umbilical artery flow velocity waveforms, end-diastolic flow velocities are present in intracerebral arteries in approximately 50 percent of waveforms collected at 11 to 12 weeks (Fig. 9-14). This suggests a relatively low vascular resistance at cerebral level, which may not be surprising when taking into account head to body size at that time of gestation. A gradual reduction in PI occurs with advancing gestational

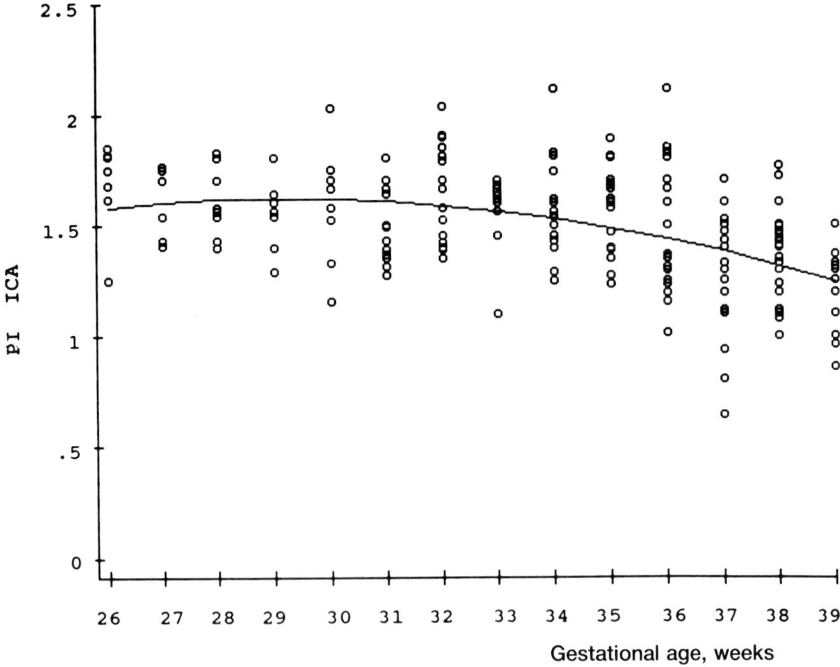

Figure 9-15 Normal pulsatility index (PI) values from the internal carotid artery between 26 and 39 weeks of gestation. *(By permission of Pediatric Research.[21])*

age as a result of increased end-diastolic flow velocities, with a marked drop during the latter 6 to 8 weeks of pregnancy (Fig. 9-15).[21]

The physiologic mechanism responsible for these flow-velocity waveforms changes is still unknown. A reduction in P_{O_2} has been established during this period of gestation.[26] On the basis of this P_{O_2} reduction, it was postulated that the aforementioned increase in end-diastolic flow velocity may reflect a hemo-dynamic redistribution favoring blood supply to the brain.

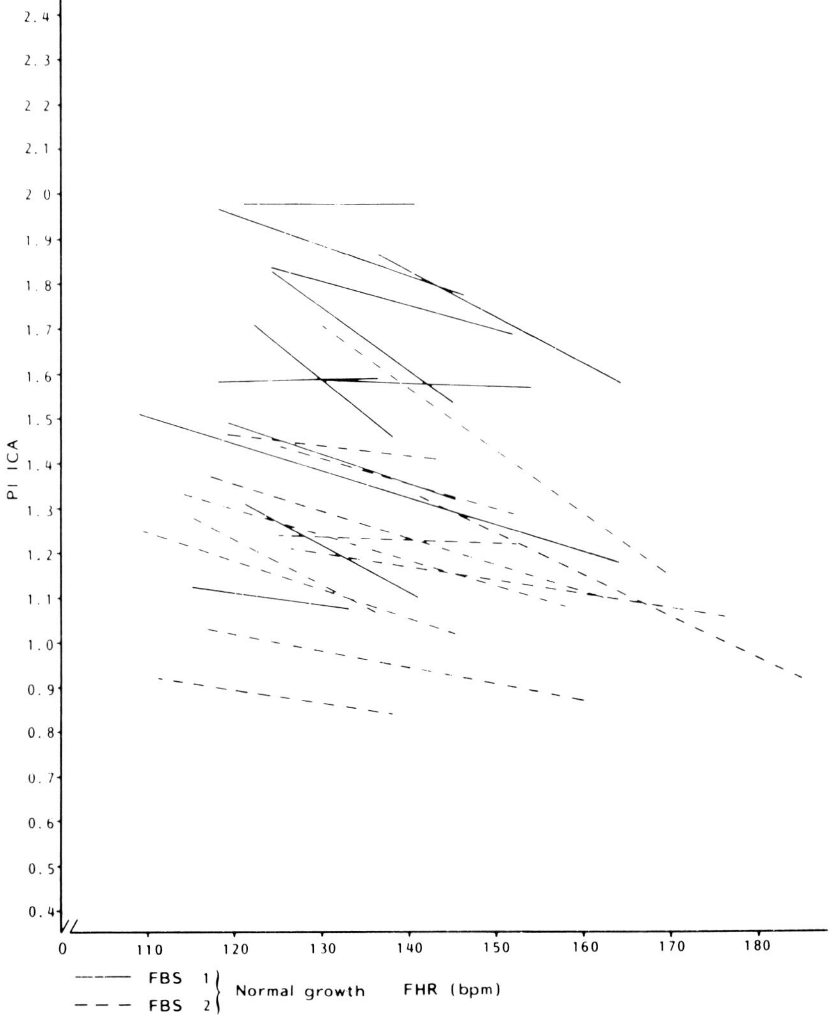

Figure 9-16   Regression lines for the pulsatility index (PI) values from the internal carotid artery relative to fetal heart rate (BPW) during quiet sleep (fetal behavior state 1F; *continuous lines*) and active sleep (behavior state 2F; *dotted lines*) in normal pregnancies at 37–38 weeks of gestation. *(By permission of the British Journal of Obstetrics and Gynaecology.[22])*

PI values are markedly higher in the middle cerebral artery than in the other intracerebral vessels. This may be explained by the rapid systolic upstroke in the flow-velocity waveform followed by a sharp velocity decline during diastole.

Behavioral state dependency has also been observed in intracerebral flow-velocity waveforms.[27] As in the descending aorta, a marked reduction in PI was observed in the internal carotid artery during active sleep (Fig. 9-16). In fetal lamb this behavioral state is characterized by increased electrocortical activity requiring increased oxygen supply to the brain.[28]

CONCLUSION

During late first and early second trimester of pregnancy, the fetus and placenta display a clear transition from a high-resistance into a low-resistance vascular system. This is characterized by the appearance of end-diastolic velocities in all fetal arterial vessels studied. Apart from the descending aorta, all other arterial vessels studied display a further rise in end-diastolic flow velocity (and therefore a drop in pulsatility index) with advancing gestational age.

Throughout pregnancy venous flow velocities are the highest in the ductus venosus. Inferior vena cava flow-velocity waveforms suggest a low cardiac ventricular compliance (stiff ventricles) in early pregnancy.

REFERENCES

1. Rudolph AM: Hepatic and ductus venosus blood flows during fetal life. Hepatology 3:254–258, 1983.
2. Edelstone DI, Rudolph AM: Preferential streaming of ductus venosus blood to the brain and heart in fetal lambs. Am J Physiol 237:H724–729, 1979.
3. Itskovitz J, LaGamma EF, Rudolph AM: Effects of cord compression on fetal blood flow distribution and O_2 delivery. Am J Physiol 252:H100–109, 1987.
4. Reed KL, Appleton CP, Anderson CF, Shenker L, Sahn DJ: Doppler studies of vena cava flows in human fetuses—insight into normal and abnormal cardiac physiology. Circulation 81:498–505, 1990.
5. Trudinger BJ, Giles WB, Cook CM: Flow velocity waveforms in the maternal uteroplacental and fetal umbilical placental circulations. Am J Obstet Gynecol 152:155–160, 1985.
6. Gosling RG, King DH: ''Ultrasound angiology,'' in Marcus AW, Adamson L (eds), *Arteries and Veins*. Edinburgh, England, Churchill-Livingstone, 1975, pp 61–98.
7. Den Ouden M, Cohen-Overbeek TE, Wladimiroff JW: Uterine and fetal umbilical artery flow velocity waveforms in normal first trimester pregnancies. Br J Obstet Gynaecol 97:716–719, 1990.
8. Van den Wijngaard JAGW, Van Eyck J, Wladimiroff JW: The relationship between fetal heart rate and Doppler blood flow velocity waveforms. Ultrasound Med Biol 14:593–597, 1988.
9. Lingman S, Marsal K: Fetal central blood circulation in the third trimester of normal pregnancy. I. Aortic and umbilical blood flow. Early Hum Dev 13:137–150, 1986.
10. Van Eyck J, Wladimiroff JW, Noordam MJ, Prechtl HFR: The blood flow velocity waveforms in the fetal descending aorta; its relationship to fetal behavioral states in normal pregnancy at 37–38 weeks. Early Hum Dev 12:137–143, 1985.

11. Nijhus JG, Prechtl HFR, Martin LB Jr, Bots R: Are there behavioral states in the human fetus? Early Hum Dev 6:177–195, 1982.
12. Eik-Nes SH, Brubakk AO, Ulstein MK: Measurement of human fetal blood flow. Br Med J 280:283–284, 1980.
13. Lindström K, Marsal K, Gennser G: Device for monitoring fetal breathing movements. I. TD recorder. A new system for recording the distance between two echo-generating structures as a function of time. Ultrasound Med Biol 3:143–151, 1977.
14. Sindberg Eriksen P, Gennser G, Lindström G: "Characteristics of pulse waves in the fetal aorta descendence," in Kurjak A, Kratochwil A (eds): *Recent Advances in Ultrasound Diagnosis 3.* Amsterdam, Excerpta Medica, 1981, pp 234–240.
15. Tonge HM, Struyk PC, Custers P, Wladimiroff JW: Vascular dynamics in the descending aorta of the human fetus in normal late pregnancy. Early Hum Dev 9:21–26, 1983.
16. Vyas S, Nicolaides KH, Campbell S: Renal artery flow-velocity waveforms in normal and hypoxemic fetuses. Am J Obstet Gynecol 161:168–172, 1989.
17. Campbell S, Wladimiroff JW, Dewhurst CJ: The antenatal measurement of fetal urine production. J Obstet Gynaecol Br Commonw 80:680–686, 1973.
18. Stewart PA, Wladimiroff JW, Stijnen T: Blood flow velocity waveforms from the fetal external iliac artery as a measure of lower extremity vascular resistance. Br J Obstet Gynaecol 97:425–430, 1990.
19. Griffin D, Bilardo K, Masiui L, Diaz-Recasens J, Pearce M, Wilson K, Campbell S: Doppler blood flow waveforms in the descending aorta on the human fetus. Br J Obstet Gynaecol 93:471–475, 1984.
20. Reuwer PJHM, Sijmons EA, Rietman GW, Van Tiel MWM, Bruinse HW: Intrauterine growth retardation: prediction of perinatal distress by Doppler ultrasound. Lancet ii:415–418, 1987.
21. Wladimiroff JW, Noordam MJ, Van den Wijngaard JAGW, Hop WCJ: Fetal internal carotid and umbilical artery blood flow velocity waveforms as a measure of fetal well-being in intrauterine growth retardation. Ped Res 24:609–612, 1988.
22. Wladimiroff JW, Tonge HM, Stewart PA: Doppler ultrasound assessment of cerebral blood flow in the human fetus. Br J Obstet Gynaecol 93:471–475, 1986.
23. Arbeille Ph, Roncin A, Berson M, Patat F, Pourcelot L: Exploration of the fetal cerebral blood flow by duplex Doppler-linear array system in normal and pathological pregnancies. Ultrasound Med Biol 13:329–337, 1987.
24. Woo JSK, Liang ST, Lo RLS, Chan FY: Middle cerebral artery Doppler flow velocity waveforms. Obstet Gynecol 70:613–616, 1987.
25. Kirkinen P, Müller R, Huch R, Huch A: Blood flow velocity waveforms in human fetal intracranial arteries. Obstet Gynecol 70:617–621, 1987.
26. Soothill PW, Nicolaides KH, Rodeck CH, Campbell S: Effect of gestational age on fetal and intervillous blood gas and acid-base values in human pregnancy. Fetal Ther 4:168–175, 1986.
27. Van Eyck J, Wladimiroff JW, Van den Wijngaard JAGW, Noordam MJ, Prechtl HFR: The blood flow velocity waveform in the fetal internal carotid and umbilical artery; its relationship to fetal behavioral states in normal pregnancy at 37–38 weeks of gestation. Br Obstet Gynaecol 94:736–741, 1987.
28. Richardson BS, Patrick JE, Abduljabbar H: Cerebral oxidative metabolism in the fetal lamb: relationship to electrocortical state. Am J Obstet Gynecol 153:426–431, 1985.

VENOUS FLOW VELOCITIES IN THE FETUS

KATHRYN L. REED

Blood flow to the fetal brain is supplied by the left ventricle, just as in the adult. The organ of oxygenation in the fetus, however, is not the lungs, but rather the placenta. The path of oxygenated blood flow in the fetus is therefore more complex than in the adult. Umbilical venous blood flows from the placenta, through the ductus venosus, into the inferior vena cava, and across the right atrium, through the foramen ovale, into the left atrium and ventricle.[1]

Venous blood flow, therefore, is significant to fetal health, and changes in venous flow may correlate with fetal well-being. We have investigated the association of Doppler-detected umbilical venous and inferior vena caval blood flow velocities with fetal outcome.

METHODS

The fetus is examined initially with two-dimensional ultrasound, to establish position, size, anatomy, amniotic fluid volume, and placental location. Pulsed Doppler interrogation is performed by placing the sample volume immediately proximal to the right atrium at the entrance of the inferior vena cava, using two-dimensional ultrasound guidance. Strip chart recordings are obtained for off-line analysis. Umbilical arterial and venous waveform tracings are obtained by placing the sample volume over the umbilical cord outside the fetal body, again using two-dimensional ultrasound guidance.

Peak velocities and time-velocity integrals of each phase of blood flow in the inferior vena cava during the cardiac cycle are measured. In the inferior vena

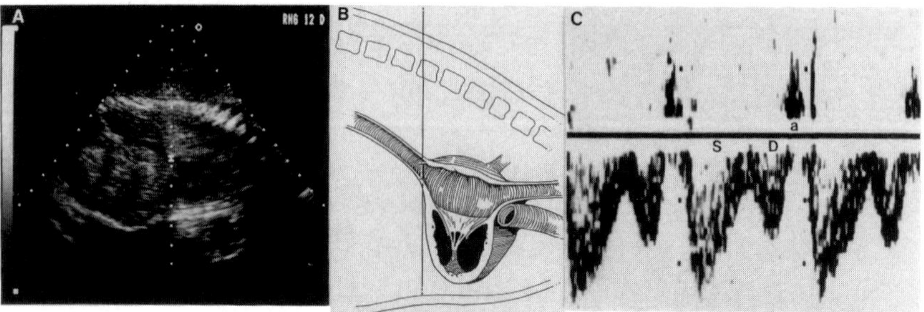

Figure 10-1   Two-dimensional Doppler flow-velocity waveform of fetal inferior vena cava in a normal fetus. *A.* Two-dimensional ultrasound image of the inferior vena cava; the Doppler gate is immediately proximal to the right atrium. *B.* Diagram of the image in panel *A*. *C.* Doppler flow-velocity waveform from the fetal inferior vena cava. S = systole; D = diastole; a = atrial contraction. *(Reproduced with permission from Reed KL, Appleton CP, Anderson CF, Shenker L, Sahn DJ: Doppler studies of vena cava flows in human fetuses. Circulation 81:498–505, 1990.)*

cava, flow occurs in three phases. During systole, forward flow occurs as the atrium relaxes and the valve ring descends. During diastole, a second peak occurs as the atrioventricular valves open and blood flows directly through the atrium. With atrial contraction during late diastole, blood flows both into the ventricles and in a reverse direction into the superior and inferior venae cavae (Fig. 10-1).[1–3] Peak velocity is measured from the zero line to the highest detectable velocity. Time-velocity integrals are measured as the area under the peak for that phase of the cycle.

The angle of incidence between the ultrasound beam and the direction of blood flow is difficult to measure in the inferior vena cava of the fetus, both because of the position of the fetus and because blood flow direction is not completely predictable at this juncture of several veins and the funneling of the inferior vena cava walls. For this reason, we do not report velocities and time-velocity integrals other than in relative terms; that is, we compare systolic and diastolic peaks and create ratios, and compare systolic and diastolic time-velocity integrals and create ratios. Reverse flow during atrial contraction can also be measured in terms of peak velocities and time-velocity integrals. In order to compare reverse flow velocities of different fetuses, or in the same fetus at different times, the time-velocity integral of reverse flow during atrial contraction is expressed as a percent of forward flow. Forward flow is defined as the sum of the time-velocity integrals during systole and diastole.

Inferior vena caval waveforms in fetuses with abnormally fast, slow, or irregular heart rates were also examined. In fetuses with both normal and abnormal heart rates, values were compared with normal in the same fetus. In fetuses with persistently abnormal heart rates (e.g., complete heart block) values obtained were compared with results from normal fetuses.

RESULTS

In the normal fetus, the highest peak and largest time-velocity integral of flow occur during systole. This is followed by a smaller peak and time-velocity integral during diastole (Fig. 10-1). Reverse flow during atrial contraction is detectable in 87 percent of fetuses.[3] In 15 normal fetuses between 25 and 36 weeks gestation, the ratio of systolic-to-diastolic time-velocity integral (average 3.31 ± 0.21) decreased with advancing gestational age ($r = -0.06$, $p < 0.05$).[3]

Fetuses with premature atrial contractions ($n = 13$) had large increases in reverse flow with the premature atrial contraction, from 4.5 ± 0.3 percent to 28.3 ± 3.7 percent.[3] The diastolic time-velocity integral increased during the following beat; reverse flow during atrial contraction was also increased (8.2 ± 0.8 percent) following the prolonged diastolic pause.[3]

Fetuses with abnormally fast heart rates ($n = 4$) had increases in reverse-flow velocities with atrial contraction, and the percentage of reverse flow increased with heart rate ($r = 0.96$, $p < 0.01$, slope $= 0.4$, Fig. 10-2).[3] Fetuses with sinus bradycardia ($n = 3$) also had increases in reverse-flow velocities with atrial contraction (from 5.2 ± 0.9 percent to 14.0 ± 2.1 percent, $p < 0.02$); again, reverse flow increased as the heart rate decreased ($r = -0.99$, $p < 0.001$, slope $= -0.7$, Fig. 10-2).[3] In the presence of complete heart block, reverse flow with atrial contraction was in the normal range (5.4 ± 1.0 percent) unless

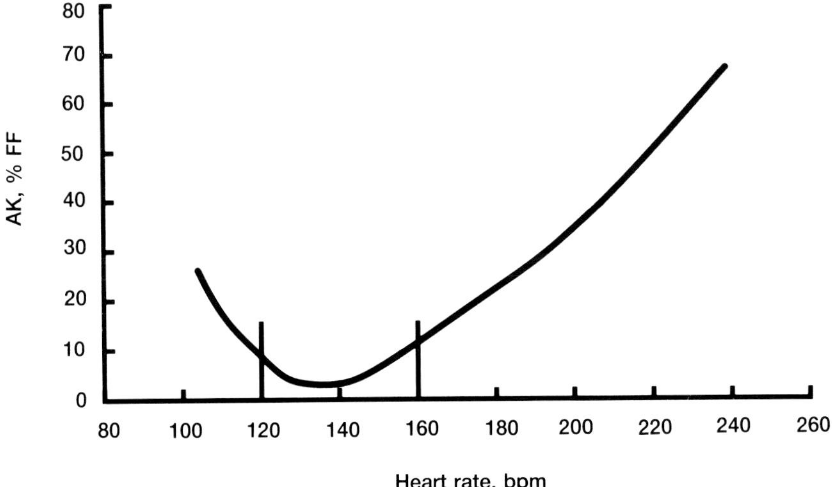

Figure 10-2   Comparison of heart rate with percent of forward flow (%FF) in the inferior vena cava, which moves in a reverse direction with atrial contraction (AK). Normal fetal heart rate is between 120 and 160 beats/min. *(Reproduced with permission from Reed KL, Appleton CP, Anderson CF, Shenker L, Sahn DJ: Doppler studies of vena cava flows in human fetuses. Circulation 81:498–505, 1990.)*

a "cannon *a*" wave (when atrial contraction occurred during ventricular systole) was present.[3]

Inferior vena caval waveforms were also examined in 15 fetuses with absent umbilical artery end-diastolic velocities. Reverse-flow velocities (13.8 ± 2.3 percent) were increased compared with normal ($p < 0.01$).[3] All fetuses in this group had intrauterine growth retardation (birthweight < tenth percentile).

In 74 fetuses, umbilical venous waveforms were obtained simultaneously with umbilical arterial waveforms.[4] In 32 normal fetuses from this group, no decreases in velocity in the umbilical vein were detectable in the absence of fetal breathing or movement. Decreases in velocity in the umbilical vein in the absence of fetal breathing were detectable in some subgroups of the remaining fetuses. In fetuses with regular heart rates, the decreases in velocity corresponded with the time of atrial contraction. These decreases in velocities are referred to as *venous pulsations*.

In 15 fetuses with premature atrial contractions, venous pulsations occurred if the diastolic pause lasted longer than 0.05 s ($n = 8$).[4]

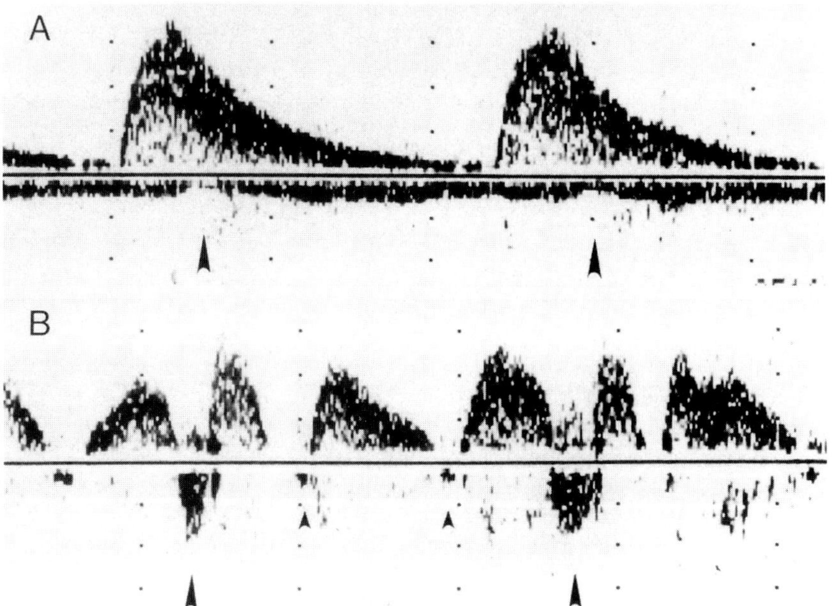

Figure 10-3 Umbilical venous and arterial waveforms (*A*) and inferior vena caval waveforms (*B*) in a fetus with complete heart block. Umbilical venous pulsations occur at varying times during arterial (ventricular) systole. This is explained by inferior vena caval reverse-flow velocities that occur when the atrium contracts against closed atrioventricular valves, during ventricular systole. Atrial rate is 150 beats/min (*small arrowheads*); ventricular rate is 50 beats/min (*large arrowheads*). *(Reproduced with permission from Indik JH, Chen V, Reed KL: Association of umbilical venous with inferior vena cava blood flow velocities. Obstet Gynecol 77:551–557, 1991.)*

Fetuses with abnormally fast heart rates (>160 beats/min, $n = 6$) or abnormally slow heart rates (< 120 beats/min, $n = 6$, three with sinus bradycardia and three with complete heart block) also demonstrated umbilical venous pulsations.[4]

Umbilical venous pulsations were detected in the three fetuses with complete heart block at a time that corresponded to the cannon *a* wave produced by atrial contraction against closed atrioventricular valves during ventricular contraction (Fig. 10-3).[4]

Fetuses with absent end-diastolic velocities in the umbilical artery could be divided into two groups on the basis of the presence or absence of umbilical venous pulsations. The group with venous pulsations ($n = 11$, Fig. 10-4) had a higher mortality (55 percent) when compared with the group without venous pulsations ($n = 10$, 10 percent, $p < 0.05$).[4] Reverse flow in the inferior vena cava was also greater in the group with umbilical venous pulsations (27.5 ± 14.9 percent) than in the group without umbilical venous pulsations (7.5 ± 5.7 percent, $p < 0.001$).[4]

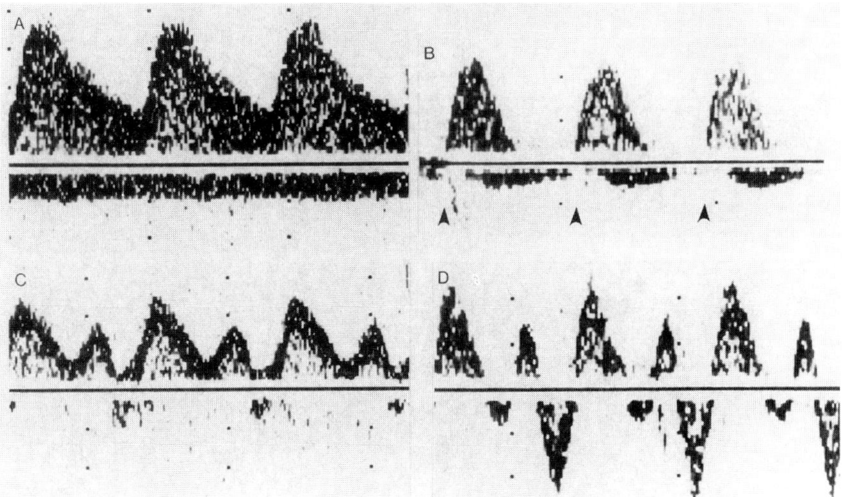

Figure 10-4   Umbilical arterial, venous, and inferior vena caval velocities in a normal 38-week fetus and in a 34-week fetus with absent end-diastolic velocities in the umbilical artery. *A.* Umbilical arterial and venous velocity in the normal fetus. *B.* Umbilical arterial and venous velocity in the fetus with absent end-diastolic velocities in the umbilical artery. Umbilical venous pulsations are marked. *C.* Inferior vena caval waveform from the fetus in *A.* *D.* Inferior vena caval waveform from the fetus in *B.* In the inferior vena caval waveforms, the largest peak is during systole, the second peak is during early diastole, and reverse flow occurs during atrial contraction. Dots are 0.5 s apart. *(Reproduced with permission from Indik JH, Chen V, Reed KL: Association of umbilical venous with inferior vena cava blood flow velocities. Obstet Gynecol 77:551–557, 1991.)*

DISCUSSION

Supply of the fetal brain with oxygenated blood requires flow of blood from the umbilical vein to the ascending aorta. In the fetus, this is accomplished via the ductus venosus, inferior vena cava, and foramen ovale. Streaming of blood through the right atrium has been described in the fetal lamb[1] and is presumed to occur in the human fetus. Studies of changes in inferior vena caval blood flow with fetal manipulation have been performed in fetal lambs.[5]

Perturbation of the flow through the right atrium, either by abnormal heart rates or by abnormal ventricular filling, would result in potentially adverse consequences for the fetus. Abnormally high reverse flow into the inferior vena cava with atrial contraction would appear to be a marker for this perturbed flow and was seen both in fetal lamb studies and in human fetal Doppler studies.[3,5]

Sustained abnormally rapid or slow heart rates are accompanied by fetal morbidity, and increases in reverse flow with atrial contraction are seen in these conditions. It is interesting to note that reverse flow in the inferior vena cava is lowest at the normal heart rates of 120 to 160 beats/min (Fig. 10-2). Fetuses with absent end-diastolic flow velocities in the umbilical artery have an increase in perinatal morbidity and mortality[6]; reverse flow in the inferior vena cava is also increased in this group.

Umbilical venous pulsations are seen in fetuses with increases in reverse flow with atrial contraction in the inferior vena cava. While detection of reverse flow in the inferior vena cava requires pulsed Doppler and relatively sophisticated imaging techniques, umbilical artery and venous velocity detection is relatively simple. It appears that venous pulsations can be used as an indicator of perturbed inferior vena caval flow and therefore right atrial flow.

An association of umbilical venous pulsations with adverse perinatal outcome in fetuses with hydrops has been reported; inferior vena cava reverse-flow velocities were also increased in these fetuses.[7]

In summary, Doppler studies of venous flow in the fetus may be used to detect alterations in the circulation that may result in adverse fetal outcomes.

REFERENCES

1. Reuss ML, Rudolph AM, Heymann MA: Selective distribution of microspheres injected into the umbilical veins and inferior venae cavae of fetal sheep. Am J Obstet Gynecol 141:427–432, 1981.
2. Appleton CP, Hatle LK, Popp RL: Superior vena cava and hepatic vein Doppler echocardiography in healthy adults. J Am Coll Cardiol 10:1032–1039, 1987.
3. Reed KL, Appleton CP, Anderson CF, Shenker L, Sahn DJ: Doppler studies of vena cava flows in human fetuses. Circulation 81:498–505, 1990.
4. Indik JH, Chen V, Reed KL: Association of umbilical venous with inferior vena cava blood flow velocities. Obstet Gynecol 77:551–557, 1991.

5. Reuss ML, Rudolph AM, Dae MW: Phasic blood flow patterns in the superior and inferior venae cavae and umbilical vein of fetal sheep. Am J Obstet Gynecol 145:70–78, 1983.
6. Reed KL, Anderson CF, Shenker L: Changes in intracardiac Doppler blood flow velocities in fetuses with absent umbilical artery diastolic flow. Am J Obstet Gynecol 157:774–779, 1990.
7. Gudmundsson S, Huhta JC, Wood DC, Tulzer G, Cohen AW, Weiner S: Venous Doppler ultrasonography in the fetus with nonimmune hydrops. Am J Obstet Gynecol 164:33–37, 1991.

ELEVEN

COLOR DOPPLER STUDIES OF FETAL CIRCULATION IN INTRAUTERINE GROWTH RETARDATION

DOMENICO ARDUINI
GIUSEPPE RIZZO

An impaired fetal growth can be secondary to multiple and various etiologies including chromosomal aberrations, structural abnormalities, constitutionally low growth potentialities, or the so-called uteroplacental insufficiency.[1] One of the main challenges of the management of these fetuses is to identify and properly monitor those in which the growth retardation is secondary to uteroplacental insufficiency, as these fetuses have an increased risk to develop perinatal mortality and morbidity.[2,3] Besides, small fetuses secondary to constitutional factors do not show any significant increase in perinatal complications,[4] while the prognosis of fetuses with chromosomal and structural abnormalities is related to the severity of the underlying disease.[1] This chapter is therefore restricted to fetuses in which the growth retardation (IUGR) is secondary to uteroplacental insufficiency.

Much of the understanding and present knowledge of this phenomenon are derived from both animal research and pathologic studies of human placenta or uterine biopsies. Moreover the advent of pulsed and color Doppler ultrasonography has allowed physicians to obtain noninvasive hemodynamic measurements from several vascular beds of uterine, placental, and fetal circulation in humans. Thus, it has been possible to further improve the understanding of the pathophysiology of fetal circulation in IUGR. After a brief summary of the pathophysiology of uteroplacental insufficiency, this chapter reviews the application of Doppler ultrasonography to the study of IUGR and considers its potential clinical role.

PATHOPHYSIOLOGY

The underlying pathophysiology of uteroplacental insufficiency is a reduction in the supply of nutrients provided from the mother to the fetus through the placenta. In normal pregnancies the blood supply to the uterus remarkably increases from 50 mL/min in early pregnancy to approximately 500 mL/min at term.[5] It has been clearly demonstrated that fetal growth is directly related to the normal incremental increases in uterine blood flow through pregnancy[6] and that in cases of prolonged reduction of uterine blood flow fetal growth is slowed.[7] Systemic events occurring during pregnancy such as the expansion in maternal blood volume and the rise of cardiac output have a partial role in this increase of uterine blood flow, but its main origin may be found in local factors causing the decrease of uterine vascular resistance.

In normal early pregnancy the trophoblastic cells invade the placental bed and migrate through the spiral arteries of the uterine circulation. The invading trophoblast destroys the elastic lamina and replaces the smooth-muscle cells of the vascular wall of the spiral arteries. This transformation, completed by 20 weeks of gestation, leads to the formation of a low-vascular-resistance system in which relatively large arteries pump blood directly to the placental intervillous space.[8] Failure or impairment of trophoblast invasion does not allow the fall of uterine vascular resistance and impairs the maternal-fetal exchange of nutrients and oxygen, thus leading to IUGR and/or maternal hypertension.[9]

Moreover IUGR might occur also in presence of normal uterine blood supply associated with an abnormal placental function. The difficulties in studying the placental function have limited the present knowledge. However, it has been shown that the number of small muscular arteries in the tertiary stem villi is reduced in IUGR fetuses, thus resulting in an impaired supply of oxygen and nutrients from the mother to the fetus. There has been debate as to whether this reduction is secondary to a developmental arrest of placental angiogenesis[10] or to an obliterative process of small muscular arteries[11]; however, it can be suggested that both phenomena might occur.

The decrease of uterine blood flow and/or placental exchange capability leads to a reduced supply to the fetus of oxygen, glucose, and essential nutrients.[12–14] This limitation of substrates causes concomitant adaptatory circulatory responses.

Umbilical blood venous flow that passes through the ductus venosus increases, whereas the passage to the liver decreases, thus improving the impaired concentration of oxygen and nutrients in the inferior vena cava and consequently in the heart.[15] Concomitantly there is a change of arterial vascular resistances in fetal circulation with a vasodilatation at the level of the brain and myocardium and a constriction at the level of muscles and viscera.[16] Therefore a redistribution of cardiac output occurs (the so-called brain sparing effect) in favor of the priority organs (i.e., brain and heart) with a reduction of flow to the other organs that are less essential for the immediate survival of the fetus and a consequent impairment of their growth. The persistence or the worsening of this condition of nutritional deprivation leads to a progressive deterioration of fetal conditions with further hemodynamic changes mainly characterized by a reduction of cardiac output and an impairment of cardiac function.[17] Further modifications include abnormalities in fetal motor behavior and heart rate patterns.[18] Finally if the fetus is not delivered in due course, death will occur.

DOPPLER STUDIES

Since the earlier signs of fetal impairment secondary to reduced nutrient and oxygen supplies are adaptive circulatory responses, Doppler ultrasound provides a unique tool to examine these changes noninvasively. Particularly the combined use of color and pulsed Doppler techniques in obstetrics has greatly enhanced the possibilities of studying IUGR. The combined use of these techniques improves the recordings of flow-velocity waveforms from uteroplacental and fetal vessels for different reasons such as (1) the higher reproducibility and the shorter recording time,[19] (2) the possibility of having recordings from vessels of small dimension in uteroplacental and fetal circulations which are difficult or impossible to obtain with pulsed or continuous wave Doppler equipments, (3) the visualization of low-velocity flows in venous circulation and their correct recording, and (4) the clear identification of flow direction, which allows the optimization of the angle of insonation between flow and Doppler beam and makes it possible to obtain quantitative analysis of blood flow in some vascular regions.

By these techniques it is therefore possible to study the vascular regions as shown in the following sections.

Uterine Circulation

Velocity waveforms from uterine vessels can be recorded at different levels. In particular, the advent of transvaginal color Doppler ultrasonography has allowed visualization in early pregnancy of the main uterine arteries, arcuate arteries, radial arteries, and flows near the trophoblastic area representing spiral arteries.[20,21] The small dimensions of uterine vessels and the difficulties in obtaining a low angle of insonation have limited the analysis of blood flow-velocity waveforms mainly to a qualitative angle-independent indices considered directly related to vascular resistances such as the S/D ratio (systolic velocity to diastolic velocity) or resistance index [RI = (systolic velocity-diastolic velocity)/systolic velocity]. Attempts to record absolute uterine blood flow have recently been performed with the aid of color Doppler.[22] Their reproducibility and clinical significance still remain to be defined.

In normal pregnancy a progressive decrease of Doppler-measured vascular resistance is present at the level of both uterine arteries and their branches.[20,21,23]

There are no particular advantages in obtaining recordings from the peripheral regions of the uterine circulation, and the main uterine artery is the most commonly analyzed vessel.[23] This choice is based on two factors. The first is the higher reproducibility of the recordings due to the easier identification of this vessel when compared with a single arcuate or spiral artery. Furthermore as the indices measured reflect the vascular resistance of the downstream circulation, the main uterine artery provides information on the whole uterine circulation, while an arcuate or spiral artery provides information on only a limited vascular area that may differ from the general situation.

The use of color Doppler by means of a parasagittal scan of the pelvis lateral to the uterus allows an easy identification of the main uterine artery from its origin at the level of the hypogastric artery to its first branching inside the myometrium.[19] By placing the sample volume of the pulsed Doppler in the main uterine artery just medial to the external iliac artery, it is possible to obtain in short time and with a high reproducibility velocity waveforms from both sides of the uterus (Fig. 11-1). In normal pregnancies the S/D and RI values significantly decrease with advancing gestation until 24 to 26 weeks, when a plateau is reached[23] (Fig. 11-1*A*). In the absence of this physiologic decrease, a higher incidence of hypertensive diseases and/or IUGR has been widely documented[23–26] (Fig. 11-1*B*). On the other hand, as previously described, several IUGR fetuses present normal uterine artery waveforms despite severe compromise of the maternal-fetal exchange of substrates because of a pathologic disease limited to the fetal side of the uteroplacental circulation.

Umbilical Artery

Similarly to the uterine circulation, velocity waveforms from the umbilical artery are usually analyzed by angle-independent indices, mainly S/D ratio or pulsatility index [PI = (systolic velocity-diastolic velocity)/mean velocity]. The latter index is preferred by several authors as it allows evaluation of the waveforms also in the absence of end-diastolic flow. Normal pregnancies show a progressive decrease of S/D and PI values mainly due to an increase of the end-diastolic velocities.[27] End-diastolic velocities are physiologically absent in the first trimester while they are always present from 16 weeks of gestation onward[28] (Fig. 11-2*A*). These changes in Doppler indices are considered an expression of the physiologic decrease of placental resistances (i.e., progressive opening and merging of small muscular arteries in the tertiary stem villi).

In IUGR fetuses there is an increase of these indices secondary to the decrease (Fig. 11-2*B*), absence (Fig. 11-2*C*), or reversal (Fig. 11-2*D*) of end-diastolic flow. The changes in these waveform patterns are thought to be indicative of increased placental resistances. However, other explanations such as an increase in blood viscosity or a reduction in arterial blood pressure have not been excluded. There is no account as to whether the abnormalities in the umbilical artery occur earlier, simultaneously, or later than those in fetal vessels. As already

(*Text continues on page 190.*)

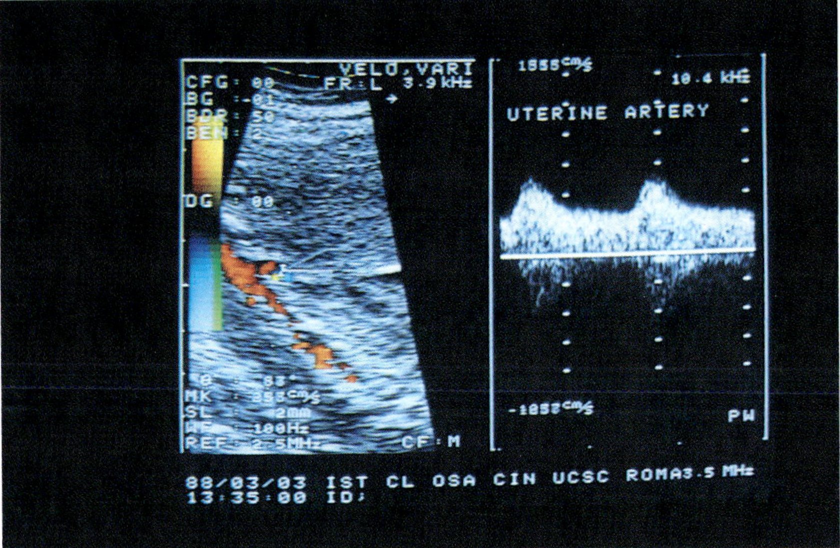

A

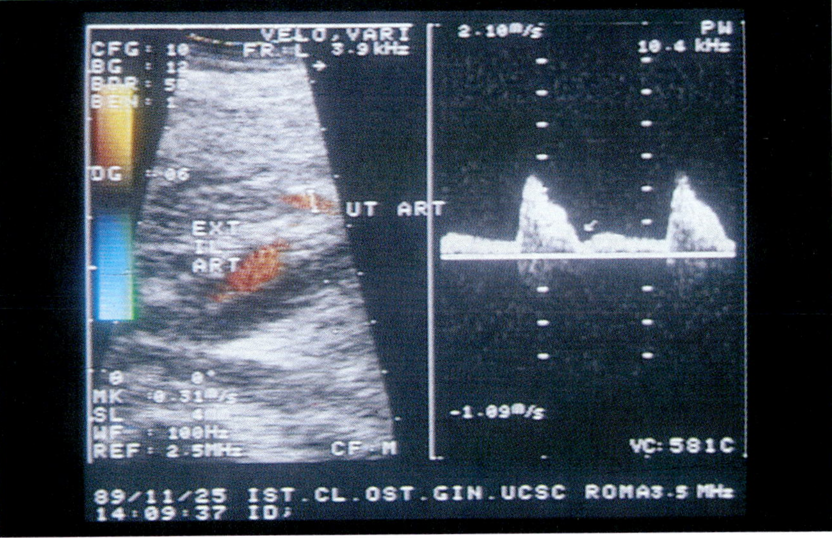

B

Figure 11-1   Velocity waveforms from uterine artery. The sample volume is placed in the portion of the main uterine artery close to the external iliac artery. Velocity waveforms were recorded at 22 weeks of gestation in a normal pregnancy (*A*) and in a complicated pregnancy that later developed preeclampsia and IUGR (*B*). In the latter case the end-diastolic velocity is reduced and a diastolic notch is evident.

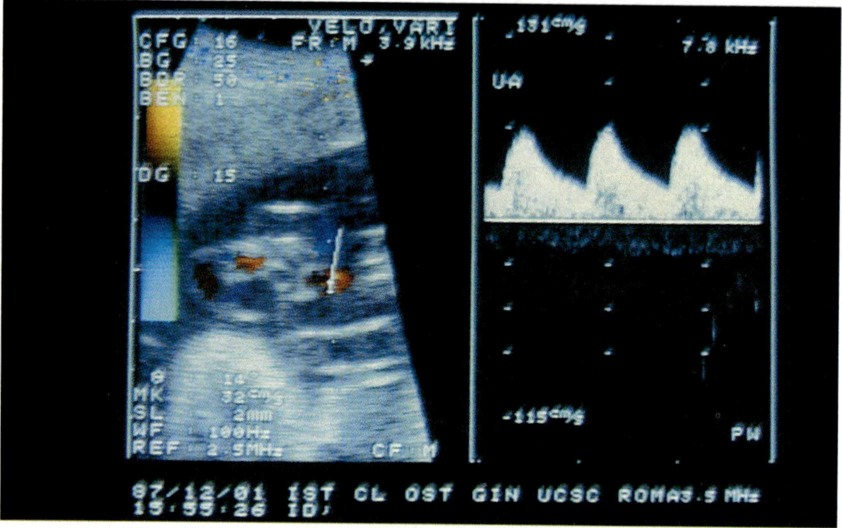

A

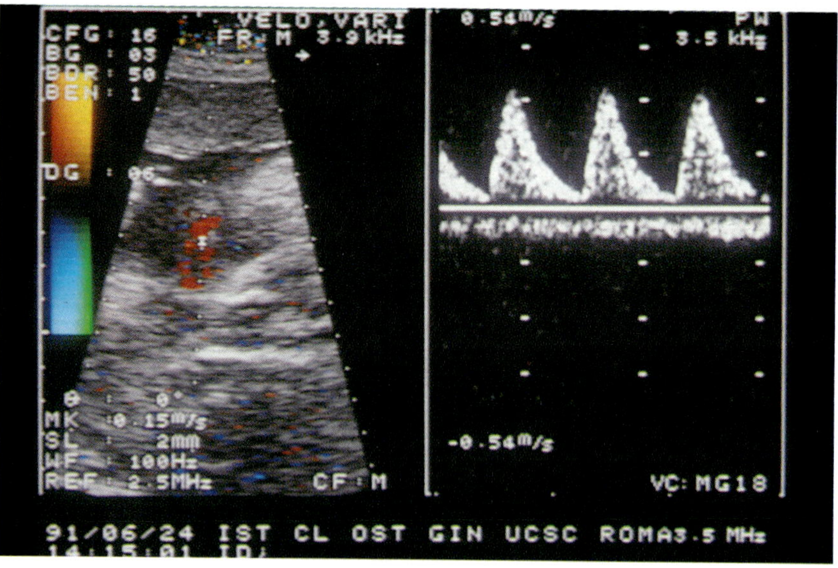

B

Figure 11-2 Velocity waveforms from umbilical artery in a normal pregnancy at 33 weeks (*A*) and in pregnancies complicated in IUGR (*B, C, D*) in which the end-diastolic velocities are reduced (*B*), absent (*C*), and reversed (*D*).

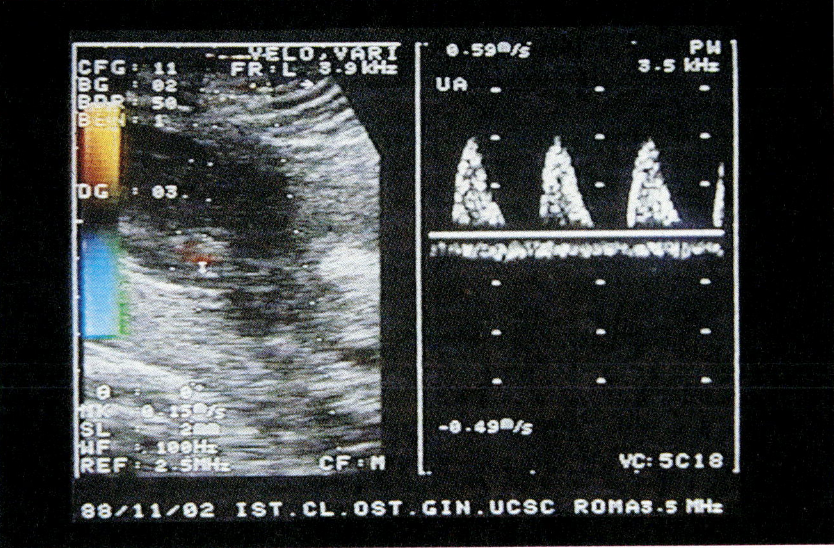

C

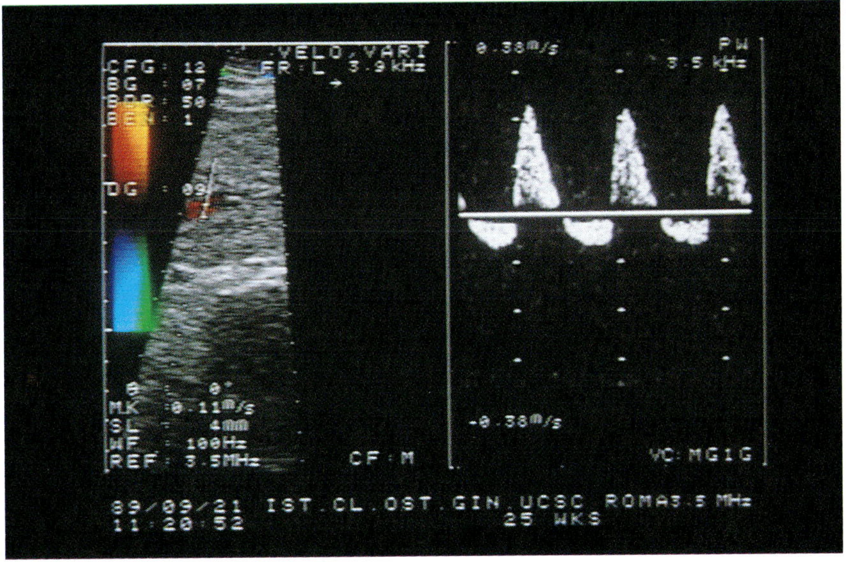

D

Figure 11-2 (*Continued*).

described, despite the common denominator of a reduced supply of nutrients, IUGR has multiple etiologies which may involve the placenta primarily with an early increase of its vascular resistance. On the other hand, different causes (e.g., impaired uterine circulations) might primarily induce the brain-sparing phenomenon with a consequent reduction of the blood supply to the placenta and secondary obliterative and degenerative phenomena leading to increased vascular resistances.

The absent or reverse end-diastolic flows are strongly associated with an abnormal course of pregnancy and a higher incidence of perinatal complications as compared to IUGR fetuses of similar severity but characterized by the presence of end-diastolic flow.[29]

Fetal Descending Aorta

Velocity waveforms from the fetal descending aorta are usually recorded at the lower thoracic level, keeping the angle of insonation of the Doppler beam below 45°. Diastolic velocities are always present during the second and third trimester of normal pregnancy, and the PI remains constant through gestation[27] (Fig. 11-3A). Flow-velocity waveforms in the descending aorta represent the summation of flows to the kidneys, other abdominal organs, femoral arteries, and placenta. The absence of modifications of PI during pregnancy suggests that despite the decrease of placental and renal (see later) resistances with advancing gestation, aortic resistances remain constant, implying a concomitant increase of vascular resistances in other regions such as the extremities.

IUGR fetuses show an increase of PI with reduction, absence, or reversal of diastolic velocities[3] (Fig. 11-3B). The absence of end-diastolic velocities, suggestive of profound vascular changes causing a severe reduction of flow to splanchnic organs, has been associated with a higher incidence of neonatal complications, particularly necrotizing enterecolitis, when compared with matched controls with presence of end-diastolic flow.[3]

Fetal Renal Artery

Color Doppler allows easy identification in a longitudinal view of the fetal renal artery from its origin as a lateral branch of the abdominal aorta to the hilus of the kidney[27] (Fig. 11-4A). Diastolic velocities are physiologically absent until 34 weeks, and the PI significantly decreases with advancing gestation[27,30] (Fig. 11-4B). If it is assumed that arterial pressure remains constant through gestation; then fetal renal perfusion increases. This may offer an explanation for the increase of fetal urine production that occurs with advancing gestation.

IUGR fetuses show higher PI values from the renal artery, and this increase is proportional to the severity of fetal hypoxemia.[30] Furthermore, the abnormalities of renal artery PI are inversely related to the amount of amniotic fluid volume.[31]

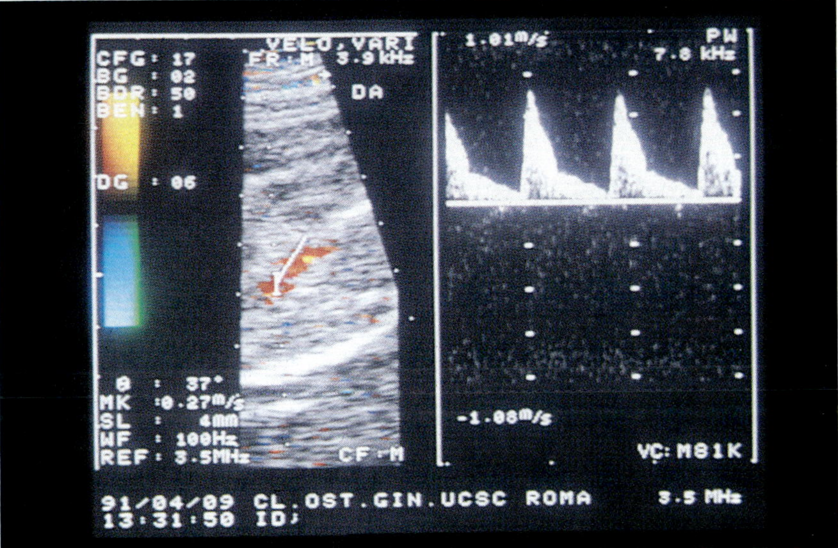

A

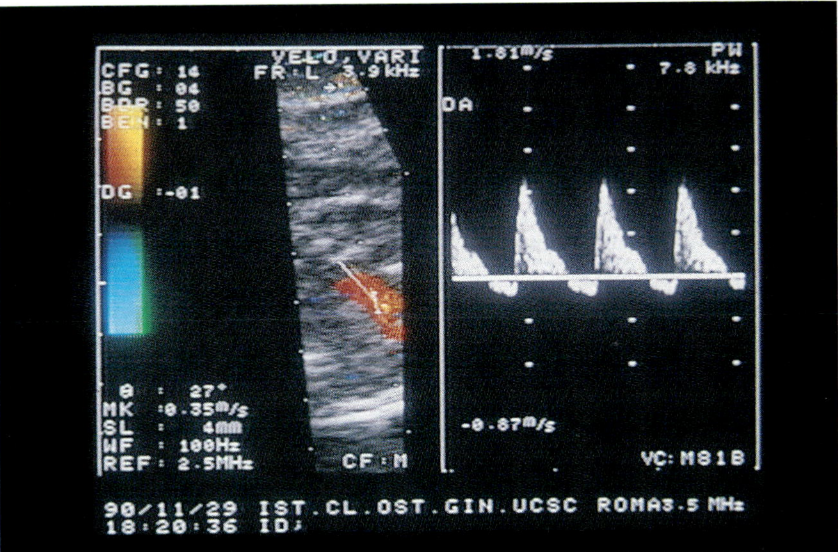

B

Figure 11-3   Velocity waveforms from the fetal descending thoracic aorta in a normal fetus (*A*) with presence of end-diastolic velocities and in a IUGR fetus with reverse end-diastolic velocities (*B*).

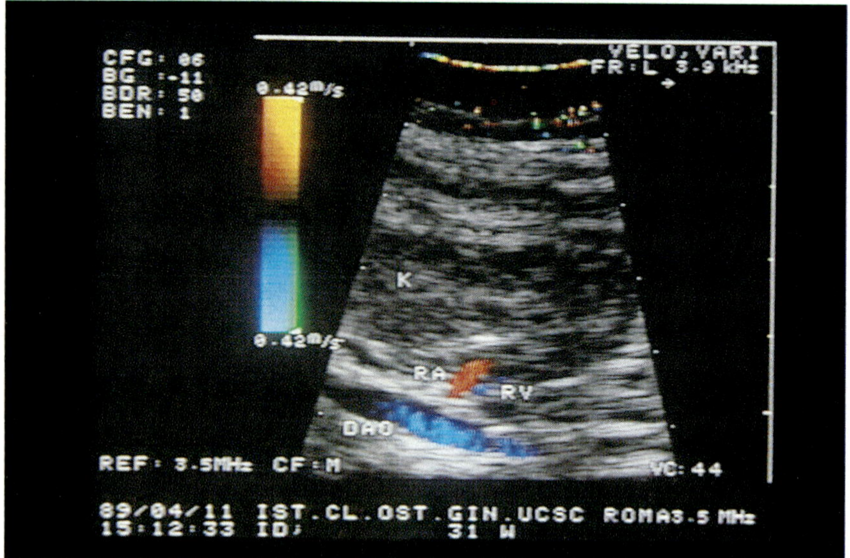

A

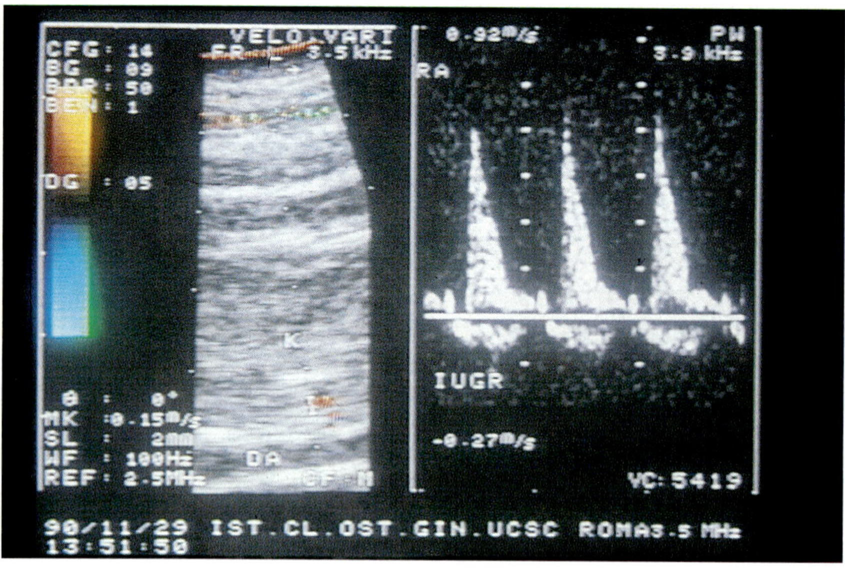

B

Figure 11-4 Longitudinal view of the fetal trunk with the renal artery branching from the abdominal aorta (*A*). Velocity waveforms from the renal artery in an IUGR fetus at 35 weeks of gestation (*B*). The end-diastolic velocities are absent, and the PI is 3.46 (normal mean at 35 weeks = 2.19).

This suggests that the PI from renal artery can be considered a good marker of renal perfusion and may be used to monitor fetal adaptatory response to hypoxemia.

Fetal Cerebral Circulation

With the color Doppler technique it is possible to investigate the main cerebral arteries such as the internal carotid artery, the middle cerebral artery, and the anterior and the posterior cerebral arteries and to evaluate the vascular resistances in the different areas supplied by these vessels (Fig. 11-5A and B). In healthy fetuses the Doppler-measured vascular resistances remain constant during the second and early third trimester of pregnancy, whereas they significantly decrease during the late third trimester.[27] The PI is significantly higher in the middle cerebral artery than in internal carotid artery or in the anterior and posterior cerebral arteries. It is therefore important to know exactly which cerebral vessel is sampled during a Doppler examination, as a PI value that might be normal for the internal carotid artery may be abnormal for the middle cerebral artery.[32] The use of color Doppler greatly improves the identification of the cerebral vessels, thus limiting the possibility of sampling errors.

The middle cerebral artery is usually considered the vessel of choice in the evaluation of the fetal cerebral circulation, as it is possible to obtain easily velocity waveforms with angle of insonation near 0° and with a high reproducibility (Fig. 11-5C). However, the physiologic differences between the cerebral vessels still remain to be clarified.

In IUGR fetuses the PI from cerebral arteries decreases (Fig. 11-5D), and these changes are secondary to a vasomotor response (vasodilatation) occurring during the brain-sparing phenomenon.[33] Comparison between cerebral PI and the measurement of umbilical P_{O_2}, CO_2, pH, and O_2 content obtained by cordocentesis or at birth has evidenced significant correlations between these parameters.[34,35] However, these correlations do not appear sufficiently strong to use the cerebral Doppler indices in clinical practice to quantify the compromise of fetal acid-base status and to decide on the time of delivery. Nevertheless, a satisfying relationship has been found between the existence of significantly decreased fetal cerebral resistances and the development in the newborn of postasphyxial encephalopathy, thus suggesting an important prognostic role of cerebral Doppler velocimetry.[36]

Fetal Cardiac Flows

Doppler velocimetry allows the study of intracardiac hemodynamics at the level of the atrioventricular valves and outflow tracts. In normal pregnancies a progressive improvement of the cardiac performance occurs. The E/A ratio [where E = early phase of atrioventricular velocity waveform (passive venous filling of

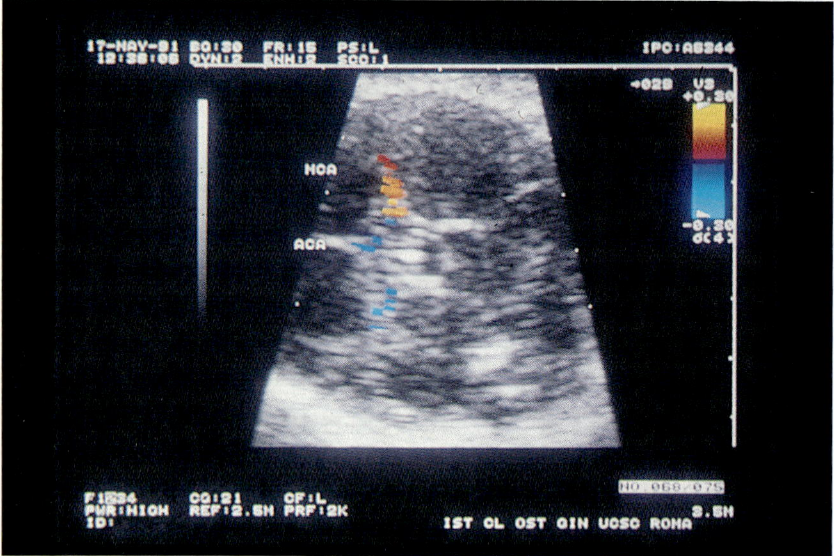

A

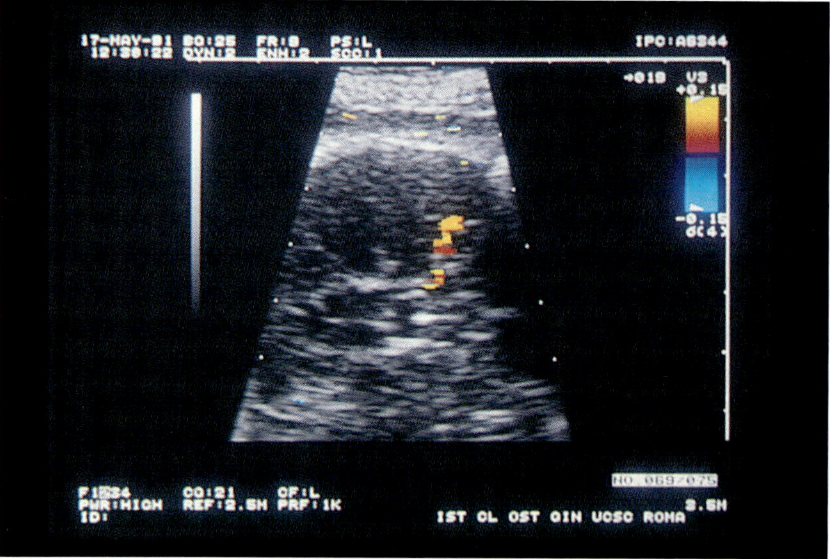

B

Figure 11-5 Cross-sectional view of the fetal head at the level of cerebral peduncles showing the division of the internal carotid artery into the middle cerebral artery (red) and anterior cerebral artery (blue) (A). More caudal plane of the fetal head at the level of the greater wings of the sphenoid showing the middle cerebral artery (B).

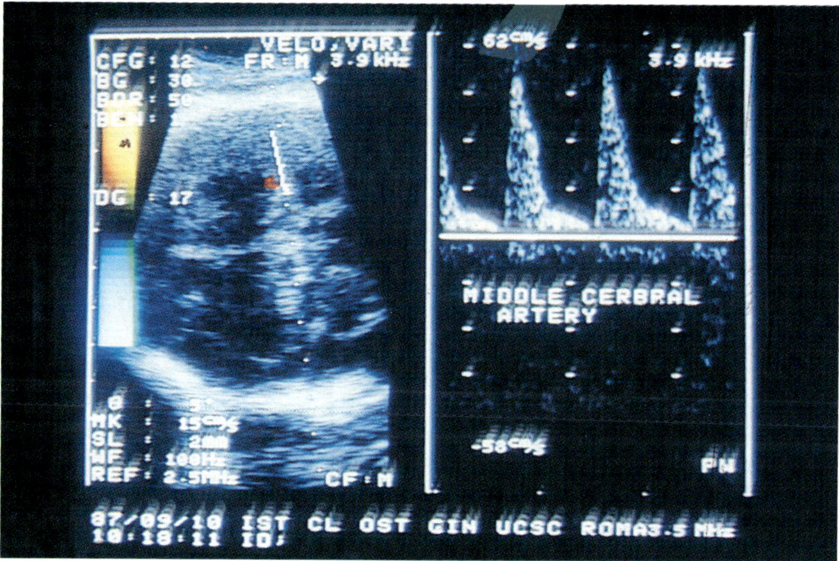

C

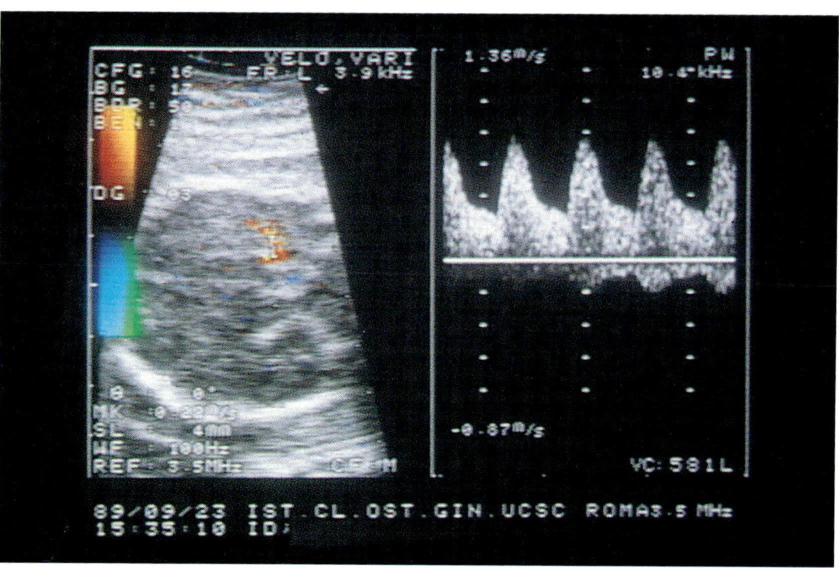

D

Figure 11-5 (*Continued*)   Velocity waveforms from middle cerebral artery in a normal fetus (*C*) and in an IUGR fetuses (*D*) showing an evident increase of diastolic velocities.

ventricle), and A = late phase of atrioventricular velocity waveform (active ventricular filling)], a widely accepted index of ventricular diastolic function,[37] significantly increases during gestation at the level of both mitral and tricuspid valves, changes believed to be secondary to the progressive maturation of ventricular compliance[37,38] (Fig. 11-6A). Similarly there is an increase of aortic and pulmonary peak velocities and of left and right stroke volumes[39,40] (Fig. 11-7A). These changes are secondary to several factors including a progressive improvement in myocardial contractility, a reduction of cardiac afterload, and an increase in cardiac preload. Study of the time-to-peak velocity (TPV), a parameter inversely related to blood pressure, suggests that in healthy fetuses, the mean pressure is slightly higher in the pulmonary artery than in the ascending aorta.[41] Finally, it has been shown that cardiac output increases progressively with gestation and that the right cardiac output (RCO) is slightly higher than the left cardiac output (LCO) with an RCO/LCO ratio of about 1.3.[42]

Secondary to the brain-sparing effect, selective changes in cardiac afterload occur in IUGR fetuses (i.e., decreased left ventricle afterload due to the cerebral vasodilatation and increased right ventricle afterload due to the systemic vasoconstriction). Furthermore hypoxemia might impair myocardial contractility while the polycythemia usually present[12] might alter blood viscosity and therefore preload. As a consequence IUGR fetuses show impaired ventricular filling properties[38,43] (Fig. 11-6B), lower peak velocities in the aorta and pulmonary arteries[44,45] (Fig. 11-7B), increased aortic and decreased pulmonary TPV,[46] and a relative increase of LCO associated with decreased RCO.[46,47] These hemodynamic intracardiac changes are compatible with a preferential shift of cardiac output in favor of the left ventricle leading to improved perfusion to the brain. Thus, the supply of substrate and oxygen can be maintained at near normal despite any absolute reduction of placental transfer.

The longitudinal studies of progressively deteriorating IUGR fetuses have allowed elucidation of the natural history of these hemodynamic modifications during uteroplacental insufficiency.[45] Since TPV and the ratios between right and left ventricle outputs remain stable during repeated recordings in such fetuses, it appears that there are no other significant changes in outflow resistances and cardiac output redistribution after establishment of the brain-sparing mechanism. However, in deteriorating IUGR fetuses peak velocities and cardiac output decline progressively rather than the expected rise with gestation. The physiologic significance of these longitudinal changes is subject to several interpretations. However, as they are closely followed by the onset of abnormal heart rate patterns, one might speculate that the fall in cardiac output terminally may reflect a decompensation of a normally protective mechanism responsible for the brain-sparing effect.

According to this model, the fetal heart adapts to placental insufficiency in a manner which helps to maximize brain substrate and oxygen supply. With progressive deterioration of fetal conditions, this protective mechanism is overwhelmed by the fall of cardiac output, and fetal distress occurs.

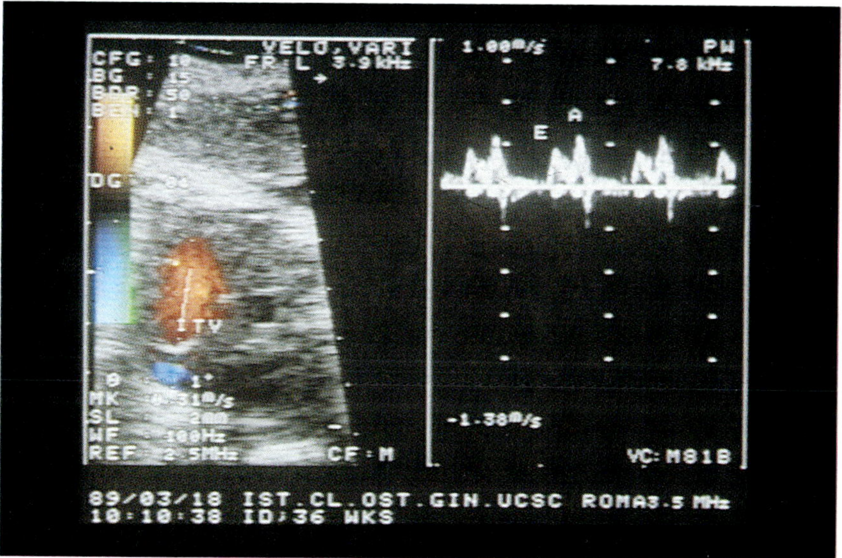

A

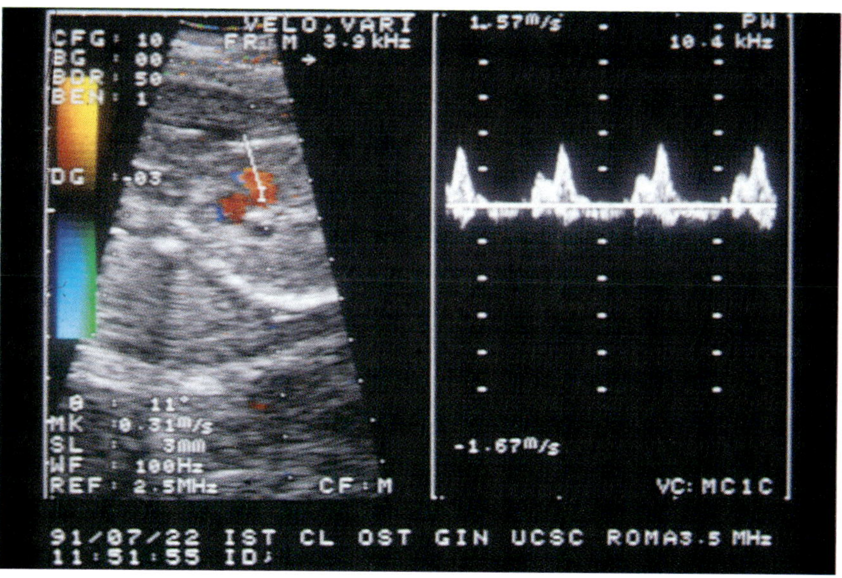

B

Figure 11-6   Velocity waveforms recorded at the level of tricuspid valve in a normal fetus (*A*) and in an IUGR fetus (*B*) at 34 weeks of gestation. The E/A ratios are 0.85 in the former and 0.54 in the latter.

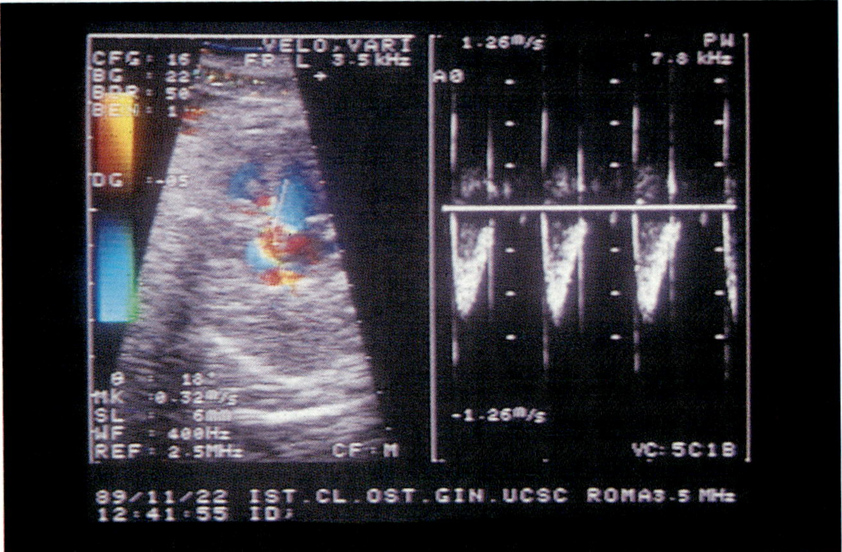

A

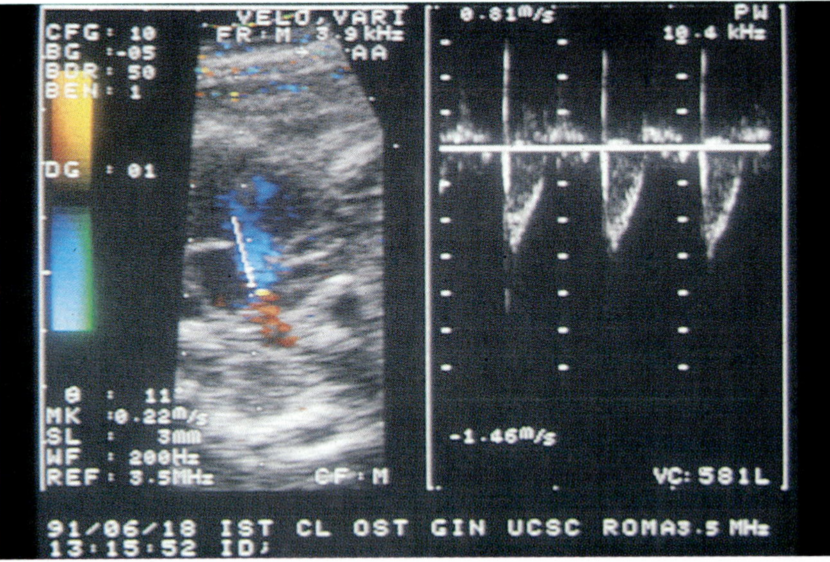

B

Figure 11-7 Velocity waveforms recorded at the level of the ascending aorta (outflow tract of the left ventricle) in a normal fetus (*A*) and in an IUGR fetus (*B*) at 33 weeks of gestation. The peak velocity is 83 cm/s in the former and 56 cm/s in the latter.

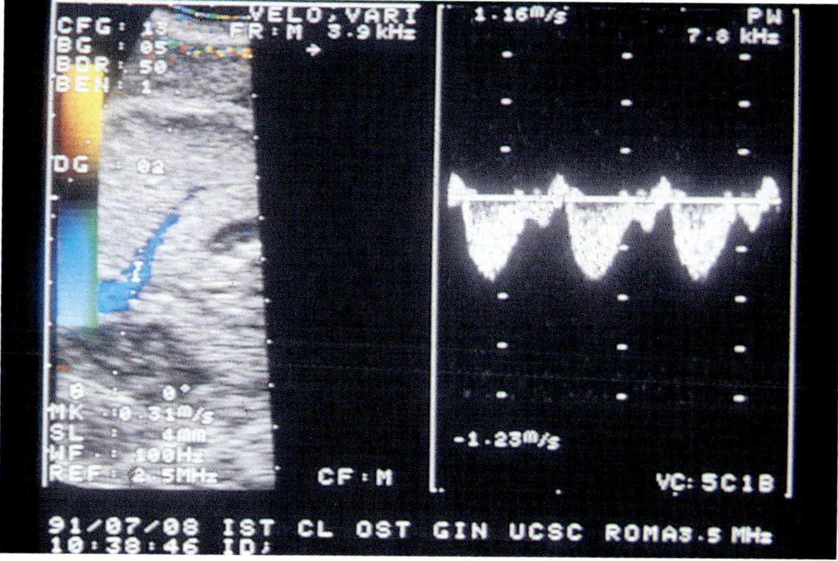

A

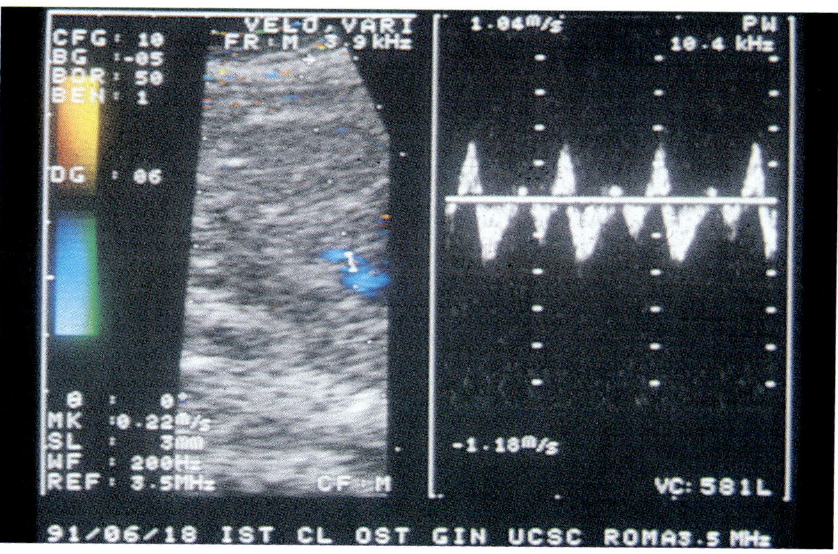

B

Figure 11-8   Velocity waveforms from the inferior vena cava in a normal fetus (*A*) and in an IUGR fetus (*B*). The reverse flow during atrial contraction (*top channel*) is increased in the IUGR fetuses and the percent of reverse flow is 21.4 (normal mean for gestation = 8.1).

Fetal Venous Blood Flow

Fetal supply of oxygen and nutrients depends on blood returning to the heart from the placenta via the umbilical vein, ductus venosus, and inferior vena cava. In the human fetus the inferior vena cava blood flow has a triphasic pulsatile pattern.[48] The *first forward wave* begins to increase with atrial relaxation, reaches the peak during ventricular systole, and then falls to reach the nadir at the end of ventricular systole. The *second forward wave* occurs during early diastole, while the *third wave,* characterized by a reverse flow, is present in late diastole with atrial contraction. In healthy fetuses a significant decrease of reverse flow during atrial contraction is present with advancing gestation[49] (Fig. 11-8*A*). As the amount of reverse flow is proportional to the pressure gradient present between the right atrium and the right ventricle at the end diastole, these changes are considered related both to the improvement of ventricular compliance and to the reduction of right ventricular afterload due to the fall of placental resistances occurring with gestation.

In IUGR fetuses an increase of reverse flow during atrial contraction might be present in the most severely compromised fetuses[48,49] (Fig. 11-8*B*). As a consequence of these venous abnormal flow patterns, the return of blood from the placenta to the heart is impaired, thus further reducing the supply of oxygen and nutrients. These findings are compatible with the fall of both cardiac output and aortic and pulmonary peak velocities described in progressively deteriorating

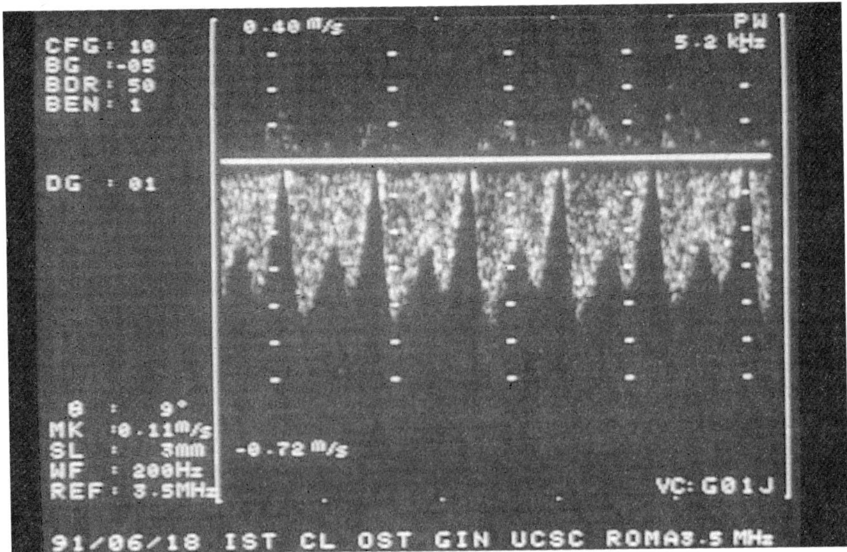

Figure 11-9 Velocity waveforms from the ductus venosus in an IUGR fetus. The mean velocity is increased (47 cm/s normal mean for gestation = 32 cm/s).

IUGR fetuses.[45] All these changes are the expression of the same phenomenon, namely, cardiac decompensation, which impairs both the filling and the output of the heart.

Up to now few data have been available on blood flow velocity waveforms in the ductus venosus, but preliminary observations from our laboratory suggest increased mean temporal velocities and reverse flow during end-diastole in this vascular region in IUGR fetuses. These changes are compatible with the increased blood flow through the ductus venosus present in animal models during hypoxemia (Fig. 11-9).

Umbilical venous blood flow is usually continuous (Fig. 11-10*A*). However, in the presence of a relevant amount of reverse flow during atrial contraction in the inferior vena cava, pulsations with heart rate in umbilical venous flows occur. In normal pregnancies these pulsations occur only before the 12th week of gestation, and they are secondary to the stiffness of the ventricles present at this gestational age causing a high percentage of reverse flow in the inferior vena cava. Later in gestation the presence of pulsations in the umbilical vein expresses severe cardiac compromise and has a significance similar to that of increased reverse flow in the inferior vena cava (Fig. 11-10*B*). Particularly in IUGR fetuses, the presence of pulsation in the umbilical vein is associated with a fivefold increase in perinatal mortality when compared with IUGR fetuses with continuous umbilical flow.[50]

CLINICAL APPLICATIONS

Prediction of IUGR

The possibility of predicting IUGR before the clinical or ultrasonographic identification of the growth defect has been tested by several authors.[24,26,51–60] The rationale of these studies was based on the earlier onset of the hemodynamic changes with respect to the development of the growth defect. Most of the investigations have limited the analysis to uterine arteries and/or umbilical artery as velocity waveforms from these vessels may be recorded with low-cost continuous Doppler equipment, thus allowing the examination of a large number of subjects. The results obtained with uterine and umbilical arteries in the prediction of IUGR are summarized in Tables 11-1 and 11-2. Despite the good specificity obtained in all the studies, the sensitivity (the proportion of abnormal fetal outcome detected by the test) was disappointingly low, and this was particularly evident when low-risk populations were studied in which the prevalence of IUGR fetuses is low.

Therefore a screening with Doppler velocimetry does not seem to be justified in a general population. On the other hand, there is no doubt that the findings of abnormal velocity waveforms in a high-risk population identify those fetuses at risk to develop IUGR and perinatal complications.

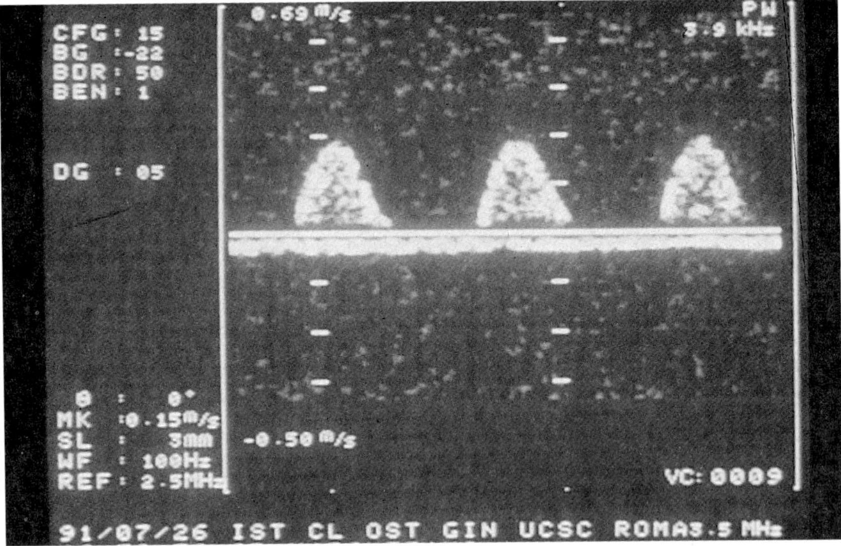

A

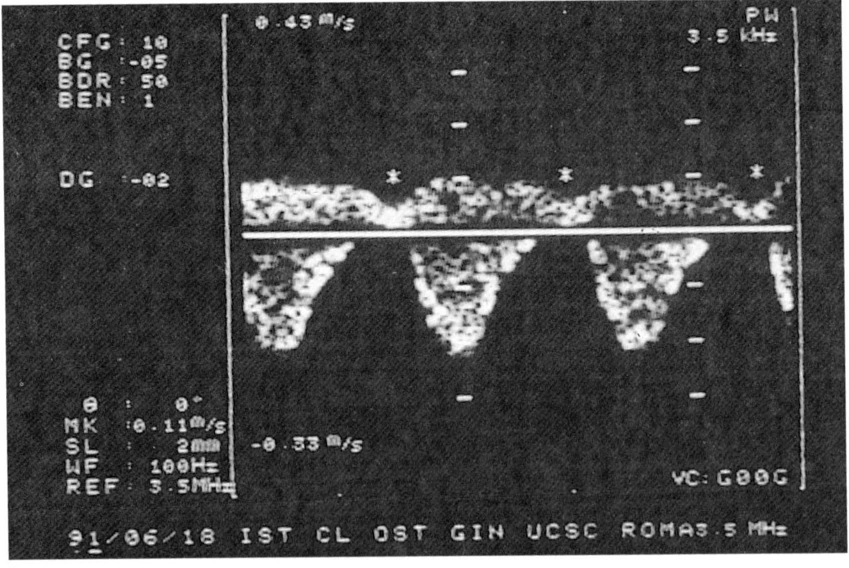

B

Figure 11-10 Velocity waveforms from the umbilical artery and vein in two IUGR fetuses with absence of end-diastolic flow in the umbilical artery. Despite the similar values of PI, the umbilical vein shows a continuous pattern in one case (*A*) and pulsations in the other (*B*). This is consistent with a more severe impairment of cardiovascular function in the latter fetus.

Table 11-1   Predictive value of uterine blood flow velocity waveforms for growth retardation at birth

Author	Type of population	Prevalence of IUGR, %	Sensitivity, %	Specificity, %
Trudinger 1985[24]	High risk	27	60	80
Campbell 1986[25]	High risk	10	64	66
Arduini 1987[26]	High risk	15	50	68
Chambers 1989[51]	High risk	59	29	80
Jacobson 1990[52]	High risk	18	70	64
Newnham 1990[53]	Low risk	8	5	96

Differential Diagnosis of IUGR

Since hemodynamic modifications of fetal and placental circulations are present in IUGR fetuses secondary to uteroplacental insufficiency, it is logical to predict a role for Doppler velocimetry as a secondary diagnostic test to identify among small fetuses those malnourished and therefore at risk for perinatal complications.[61] Several studies have tested the ability of Doppler recordings limited to the umbilical artery in predicting adverse outcome in high-risk fetuses. Despite the high specificity achieved, all these studies have shown a relatively low sensitivity, thus limiting the clinical application of umbilical artery velocimetry.[62,63] When different vascular regions of the fetal circulation were tested singularly, only a slight improvement was evident when comparing PI values of the middle cerebral artery to predict adverse fetal outcome.[64] Besides, when different vessels were considered in combination and ratios were calculated between PI from umbilical or fetal peripheral vessels and PI from cerebral vessels, an evident

Table 11-2   Predictive value of umbilical artery velocity waveforms for growth retardation at birth

Author	Type of population	Prevalence of IUGR, %	Sensitivity, %	Specificity, %
Fleisher 1985[54]	High risk	24	100	88
Giles 1986[55]	High risk	16	78	83
Arduini 1987[56]	High risk	31	61	73
Divon 1988[57]	High risk	35	49	94
Dempster 1989[58]	High risk	40	41	82
Beattie 1989[59]	Low risk	10	22	92
Sijmons 1989[60]	Low risk	22	22	94
Newnham 1990[53]	Low risk	8	17	95

improvement of the diagnostic capabilities was obtained.[64] These findings suggest that the PI ratios reflect better than a single vessel the underlying hemodynamic modifications present during the brain-sparing phenomenon. This hypothesis is supported by the results of previous studies showing a higher accuracy of the PI ratios in predicting either the development of growth retardation[56] or the severity of fetal hypoxia.[34]

In our experience the most efficient ratio available is the umbilical artery/middle cerebral artery PI ratio.[64] Possible explanations of this finding include either the higher reproducibility of the measurements from these two vessels when compared to the other vascular districts[19] or a delayed onset of Doppler-detectable abnormalities in the aortic or renal circulations with respect to placental or cerebral circulations. The latter explanation is validated by animal studies showing that in the presence of moderate hypoxemia blood flow remains constant at the level of kidneys, viscera, and carcass, whereas it is significantly modified at the level of cerebral and umbilical circulations.[16]

Umbilical artery velocity waveforms can be recorded by means of simple and low-cost continuous-wave Doppler equipment, whereas the evaluation of fetal cerebral regions requires pulsed and/or color Doppler equipments, thus adding to the cost of the Doppler examination. Therefore the examination of both umbilical and middle cerebral artery cannot be considered a routine test. Nevertheless, in presence of a small fetus a second-level ultrasonographic examination is required to rule out the presence of structural abnormalities. The ultrasound machines employed for this kind of study are of high level and therefore frequently equipped with pulsed and/or color Doppler functions. In this situation the recording of velocity waveforms from umbilical and middle cerebral arteries might be easily obtained with minimal effects on the cost of the examination but significant improvements in the diagnosis.

Timing of Delivery

The occurrence of antepartum abnormal heart rate patterns is mandatory for early delivery in IUGR fetuses. This condition reflects, as indicated above, a severe compromise of fetal conditions. Furthermore on the basis of a clear relationship existing between the presence of antepartum heart rate decelerations and neurologic morbidity, it has been suggested that IUGR fetuses should be delivered before abnormal heart rate patterns occur.[65] In IUGR fetuses abnormal Doppler findings generally precede by several weeks the occurrence of antepartum decelerations. The duration of the time interval elapsing between the first Doppler changes and the onset of abnormal heart rate patterns varies considerably among fetuses. This variability depends on the severity of uteroplacental impairment and on the ability of the fetus to compensate for the reduction in metabolic supply. Cross-sectional Doppler measurements are therefore unlikely to give precise indications on the actual degree of fetal compromise and on the extent of fetal reserve. This concept is supported by cordocentesis data[66] showing that even with severely abnormal waveforms patterns (i.e., absence of end-diastolic flow in umbilical artery), the fetal P_{O_2} and the pH are still within the (lower) normal range in 20 and 60 percent of the cases, respectively. Longitudinal Doppler measurements may lead to a more accurate definition of fetal conditions, but in clinical practice it is extremely useful to define the prognosis from the first recordings, thus allowing optimization of the perinatal management.

To this end we developed a dynamic test (oxygen test) on the fetal circulation finalized to evaluate the placental transfer capability and fetal vascular reactivity.[67] This test has now been applied to a large population of IUGR fetuses, and the results are of some interest. The PI of one cerebral vessel (internal carotid artery or middle cerebral artery) is measured before and after 15 min of maternal administration of 60% humidified oxygen via a face mask. On fetuses which do not develop abnormal fetal heart patterns within 7 days, maternal hyperoxygenation induces an increase of cerebral resistance as expressed by an increase of PI greater than 20 percent from the basal values. The fetuses not responding to the oxygen test (no increase of cerebral resistance) generally develop abnormal heart rate patterns in the following week. The sensitivity of the oxygen test when used as predictor of imminent heart rate abnormalities (within 7 days) is about 80 percent.[68]

The fetal hemodynamic response to maternal hyperoxygenation might therefore be considered a useful prognostic test. The absence of vascular responses to the oxygen test means that either the placental transfer and/or the vascular reactivity are impaired. This condition is associated with an early development of fetal jeopardization, and an early delivery might be considered. Besides, the positive response proves a maintained placental transfer and vascular reactivity, and this condition could justify an expectant management.

CONCLUSION

IUGR fetuses show evident modifications of Doppler parameters in uteroplacental and fetal circulation. Doppler studies have improved our understanding of fetal cardiovascular response to uteroplacental insufficiency. These data may prove useful in improving the methods of identifying, monitoring, and treating those fetuses.

REFERENCES

1. Lin CC, Evans MI: *Intrauterine Growth Retardation. Pathophysiology and Clinical Management.* New York, McGraw-Hill, 1984.
2. Dobson PC, Abell DA, Beisher NA: Mortality and morbidity of fetal growth retardation. Aust NZ J Obstet Gynaecol 21:69–72, 1981.
3. Hackett GA, Campbell S, Gamsu H, Cohen-Overbeek T, Pearce JMF: Doppler studies in the growth retarded fetus and prediction of neonatal necrotising enterocolitis, haemorrhage, and neonatal morbidity. Br Med J 294:13–18, 1987.
4. Burke G, Stuart B, Crowley P, Scanail SN, Drumm J: Is intrauterine growth retardation with normal umbilical blood flow a benign condition? Br Med J 300:1044–1045, 1990.

5. Blechner JN, Stenger VG, Prystowsky H: Uterine blood flow in women at term. Am J Obstet Gynecol 120:633–638, 1974.

6. Creasy RK, Barret CT, De Swiet M, Kahanpaa KV, Rudolph AM: Experimental growth retardation in the sheep. Am J Obstet Gynecol 112:566–573, 1972.

7. Gu W, Jones CT, Parer JT: Metabolic and cardiovascular effects on fetal sheep of sustained reduction of uterine blood flow. J Physiol 368:109–121, 1985.

8. Brosens I, Robertson WB, Dixon HG: The physiological response of the vessels of the placental bed to normal pregnancy. J Phatol Bacteriol 93:569–579, 1967.

9. Sheppard BL, Bonnar J: An ultrastructural study of uteroplacental spiral arteries in hypertensive and normotensive pregnancy and fetal growth retardation. Br J Obstet Gynaecol 88:695–705, 1981.

10. Giles WB, Trudinger BJ, Baird PJ, Cook CM: Fetal umbilical artery flow velocity waveforms and placental resistance: pathological correlation. Br J Obstet Gynaecol 92:31–36, 1985.

11. Bracero LA, Beneck D, Kirshenbaum N, Peiffer M, Stalter P, Schlman H: Doppler velocimetry and placental disease. Am J Obstet Gynecol 161:388–393, 1989.

12. Soothill PW, Nicolaides KH, Campbell S: Prenatal asphyxia, hyperlactemia and erythroblastosis in growth retarded fetuses. Br Med J 294:1051–1053, 1987.

13. Economides DL, Nicolaides KH: Blood glucose and oxygen tension in small for gestational age fetuses. Am J Obstet Gynecol 160:385–389, 1989.

14. Cetin I, Corbetta C, Sereni LP, Marconi AM, Bozzetti P, Pardi G: Umbilical amino acid concentrations in normal and growth retarded fetuses sampled in utero by cordocentesis. Am J Obstet Gynecol 162:253–261, 1990.

15. Rudolph AM: Distribution and regulation of blood flow in the fetal and neonatal lamb. Circ Res 57:811–821, 1985.

16. Peeters LLH, Sheldon RF, Jones MD, Makowsky EI, Meschia G: Blood flow to fetal organ as a function of arterial oxygen content. Am J Obstet Gynecol 135:637–646, 1979.

17. Creasy RK, De Swiet M, Kahanpaa KV, Young WP, Rudolph AM: "Pathophysiological changes in the foetal lamb with growth retardation," in Comline RS, Croos KW, Dawes GS, Nathanielz PW (eds), *Foetal and Neonatal Physiology*. London, Cambridge University Press, 1973, pp 398–402.

18. Visser GHA, Bekedam DJ: "Serial observations on adaptation in the human fetus," in Dawes GS, Borruto F, Zacutti A, Zacutti Jr., A (eds), *Fetal Autonomy and Adaptation*. Chichester, England, Wiley, 1990, pp 67–80.

19. Arduini D, Rizzo G, Boccolini MR, Romanini C, Mancuso S: Functional assessment of uteroplacental and fetal circulations by means of color Doppler ultrasonography. J Ultrasound Med 9:249–253, 1990.

20. Jaffe R, Warsof SL: Transvaginal color Doppler imaging in the assessment of uteroplacental blood flow in the normal first-trimester pregnancy. Am J Obstet Gynecol 164:781–785, 1991.

21. Arduini D, Rizzo G, Romanini C: Doppler ultrasonography in early pregnancy does not predict adverse pregnancy outcome. Ultrasound Obstet Gynecol 1:180–185, 1991.

22. Thaler I, Manor D, Itskovitz J, Rottem S, Levit N, Timor Trish I, Brandes JM: Changes in uterine blood flow during human pregnancy. Am J Obstet Gynecol 162:121–125, 1990.

23. Schulman H, Fleisher A, Farmakides G, Bracero L, Rochelson B, Grunfeld L: Development of uterine artery compliance in pregnancy as detected by ultrasound. Am J Obstet Gynecol 155:1031–1036, 1986.

24. Trudinger BJ, Giles WB, Cook CM: Uteroplacental blood flow velocity time waveforms in normal and complicated pregnancies. Br J Obstet Gynaecol 92:39–45, 1985.

25. Campbell S, Pearce JMF, Hackett G, Cohen-Overbeek TE, Hernandez C: Qualitative assessment of uteroplacental blood flow: early screening test for high-risk pregnancies. Obstet Gynecol 68:649–653, 1986.

26. Arduini D, Rizzo G, Romanini C, Mancuso S: Utero-placental blood flow velocity waveforms as predictors of pregnancy-induced hypertension. Eur J Obstet Gynecol Reprod Biol 26:335–341, 1987.

27. Arduini D, Rizzo G: Normal values of pulsatility index from fetal vessels: a cross sectional study on 1556 healthy fetuses. J Perinat Med 18:165–172, 1990.

28. Arduini D, Rizzo G: Umbilical artery velocity waveforms in early pregnancy: a transvaginal color Doppler study. J Clin Ultrasound 19:335–339, 1991.

29. Rochelson B, Schulman H, Farmakides J, Bracero L, Ducey J, Fleisher A, Penny B, Winter D: The significance of absent end diastolic velocity in umbilical artery velocity waveforms. Am J Obstet Gynecol 156:1213–1217, 1987.

30. Vyas S, Nicolaides KH, Campbell S: Renal flow-velocity waveforms in normal and hypoxemic fetuses. Am J Obstet Gynecol 161:168–172, 1989.

31. Arduini D, Rizzo G: Fetal renal artery velocity waveforms and amniotic fluid volume in growth-retarded and post-term fetuses. Obstet Gynecol 77:370–374, 1991.

32. Mari G, Moise KJ, Deter RL, Kirshon B, Carpenter RJ, Hutha JC: Doppler assessment of the pulsatility index in the cerebral circulation of the human fetus. Am J Obstet Gynecol 160:698–703, 1989.

33. Wladimiroff JW, Tonge HM, Stewart PA: Doppler ultrasound assessment of cerebral blood flow in the human fetus. Br J Obstet Gynaecol 93:471–475, 1986.

34. Bilardo CM, Nicolaides KH, Campbell S: Doppler measurement of fetal and uteroplacental circulation: relationship with umbilical venous blood gases measured at cordocentesis. Am J Obstet Gynecol 162:115–121, 1990.

35. Arduini D, Rizzo G, Romanini C, Mancuso S: Are blood flow velocity waveforms related to umbilical cord acid-base status in the human fetus? Gynecol Obstet Inv 27:183–187, 1989.

36. Rizzo G, Luciano R, Arduini D, Rizzo C, Tortorolo G, Romanini C, Mancuso S: Prenatal cerebral Doppler ultrasonography and neonatal neurological outcome. J Ultrasound Med 8:237–240, 1989.

37. Reed KL, Sahn DJ, Scagnelli S, Anderson CF, Shenker L: Doppler echocardiographic studies of diastolic function in the human fetal heart: changes during gestation. J Am Coll Cardiol 8:391–395, 1986.

38. Rizzo G, Arduini D, Romanini C, Mancuso S: Doppler echocardiographic assessment of atrioventricular velocity waveforms in normal and small for gestational age fetuses. Br J Obstet Gynaecol 95:65–69, 1988.

39. Reed KL, Meijboom EJ, Sahn DJ, Scagnelli SA, Valdes-Cruz LM, Skenker L: Cardiac Doppler flow velocities in human fetuses. Circulation 73:41–56, 1986.

40. Kenny JF, Plappert T, Saltzman DH, Cartire M, Zollars L, Leatherman GF, St John Sutton MG: Changes in intracardiac blood flow velocities and right and left ventricular stroke volumes with gestational age in the normal human fetus: a prospective Doppler echocardiographic study. Circulation 74:1208–1216, 1986.

41. Machado MVL, Chita SC, Allan LD: Acceleration time in the aorta and pulmonary artery measured by Doppler echocardiography in the midtrimester normal human fetus. Br Heart J 58:15–18, 1987.

42. De Smedt MCH, Visser GHA, Meijboom EJ: Fetal cardiac output estimated by Doppler echocardiography during mid- and late gestation. Am J Cardiol 60:338–342, 1987.

43. Reed KL, Anderson CF, Shenker L: Changes in intracardiac Doppler blood flow velocities in fetuses with absent umbilical artery diastolic flow. Am J Obstet Gynecol 157:774–779, 1987.

44. Groenenberg IAL, Wladimiroff JW, Hop WCJ: Fetal cardiac and peripheral arterial flow velocity waveforms in intrauterine growth retardation. Circulation 80:1711–1717, 1989.

45. Rizzo G, Arduini D: Fetal cardiac function in intrauterine growth retardation. Am J Obstet Gynecol 165:876–882, 1991.

46. Rizzo G, Arduini D, Romanini C, Mancuso S: Doppler echocardiographic evaluation of time to peak velocity in the aorta and pulmonary artery of small for gestational age fetuses. Br J Obstet Gynaecol 97:603–607, 1990.

47. Al-Ghazali W, Chita SK, Chapman MG, Allan LD: Evidence of redistribution of cardiac output in asymmetrical growth retardation. Br J Obstet Gynaecol 96:697–704, 1989.

48. Reed KL, Appleton CP, Anderson CF, Shenker L, Sahn DJ: Doppler studies of vena cava flows

in human fetuses—insights into normal and abnormal cardiac physiology. Circulation 81:498–505, 1990.

49. Rizzo G, Arduini D, Romanini C: Inferior vena cava velocities in appropriate and small for gestational age fetuses. Am J Obstet Gynecol 166:1992 (in press).

50. Indick JH, Reed KL: Umbilical venous pulsations are associated with inferior vena cava velocities. Am J Obstet Gynecol 164:330, 1991 [abstract].

51. Chambers SE, Hoskins RS, Haddad NG, Johnstone FD, McDicken WN, Muir BB: A comparison of fetal abdominal circumference measurements and Doppler ultrasound in the prediction of small for dates babies and growth retarded pregnacies. Br J Obstet Gynaecol 96:803–808, 1989.

52. Jacobson SL, Imhof R, Manning N, Mannion V, Little D, Rey E, Redman C: The value of Doppler assessment of the uteroplacental circulation in predicting preeclampsia and intrauterine growth retardation. Am J Obstet Gynecol 162:110–114, 1990.

53. Newnham JP, Patterson LL, James RJ, Diepeveen DA, Reid SE: An evaluation of the efficacy of Doppler flow velocity waveforms analysis as a screening test in pregnancy. Am J Obstet Gynecol 162:403–410, 1990.

54. Fleisher A, Schulman H, Farmakides G, Bracero L, Blatnner P, Randolph G: Umbilical artery velocity waveforms and intrauterine growth retardation. Am J Obstet Gynecol 151:502–505, 1985.

55. Giles WB, Lingman G, Marsal K, Trudinger BJ: Fetal volume blood flow and umbilical artery velocity waveforms analysis: a comparison. Br J Obstet Gynaecol 93:461–465, 1986.

56. Arduini D, Rizzo G, Romanini C, Mancuso S: Fetal blood flow velocity waveforms as predictors of growth retardation. Obstet Gynecol 70:7–10, 1987.

57. Divon MY, Guidetti DA, Braverman JJ, Oberlander E, Langer O, Merkatz IR: Intrauterine growth retardation—a prospective study of the diagnostic value of real time sonography combined with umbilical artery flow velocimetry. Obstet Gynecol 72:611–614, 1988.

58. Dempster J, Mires GJ, Patel N, Taylor DJ: Umbilical artery velocity waveforms: poor association with small for gestational age fetuses. Br J Obstet Gynaecol 96:692–696, 1989.

59. Beattie RB, Dornan JC: Antenatal screening for intrauterine growth retardation with umbilical artery velocimetry. Br Med J 298:631–635, 1989.

60. Sijmons EA, Reuwer PJ, van Beek E, Bruinse HW: The validity of screening for small for gestational age and low weight for length infants by Doppler ultrasound. Br J Obstet Gynaecol 96:557–561, 1989.

61. Arduini D, Rizzo G: Differential diagnosis of small for gestational age fetuses by Doppler ultrasound. Fetal Ther 3:31–36, 1988.

62. Malcus P, van Beek E, Marsal K: Umbilical artery velocimetry and nonstress test in monitoring high-risk pregnancies. A comparative longitudinal study. Ultrasound Obstet Gynecol 1:95–99, 1991.

63. Trudinger BJ, Cook CM, Jones L, Giles WB: A comparison of fetal heart rate monitoring and umbilical artery waveforms in the recognition of fetal compromise. Br J Obstet Gynaecol 93:171–175, 1986.

64. Arduini D, Rizzo G, Romanini C: Prediction of fetal outcome in small for gestational age fetuses: comparison of Doppler measurements obtained from different fetal vessels. J Perinat Med 1992 (in press).

65. Visser GHA: Abnormal antepartum fetal heart rate patterns and susequent handicap. Bailliere's Clin Obstet Gynecol 2:117–139, 1988.

66. Nicolaides KH, Bilardo CM, Soothill PW, Campbell S: Absence of end diastolic frequencies in umbilical artery: a sign of fetal hypoxia and acidosis. Br Med J 297:1026–1027, 1988.

67. Arduini D, Rizzo G, Romanini C, Mancuso S: Short term effects of maternal oxygen administration on blood flow velocity waveforms in healthy and growth retarded fetuses. Am J Obstet Gynecol 159:1077–1080, 1988.

68. Arduini D, Rizzo G, Romanini C, Mancuso S: Fetal haemodynamic response to acute maternal oxygen as predictor of fetal distress in intrauterine growth retardation. Br Med J 298:1561–1562, 1989.

DOPPLER EVALUATION OF FETAL ANOMALIES

JACQUES ABRAMOWICZ
RICHARD JAFFE

Prenatal diagnosis has evolved in the last 30 years from a single-disease orientation (Rh isoimmunization) to a complex branch of medicine that includes all the latest advances in laboratory, optical, and computer technology for detection and often therapy of a multitude of fetal diseases. New technologies are constantly being developed or ameliorated, and many are useful for the assessment of the health status of the normal as well as the potentially abnormal fetus.

Doppler ultrasound is such a technology, and it has been used in obstetrics since the late 1970s. Color flow mapping is one of the latest developments of Doppler ultrasound, and its value in perinatal medicine is only burgeoning. Its most common application is for fetal cardiac evaluation (see Chap. 8).

Changes in umbilical arterial blood flow waveforms have been described in congenital anomalies.[1–7] Specific fetal abnormalities and the possible contribution of Doppler ultrasound have not been extensively addressed.

The present chapter presents a review of fetal anomalies that can benefit from the use of spectral and color Doppler, as well as some possible, but yet unpublished (as far as the authors are aware), applications of this technique.

CRANIAL-INTRACRANIAL ANOMALIES

Vein of Galen Aneurysm

The great cerebral vein (of Galen) starts by union of the two internal cerebral veins which drain deep parts of the hemispheres. It runs within the subarachnoid space to empty into the straight sinus, or more rarely, joins the inferior sagittal sinus in the posterior part of the free margin of the falx cerebri. Aneurysm of the vein of Galen is a rare vascular malformation formed by direct arterial fistula or adjacent arterial-venous malformation with enhanced flow through the vein of Galen which causes aneurysmal dilatation of a portion of the vein, contiguous with a dilated straight sinus and tortula and fed directly by anomalous branches of the carotid and/or basilar circulation.[8,9] It is often associated with other CNS anomalies such as hydrocephalus as well as polyhydramnios, nonimmune hydrops (NIH), and cardiomegaly.[10–13] Two-dimensional ultrasound is the noninvasive method of choice for diagnosis in neonates.[14,15] Prenatal diagnosis has been reported by ultrasound alone or ultrasound and elevated maternal serum alpha-fetoprotein.[16–20] The aneurysm demonstrates high and turbulent flow with Doppler in neonates[21,22] or in utero (Figs. 12-1 and 12-2).[10,23,24]

Frequent changes in flow patterns of the carotid arteries, jugular veins, and/or cerebral arteries have been demonstrated.[21,24,25] Color Doppler has been described as an adjunct in the diagnosis in newborns.[11,26–29] The method has also

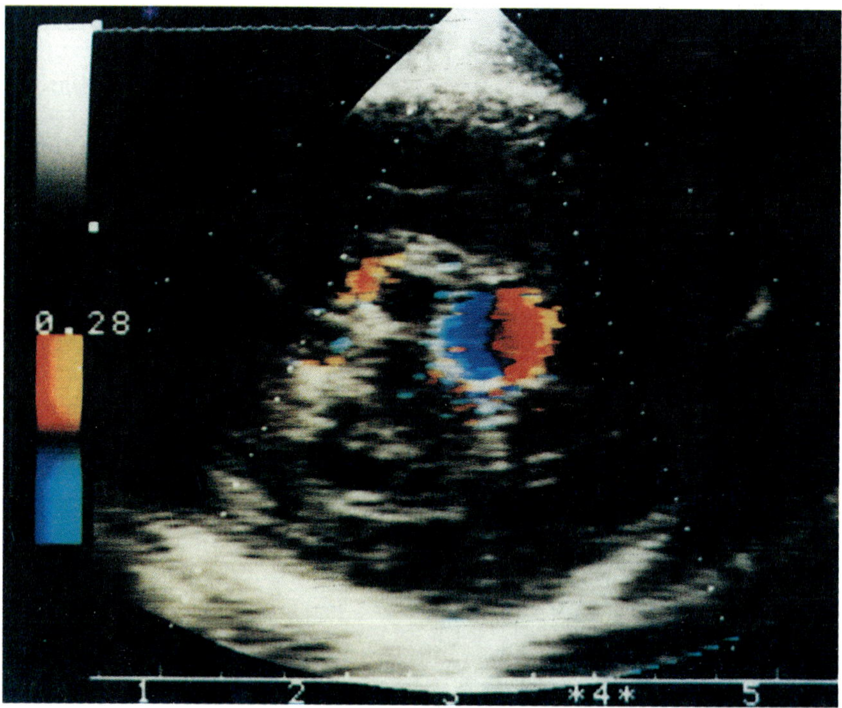

Figure 12-1 Arteriovenous malformation of the vein of Galen diagnosed by Doppler color flow mapping at 35 weeks of gestation. *(Reprinted with permission from Hata T, Hata K, Senoh D, Aoki S, Takamiya O, Yamamoto K, Kitao M: Antenatal Doppler color flow mapping of arteriovenous malformation of the vein of Galen. J Cardiovasc Ultrasonography 7:301–303, 1988.)*

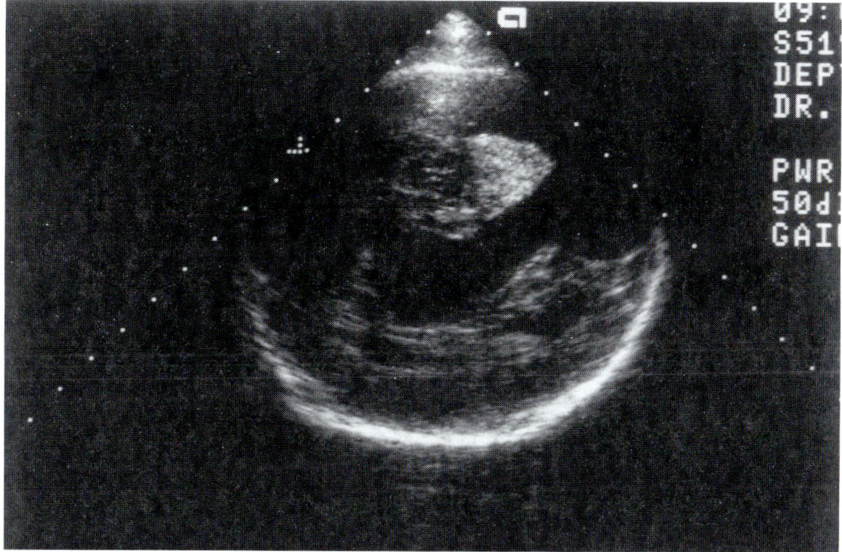

A

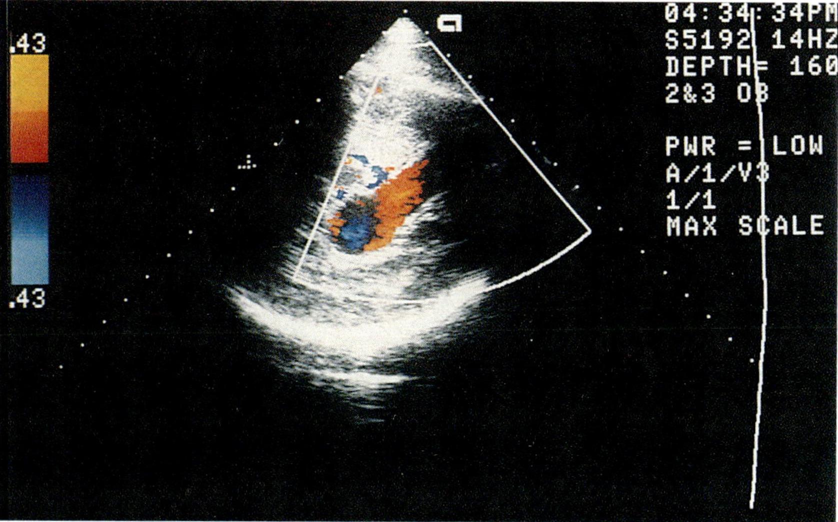

B

Figure 12-2 *A.* Vein of Galen aneurysm in a 37-week gestation. *B.* Color Doppler imaging demonstrating a vein of Galen aneurysm.

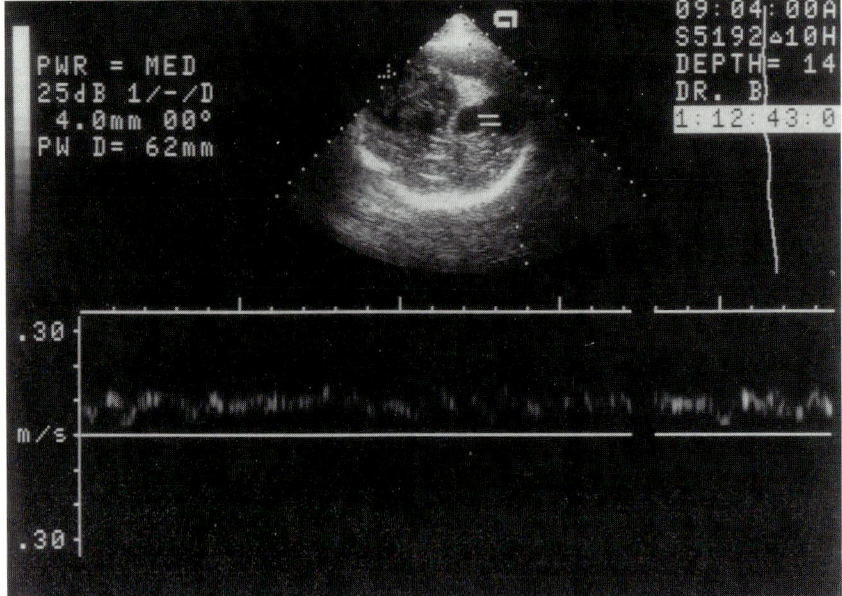

C

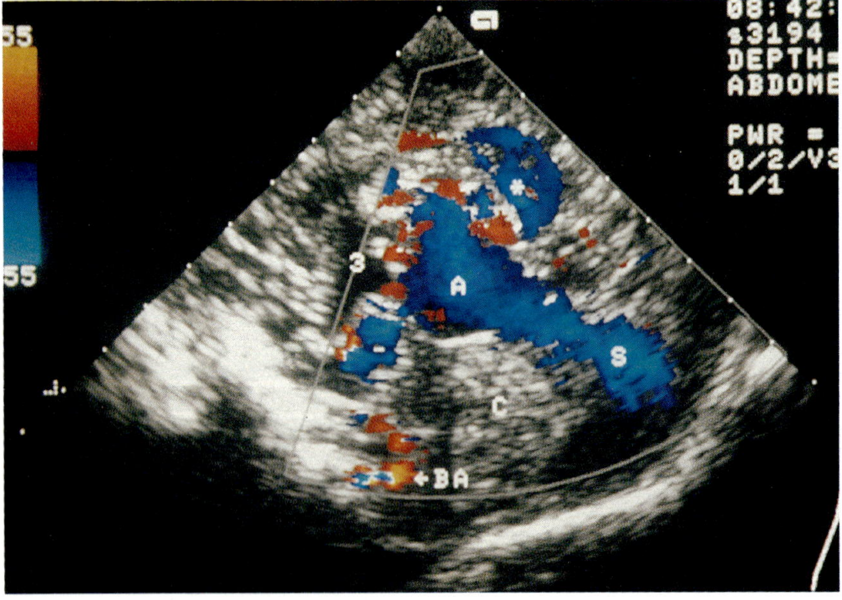

D

Figure 12-2 (*Continued*)   *C.* Spectral Doppler demonstrating flow within the vein of Galen aneurysm. (*Courtesy of Dr. Christine H. Comstock, Royal Oak, Michigan.*) *D.* Sagittal scan through the brain midline. The arteriovenous malformation (A) is clearly seen in the middle, with blood flow away from the transducer. The draining straight sinus (S) is also enlarged. 3 = third ventricle; C = cerebellum; BA = Basilar artery.

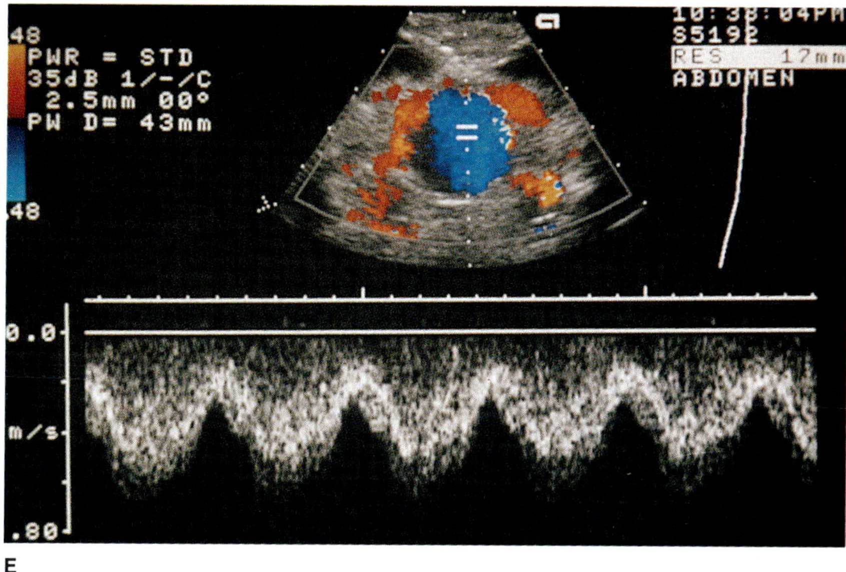

E

Figure 12-2 (*Continued*) *E.* Pulsed Doppler recording obtained from the arteriovenous malformation of the vein of Galen. The spectral waveform demonstrates increased arterial flow within the malformation. (*D* and *E* courtesy of Dr. Deeg, Pediatric Hopsital of Bamberg, Germany.)

been used in fetuses with the anomaly.[29,30] Color Doppler permits precise localization of blood vessels for exact delineation of cerebral anatomy and studies of flow patterns in suspect cases.

Abnormalities of the Circle of Willis

These have long been known to exist, but are rare.[8,31] Assessment of the circle of Willis in cases at risk of recurrence would be possible with color Doppler as has been demonstrated in neonates[32–34] and in normal pregnancies (Fig. 12-3).[35,36]

Intracranial Cysts

Several cystic conditions can affect the fetal brain: *unilateral hydrocephalus, unilateral schizencephaly, porencephalic cyst, arachnoid cyst, choroid plexus cyst, Dandy-Walker cyst, dorsal cyst of holoprosencephaly, agenesis of the corpus callosum, cystic neoplasms,* and *aneurysm of the vein of Galen*. Color Doppler may help in the delineation of these structures and the demonstration of presence (aneurysm) or absence (true cyst) of blood flow.

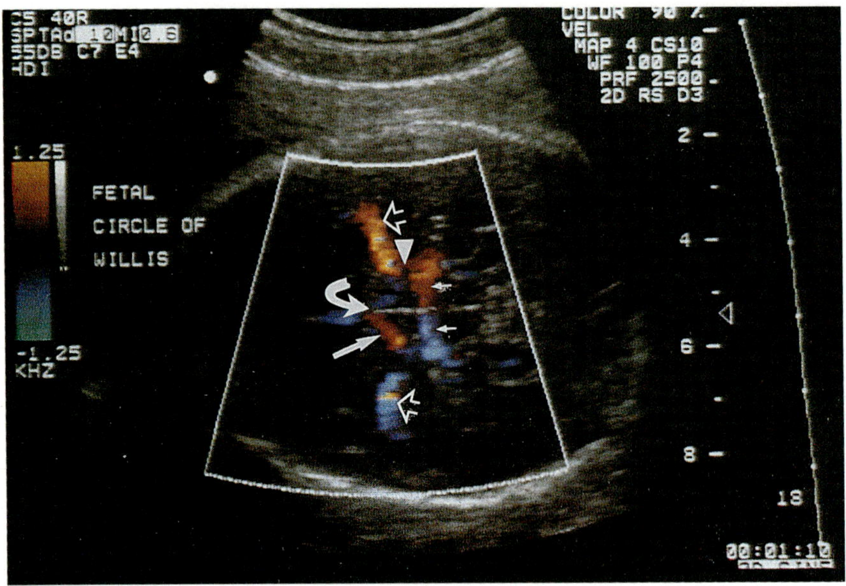

Figure 12-3 Circle of Willis in the normal fetus. The circle of Willis is formed anteriorly by parts of the anterior cerebral arteries (*large arrow*), of the internal carotid arteries that run in the horizontal plane, and of their interconnection with the anterior communicating arteries (*curved arrow*). Laterally and posteriorly, the circle is formed by connections between the posterior communicating branches (*arrowhead*) of the internal carotid arteries and the posterior cerebral branches (*small arrow*) of the basilar artery. Middle cerebral arteries (unfilled arrow heads) are also visualized. (*Courtesy of ATL, Bothel, Washington.*)

Hydrocephaly

It is beyond the scope of this chapter to go into details regarding the etiology, pathogenesis, diagnosis, and course of hydrocephaly. The reader is referred to many previously published articles.[37–41] Normal blood flow waveforms in the fetal cerebral vessels have recently been depicted[42–47] (see also Chap. 9). In neonates, correlation between hydrocephaly and changes in cerebral blood flow (elevation in resistance index) has been demonstrated.[48,49] Other authors have failed to show such changes.[32,50] In 13 fetuses with hydrocephaly (nine bilateral and four unilateral), five had elevated pulsatility index, suggesting increased resistance to cerebral blood flow. In unilateral hydrocephaly, a marked difference existed between the affected and nonaffected sides.[51] It is assumed that raised velocimetry indices are a reflection of increased resistance to cerebral blood flow and that normal blood flow would mean lower intracranial pressure and, therefore, better prognosis. But no large, definitive body of data is available at the time of this writing.

FACE AND NECK

Facial Clefting

Cleft lip and/or palate are the most common congenital facial malformations (1 per 800 to 1000 live births). Numerous syndromes have been associated with this anomaly.[52] In a large study, 63.4 percent of infants with cleft lip and/or palate had other congenital malformations.[53] The prenatal diagnosis is well established,[54,55] but shadowing, umbilical cord superimposition, or normal upper lip structures (philtrum and frenulum) may mimic the anomaly.[56] Color flow imaging of amniotic fluid movement in and out of the mouth might help to delineate the anatomy and visualize the defect, if present, but to our knowledge, this has not yet been documented.

Cystic Hygroma and Other Neck Masses

The differential diagnosis of a neck mass includes *cystic hygroma, occipital cephalocele, meningomyelocele, hemangioma, goiter, branchial cleft cyst, thyroglossal duct cyst,* and *various tumors (sarcoma, melanoma, metastatic adenopathy).*[57] Cystic hygroma is the most common cause of prenatally diagnosed neck mass. It is a benign developmental lymphangioma which arises from congenital blockage of lymphatic drainage. The in utero diagnosis is well documented.[58–61] The natural history has also been addressed.[62,63] All masses except the hemangioma will demonstrate lack of flow with Doppler. Arterial pulsations can be demonstrated in hemangiomas, and prenatal diagnosis has thus been confirmed by definition of the vascular nature of the tumor.[64–66]

Persistent Choroidal Artery

The choroidal artery is a small vessel in the eye. It originates from the main ophthalmic artery and in humans has been shown to regress in the early third trimester by 25 weeks gestational age.[67] Its persistence has been associated with fetal anomalies, particularly trisomies and CNS abnormalities.[68] Its visualization being difficult, color Doppler may help in its localization, but this has not been reported till now.

SPINE

Although spina bifida is much more common, sacrococcygeal teratoma is the only "spine" malformation that may benefit from color Doppler analysis. The teratoma is a germ cell tumor originating from embryonic multipotential cells that migrate to the sacrum-coccyx area. It always arises from the coccyx. The

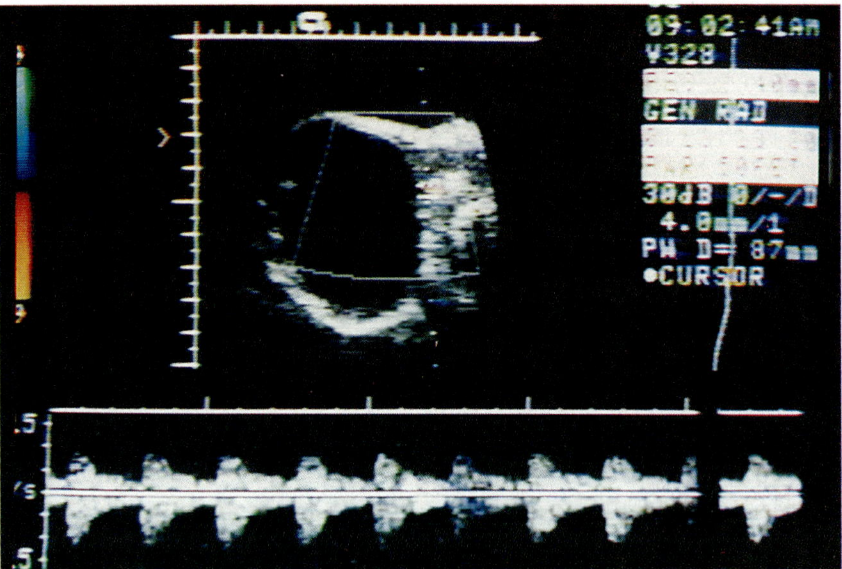

Figure 12-4 Sacrococcygeal teratoma. Color Doppler permits visualization of blood flow in tumor stalk for demonstration of arterial flow.

differential diagnosis includes myelomeningocele and other tumors.[69] Its prenatal diagnosis is well documented.[70–74] These tumors are highly vascular,[75,76] with the main source of blood alimentation originating from three sources: the *middle sacral, hypogastric (lateral sacral, gluteal, pelvic floor arteries),* or *femoral arteries.*[76] Because of the major vascular component, these tumors lend themselves to Doppler analysis. Color Doppler can be used to demonstrate arterial flow in the stalk or inside the tumor (Fig. 12-4).

Flow has been demonstrated to be pulsatile within the tumor.[77,78] Because of the large arteriovenous shunting fistula that the tumor represents, a very common complication is polyhydramnios,[79,80] hyperplacentosis,[81–83] and/or congestive heart failure.[77–79,84–86] In fact, in utero resection of the tumor has been followed by reversal of the associated hydrops.[87] Doppler ultrasound (including color-coded Doppler) is certainly of vital importance in the evaluation of cardiac function in these fetuses.

THORAX

Heart

This is addressed in detail in Chap. 8.

Other Organs

Color Doppler may help delineate the fetal aorta and other vessels to study their course and blood flow in cases of intrathoracic tumors possibly displacing surrounding anatomy, particularly cystic adenomatoid malformation of the lung, bronchogenic cyst, diaphragmatic hernia, or pericardial teratoma[88] (Fig. 12-5). In bronchopulmonary sequestration, Doppler may help in identifying the abnormal vessel arising from the descending aorta and supplying the separated portion of bronchopulmonary mass (Fig. 12-6). Anomalous pulmonary pathways have also recently been described.[89] Characterization of a chest-wall tumor by Doppler ultrasound has been reported.[90]

Diaphragmatic Hernia

Diaphragmatic hernias result from failure of fusion of the diaphragm leaves originating from the pleuroperitoneal canal and, therefore, result in communication between the thoracic and abdominal cavities. This occurs around 8 to 12 weeks gestation, by the time the intestines return to the abdomen.[91] Displacement of normally intraabdominal organs into the chest cavity ensues. Ninety percent of congenital diaphragmatic hernias are known as *Bochdalek's hernia*, and 75 percent of these are on the left side, resulting in stomach and small bowel ascending into the chest. Mediastinal structures are, therefore, displaced to the right. Right-

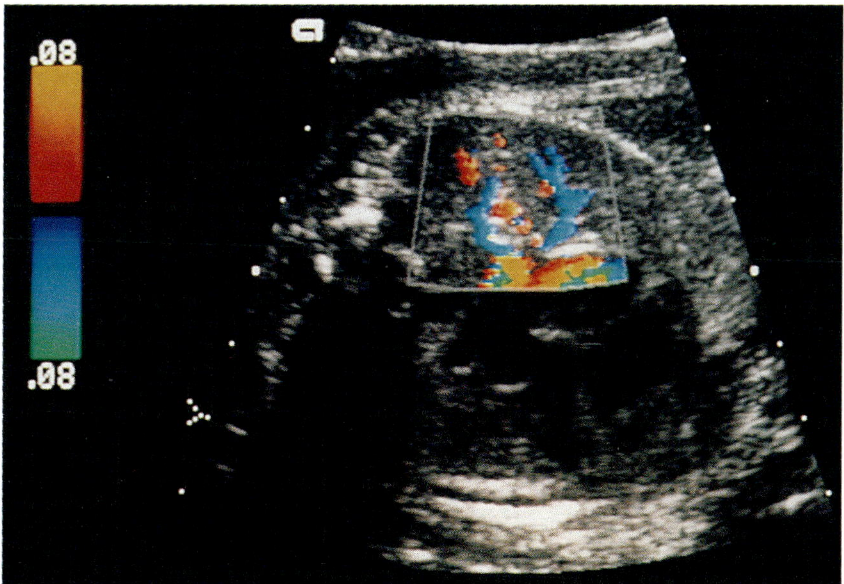

Figure 12-5   A color Doppler image demonstrating the fetal lung perfusion with the pulmonary veins entering the left atrium (blue). *(Courtesy of Acuson, Mountain View, California.)*

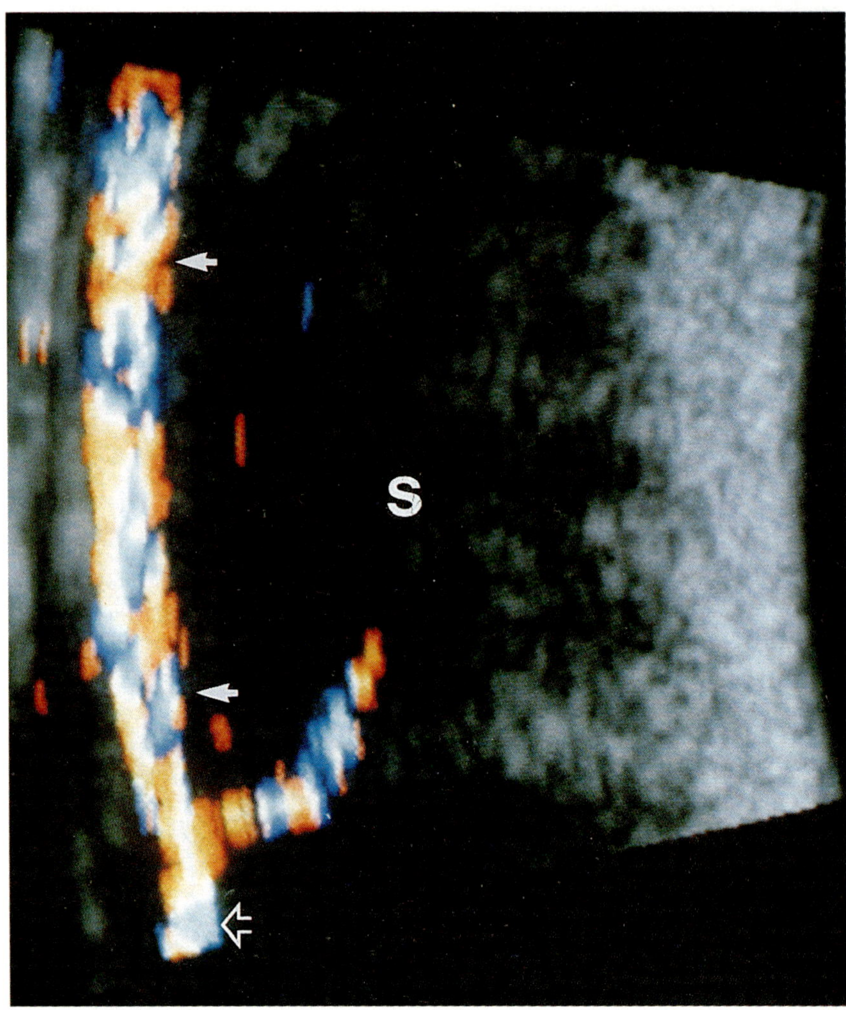

Figure 12-6 Left coronal color Doppler sonogram reveals a feeding artery through unaerated sequestration (S) arising from the left lateral aspect of the aorta, just below the diaphragm. *Solid arrow* = thoracic aorta; *open arrow* = abdominal aorta. *(Printed with permission from Hernanz-Schulman M, Stein SM, Neblett WW, Atkinson JB, Kirchner SG, Heller RM, Merrill WH, Fleischer AC. Pulmonary sequestration: diagnosis with color Doppler sonography and a new theory of associated hydrothorax. Radiology 180:817–821, 1991.)*

sided hernias are less common and, if small, are of no immediate consequence, the liver usually splinting the defect. However, with larger defects, herniation of the liver, gallbladder, or spleen can occur. This may cause major shifting of intrathoracic structures to the left.[92] *Morgagni's* (or *parasternal*) hernia is the second most common type, the liver being the usual abdominal organ involved.

Two-dimensional ultrasound is the technique of choice for prenatal diagnosis of these anomalies.[92–94] Other methods reported in the literature include amniography,[95–97] computed tomography,[98] and magnetic resonance.[99] Associated pulmonary hypoplasia is the most common cause of mortality,[100] but there may be others such as associated anomalies[101,102] and/or hemodynamic impairments.[103–105] Color Doppler will demonstrate pathways of large vessels and deviations, as well as possible increased resistance to flow, secondary to the local pressure of ''invading'' organs or generalized increased intrathoracic pressure. The liver may be difficult to differentiate from the lungs by conventional ultrasound, but the addition of color may help in definition of the organ by its vascularity or sonoelasticity. Sonoelasticity is an experimental method, allowing characterization by color-coded Doppler ultrasound of tissue from motion or mechanical response to external mechanical stimulation (Fig. 12-7).[106]

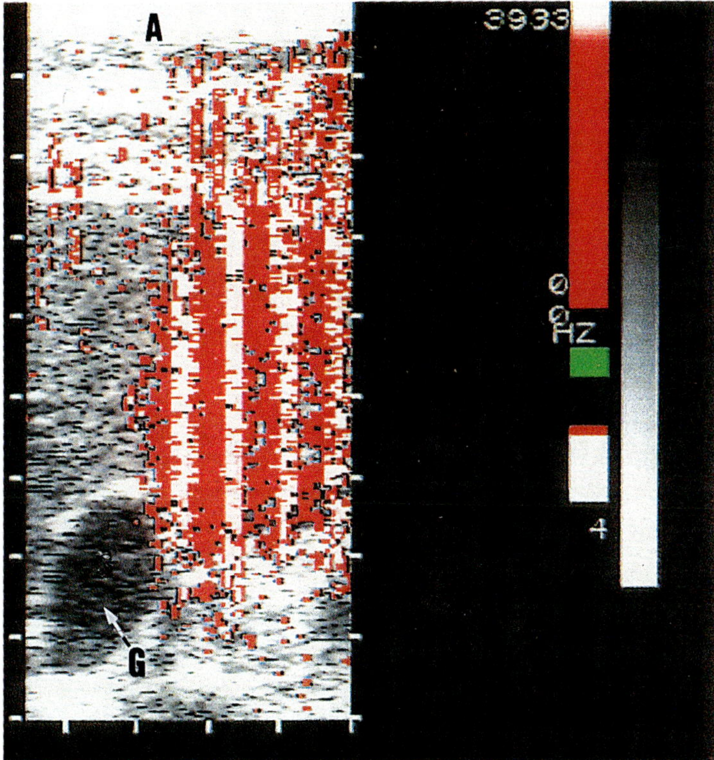

Figure 12-7   Sonoelasticity image of normal human adult liver. Abdominal wall at top (A); gallbladder on lower left (G). Vibration at 90 Hz produces a standing wave, or modal, pattern within the normal liver. Red and white overlay represent regions with vibration above 0.05 mm in displacement. Other regions depicted in conventional gray scale. *(Courtesy of Kevin J. Parker, Rochester Center for Biomedical Ultrasound, University of Rochester.)*

Vibrations at low frequencies (10 to 1000 Hz) are externally applied and induce oscillations within soft tissues. The resultant motion is detected and mapped by color Doppler. Different tissues have different periodic movements and, therefore, produce different sonoelasticity images. Deep tissues can be studied because the Doppler signal can detect very small motions.[107] This method has been applied to tumor detection and tissue differentiation in animals and, in some cases, in human diseases but, to our knowledge, not in obstetrics.

ABDOMEN

Liver

Hepatomegaly is a rarely reported prenatal diagnosis. Tumors are one of the causes of hepatomegaly that lend themselves to study by Doppler ultrasound, since most are highly vascular. Hemangioma, for instance, is essentially a cluster of capillaries.[108,109] So is a slightly different tumor, the *hemangioendothelioma*.[110,111] For both, antenatal diagnosis has been described.[112,113] Hepatoblastoma is the most common malignant hepatic tumor in infancy. It is also extremely vascular[110] and, therefore, can be studied by color Doppler. Cystic tumors such as the cavernous hemangioma and the mesenchymal hamartoma are similarly rare. Other liver tumors are the congenital neuroblastoma, metastatic tumors, and malignant hepatoblastoma, which are all solid and strongly echogenic tumors. Sonoelasticity may prove useful in cases of unexplained hepatomegaly, since normal liver tissue and tumors have been differentiated by this technique.[107]

Abdominal Wall Defects

Fetal abdominal wall defects occur in 1 per 2000 to 5000 live births. They include *omphalocele* and *gastroschisis,* which are the most common, and also *ectopia cordis, cloacal* and *bladder exstrophy,* and *limb-body wall complex* (body stalk anomaly).

Omphalocele is a midline defect resulting from failure of the embryonic abdominal folds to meet and form a normal umbilical ring. This causes failure of the intestines to become intraabdominal by not returning from their physiologic position in the umbilical cord at about 10 to 12 weeks. As a result, organs that are normally intraabdominal develop within the umbilical cord. Gastroschisis is a paraumbilical abdominal wall defect of not entirely explained origin, but anomalous involution of the right umbilical vein or disruption of the omphalomesenteric artery has been evoked. Intraabdominal contents herniate through this opening. More detailed descriptions of these defects, the differences in diagnostic features, and clinical significance can be found in numerous articles.[114–118] Differential diagnosis between omphalocele and gastroschisis is possible by ultrasound[119–122] and has also been described by magnetic resonance imaging.[123,124]

The second group of defects (ectopia cordis, cloacal exstrophy, and limb-body wall complex) is, as mentioned, much less common. They are due to abnormalities of embryonic body folding.[125] The prenatal diagnosis is documented.[126–129] Pentalogy of Cantrell is a combination of epigastric omphalocele, defective sternum, ventral diaphragmatic defect, anterior pericardial deficiency, and intrinsic cardiac disease, often ectopia cordis.[130]

Except for gastroschisis, two-thirds of cases of abdominal wall defects are associated with chromosomal (particularly trisomies 18, 13, and 21) or structural anomalies, mainly diaphragmatic hernia, neural tube defects, cleft lip and palate, gastrointestinal and/or genitourinary abnormalities, and congenital heart disease.[131]

Bladder exstrophy, although sometimes similar in appearance, has a different etiology: abnormal mesodermal migration into an area formed by appropriate embryonic body folding.[132,133] Color Doppler may allow following umbilical vessels into the fetal abdominal cavity and, thus, help in delineating the different entities in some unclear cases (Fig. 12-8).

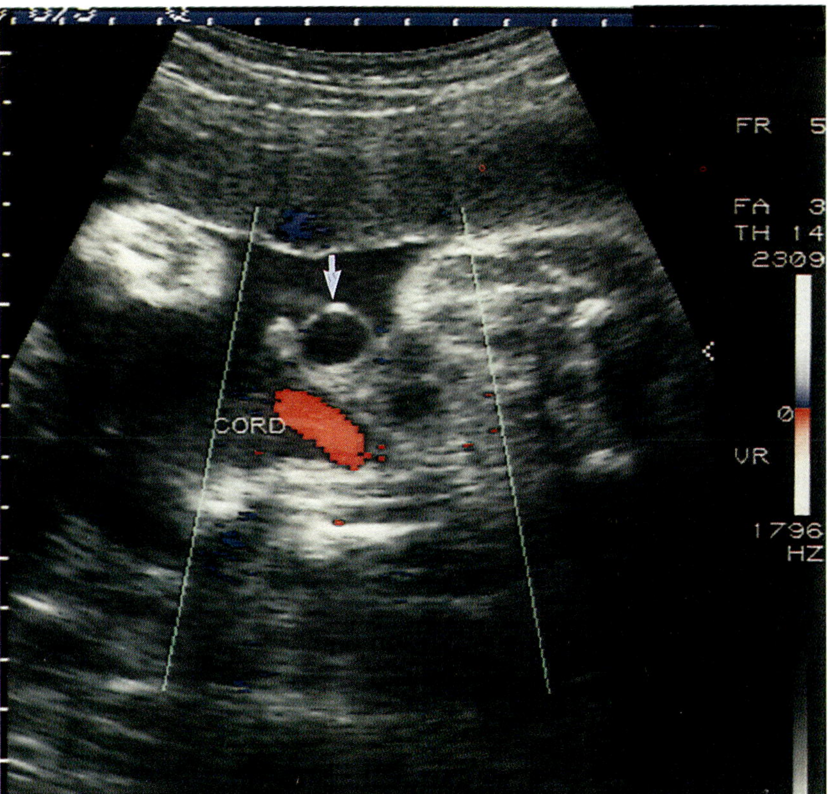

Figure 12-8 Color Doppler image demonstrating flow within the umbilical cord. Above the cord (*arrow*) are loops of small bowel with no flow detected.

The defect in omphalocele is at the site of insertion of the umbilical cord. Gastroschisis is paraumbilical, usually to the right. The defect is above the insertion of the cord in ectopia cordis and below in bladder and cloacal exstrophy. The prognosis for omphalocele has been described as depending on whether the liver is extraabdominal or not. Imaging of liver blood vessels with color Doppler may help in evaluating this issue. Doppler ultrasound has also been used to avoid confusing umbilical cord and extruded bowels.[118] Body stalk anomalies contain liver, but their location is usually lateral, and scoliosis and/or cranial and/or limb defects are present.

Others

Gastrointestinal anomalies could possibly be characterized by changes in patterns of blood alimentation as has been described in neonates.[134]

GENITOURINARY TRACT

Anomalies of the kidney and urinary tract are commonly diagnosed by ultrasound. In fact, 50 percent of ultrasound-diagnosed fetal malformations are urinary tract abnormalities.[135] These can be classified as follows:[136,137]

1. Renal agenesis or severe hypoplasia
2. Abnormal position of normal kidneys
3. Renal cystic disease (the four Potter dysplasias)
4. Renal tumors
5. Abnormal renal vasculature
6. Obstructive uropathy

Innumerable articles have been published on normal and abnormal anatomy of the fetal kidneys (we were able to uncover 413 in the last 8 years), and most of the anomalies have been diagnosed in utero.[134,138–144] Color Doppler may help in demonstrating several of these anomalies.

The diagnosis of renal agenesis, or Potter's syndrome,[145] may sometimes be relatively easy: severe oligohydramnios after 18 to 20 weeks, fetal crowding, and, naturally, absence of bladder or kidneys.[146,147] However, late in pregnancy, severe IUGR may be accompanied by some of the above-mentioned findings, such as reduced amniotic fluid, rendering identification of the kidneys extremely difficult. Adrenal hyperplasia can cause some confusion and, in the absence of kidneys, the bladder may still contain some fluid as the result of transudation and not urine production. In a study of 22 fetuses suspected of having bilateral renal malformation on the basis of oligohydramnios, the pulsatility index (PI) of the umbilical artery and the fetal aorta were measured. In cases of renal malformations, both umbilical artery and fetal aorta demonstrated normal PI.

However, when the oligohydramnios was due to severe IUGR, the PI of both vessels had abnormal values.[148] A more direct method is trying to visualize renal vessels. The renal arteries have recently been demonstrated by color Doppler ultrasound[149,150] with normal values for the different velocimetric indices (Fig. 12-9).

Color Doppler will demonstrate absence of vessels and blood flow in renal agenesis. By the same token, Doppler can allow visualization and characterization of blood flow in cases of displaced or misplaced kidneys (Fig. 12-10).

Renal tumors (mesoblastic nephroma, Wilms' tumor) are rare in fetuses, but aberrant blood flow should be demonstrated in fetal kidneys when such a tumor is present. The same holds true for vascular anomalies. Renal artery PI has been shown to be higher than normal in fetuses with intrauterine growth retardation (IUGR), possibly reflecting decreased renal perfusion.[151,152] Recently, color Doppler was used to define renal arteries in a case of Meckel's syndrome.[153]

EXTREMITIES

The list of abnormalities of fetal extremities is very extensive. It can be grossly separated into three categories: *anomalies of length, development,* and *postural deformities.*[154–156] Since large blood vessels are present in the limbs (brachial, radial, femoral, popliteal), color Doppler can be employed to demonstrate blood

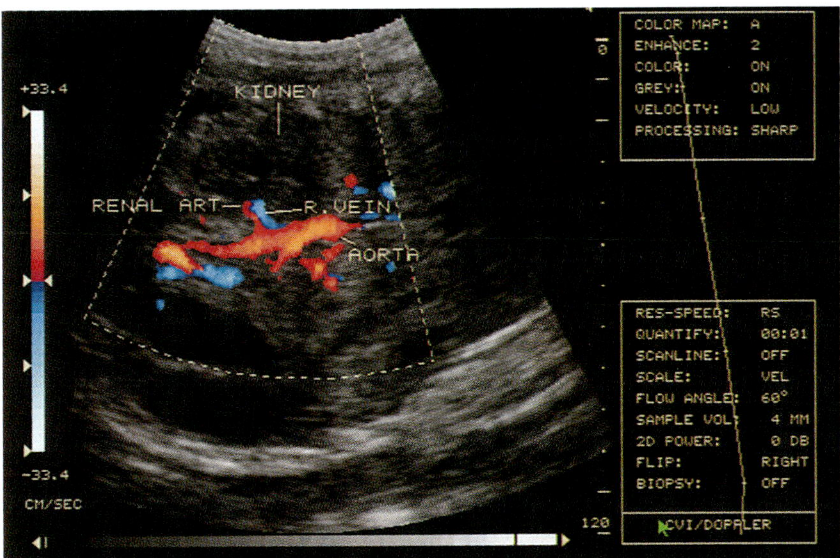

Figure 12-9 Color flow image of the lower abdomen of a 32-week-old fetus. The aorta and renal vasculature are clearly demonstrated.

flow (Fig. 12-11). This has previously been briefly addressed.[157] Anomalies of development or posture might demonstrate abnormal flow patterns. Diminution of flow may also be present in IUGR with shunting of fetal blood to vital organs at the expense of reduced flow to less important parts of the body as well as reduction in limb movements.

NONIMMUNE HYDROPS

Nonimmune hydrops (NIH) represents 90 percent of cases of fetal hydrops.[158] The etiology of NIH is extremely diverse and multiple.[158–161] A clear etiology can be exposed in more than 80 percent of cases.[162] Certain factors, because of obvious hemodynamic involvement, will lead to Doppler changes. In a recent study, 18 pregnancies with NIH were examined.[163] Cardiac or noncardiac origin for the NIH could be differentiated by looking at changes of flow pattern in the umbilical vein: venous pulsations were present only in congestive heart failure, while normal fetuses or fetuses with infectious etiology for the NIH had nonpulsatile patterns.

Doppler velocimetry needs to be implemented as a major tool in the diagnostic evaluation of a fetus with NIH. Among the most common disorders associated with NIH are congenital heart diseases[164,165] and cardiac arrhythmias.[166,167] Con-

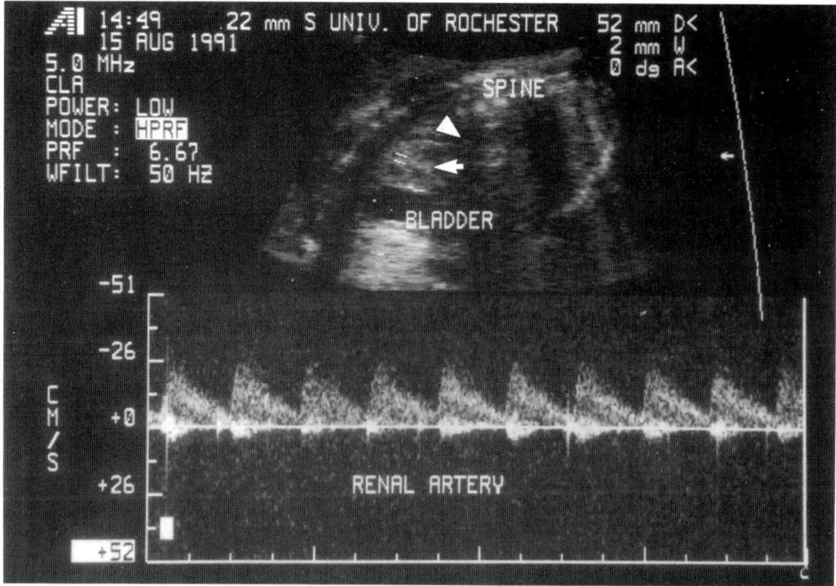

Figure 12-10 Blood flow waveform in renal artery in ectopic kidney. The pelvic kidney (*arrow*) is at the bifurcation of the aorta (*arrowhead*). The other kidney (not pictured) is in its normal location. The fetal spine and bladder are visualized as well.

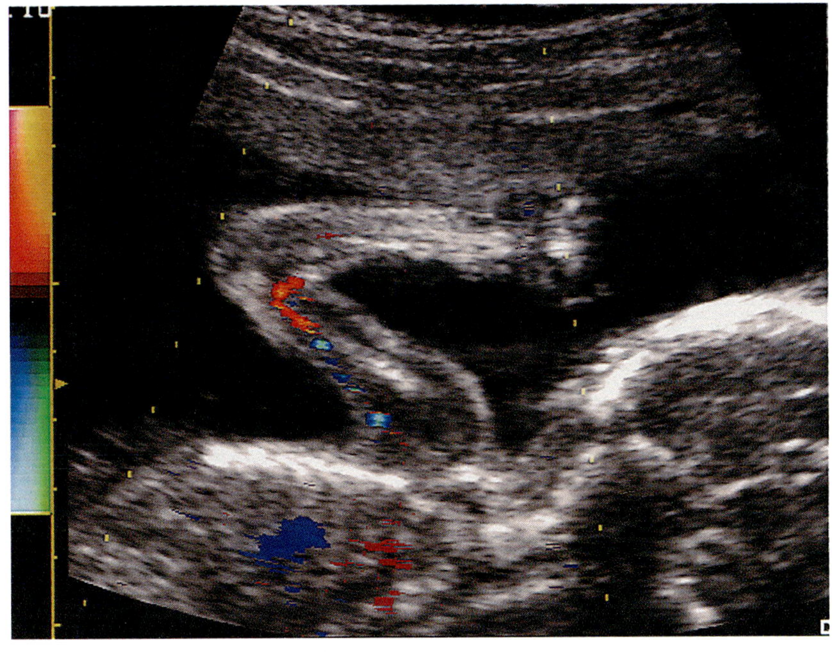

A

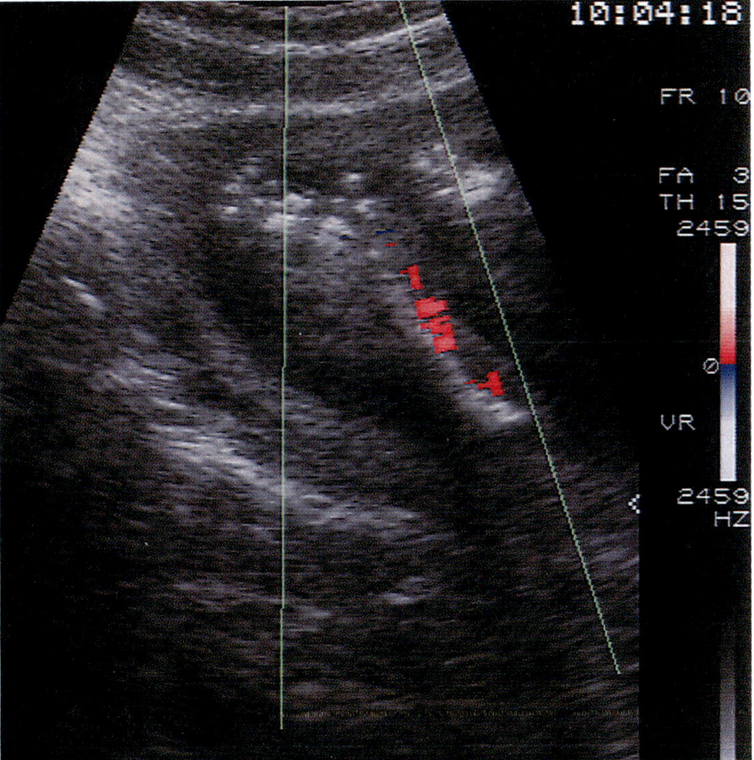

B

Figure 12-11 *A*. Color Doppler image demonstrating flow in the brachial artery. *B*. Radial artery flow in a 29-week-old fetus.

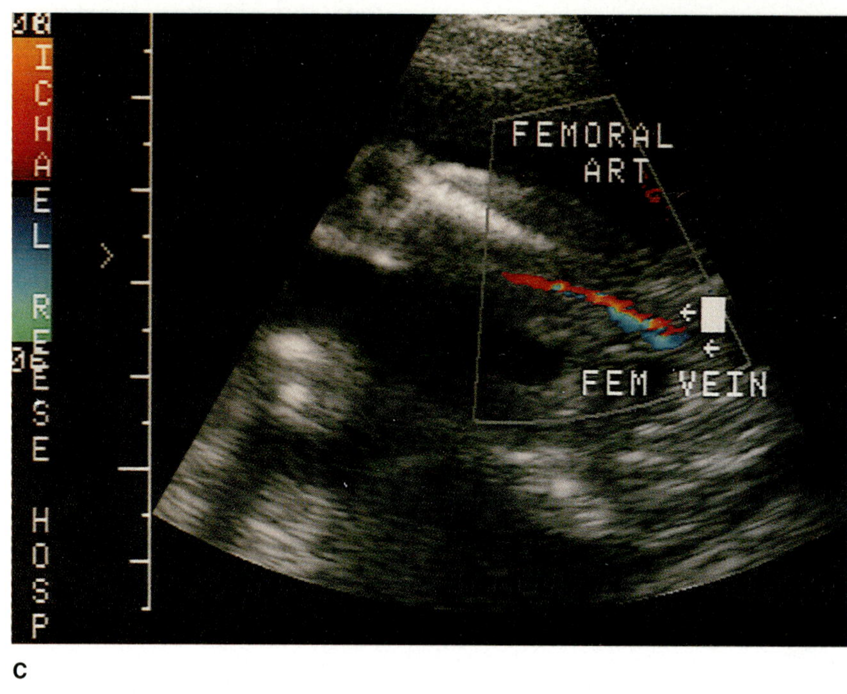

C

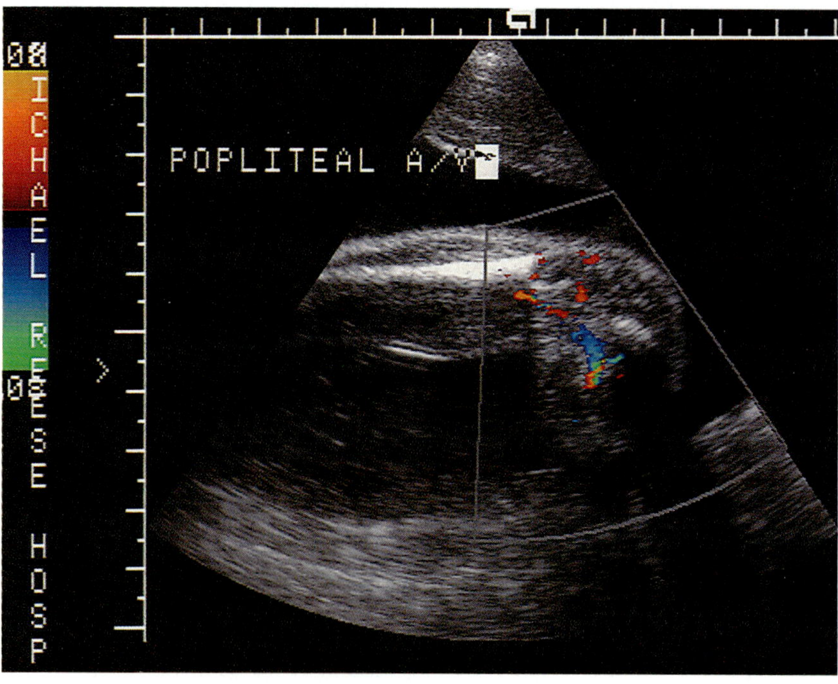

D

Figure 12-11 (*Continued*) *C* and *D*. Flow demonstrated in the femoral vessels as well as in the popliteal artery.

genital heart diseases were the main etiology in 40 percent of a group of 52 fetuses with NIH.[165] In another large study, involving 402 cases of prenatally diagnosed hydrops fetalis, cardiovascular disease was present in almost 20 percent.[168] Color Doppler is vital for the investigation of this type of derangement (Chap. 8).

Other etiologies such as vein of Galen aneurysm (with large arteriovenous shunting), renal anomalies, cystic hygroma, sacrococcygeal teratoma, and placental-umbilical cord anomalies, which may cause severe arteriovenous shunting as well, may benefit from Doppler examination as shown above. In a study of fetuses dying with congenital anomalies, four with NIH had absent diastolic flow in the umbilical artery.[169]

ANOMALIES OF MATERNAL SERUM ALPHA-FETOPROTEIN

Maternal serum alpha-fetoprotein (MSAFP) is a major protein in fetal serum with a peak level at 13 to 14 weeks. Its concentration slowly decreases thereafter. It crosses the placenta as well as amniotic fluid and, thus, reaches the maternal circulation, where it can be measured. Normal values for MSAFP have been established, and both higher and lower than normal values have been associated with certain fetal anomalies or complications of pregnancy.[170,171] Elevated levels have been found in numerous maternal-fetal conditions, the most common being open neural tube defects, abdominal wall defects, renal anomalies, gastrointestinal obstruction, and placental abnormalities.[172,173] Reduced levels were first demonstrated to be associated with chromosomal abnormalities by Merkatz et al.[174]

Several protocols have been described to follow up the findings of either elevated or reduced levels of MSAFP. They all include two-dimensional ultrasound.[175–177] Doppler ultrasound probably has a role to play by the changes occurring in the velocimetry of umbilical artery in several anomalies or chromosomal disorders. Another potential role is in the prediction by uterine artery Doppler screening of maternal complications known to be associated with elevated MSAFP in the absence of fetal disorders.[178] Also, as shown above, color-coded Doppler may assume a growing role in the definition of numerous structural anomalies.

Certainly, the finding of an elevated MSAFP with no obvious fetal anomalies requires extensive evaluation of the placenta.[179] In this evaluation, Doppler, in general, and color Doppler, in particular, play a very important role (Chap. 7).

CHROMOSOMAL ANOMALIES

Only karyotyping permits the definite diagnosis of chromosomal anomalies. In pregnancy, this will be performed after obtaining fetal cells by amniocentesis, chorionic villus sampling, placental biopsy, cordocentesis, or fetal biopsy. The role of ultrasound in the investigation of chromosomal anomalies is at two levels. Fetal chromosomal anomalies are known to be common in certain structural abnormalities such as cardiovascular malformations in 99 percent of fetuses with trisomy 13, cystic hygroma in fetuses with 45,X karyotype (Turner's syndrome), and duodenal atresia in Down's syndrome, to cite only a few. Recently, ultrasonographic signs reported to be associated with chromosomal anomalies have been described. These consist, in particular, of a shortened femur and nuchal thickness with a sensitivity of 75 percent and a specificity of 98 percent in detecting Down's syndrome in one study[180] and slightly smaller but similar indices in a second one.[181] Not all scientists agree that pathognomonic ultrasonographic signs exist in fetal chromosomal anomalies.[182] The findings of certain fetal anomalies on ultrasound should prompt further investigation of possible chromosomal derangements.[183–186]

Umbilical artery Doppler velocimetry may also have a role in the evaluation of chromosomal defects. Several authors have reported abnormal umbilical artery velocimetry in fetuses with chromosomal anomalies.[1,3,4,7,187–194] Table 12-1 represents a summary of the findings of several studies together with our own (Abramowicz et al., unpublished data). Grouping all these together yields 85 percent of abnormal Doppler velocimetry in the umbilical artery of karyotypically

Table 12-1 Umbilical artery Doppler studies in fetuses with chromosomal anomalies

Authors	Doppler[a]	
	Normal	Abnormal
Abramowicz	4	6
Al-Gazali[187]	2	4
Baton[192]		7
Berkowitz[190]		2
Brar[193]		2
Copel[223]		3
Hata[153]		1
Hsieh[3]		4
McCowan[188]		1
Reed[189]		1
Rochelson[7]	2	14
Trudinger[1]	1	6
Total	9	51

[a] Different indices used by different authors.

abnormal fetuses. The explanation for this finding can be learned in some of the cases: if IUGR is present, one can evoke it as the etiological factor. However, some of the fetuses with abnormal karyotypes have normal growth parameters. Placentas of karyotypically abnormal fetuses between 18 and 23 weeks gestation were studied at both the light and scanning electron microscopic level.[195] Particular attention was paid to the microvascularization of the tertiary stem villi in the hope of explaining some of the puzzling aspects of the Doppler findings. Lower counts in small muscular arteries and total vessels were demonstrated in 14 placentas of fetuses with abnormal karyotypes as compared with normal controls ($p < 0.01$). In a similar study, a small group of fetuses with normal karyotyping, but with physical anomalies, demonstrated decreased vascularization (Kuhlman and Abramowicz, unpublished data). This undervascularization may explain higher impedance to flow and, therefore, reduced diastolic velocities. The same conclusions were reached in another study of placental vasculature in third trimester fetuses with abnormal karyotypes.[196] Evidently, if structural anomalies are present, they can be accompanied by abnormal umbilical artery velocimetry as demonstrated above. The same holds true for abnormal velocimetry in different vascular beds (cerebral, renal, etc.) according to the specific organs involved. Abnormal umbilical artery velocimetry in the absence of a clear etiology, such as IUGR, should certainly raise the suspicion of a fetal anomaly, either structural or chromosomal, particularly if accompanied by derangements of amniotic fluid volume.

ABNORMALITIES OF AMNIOTIC FLUID VOLUME

Deviations from normal in *amniotic fluid volume* (AFV) have been shown to often be associated with fetal pathology or with complications of pregnancy. This holds true for both excess accumulation (polyhydramnios)[197] and reduced volume (oligohydramnios).[198]

Since AFV after midpregnancy is mostly regulated by fetal swallowing and voiding,[199] anomalies in AFV have mostly been correlated to interference with these processes. Several "objective" criteria have been described, but an extensive analysis is beyond the scope of this chapter.[200,201]

Congenital anomalies associated with polyhydramnios are numerous.[197,202–204] They mainly involve (1) obstructions in the fetal gastrointestinal system, (2) face, head, and neck anomalies, possibly interfering with swallowing, (3) central nervous system defects, with neural impairment of the swallowing mechanism (though often with no clear reason), and (4) many other fetal anomalies with no obvious explanation as to how, or if, they are related to increased volume of fluid,[200] such as skeletal or renal disorders, as well as fetal hydrops.

A reduced amount of amniotic fluid is diagnosed with ultrasound when fetal crowding is demonstrated with obvious lack of fluid.[205] The main causes of oligohydramnios are rupture of membranes (the most common etiology), intrauterine growth retardation, postterm pregnancies, and fetal anomalies. Fetal anomalies resulting in oligohydramnios will be those causing a reduction in the amount of urine voided: bilateral renal agenesis, severe dysplasia with diminished function, or urinary tract obstruction. However, severe IUGR will also be accompanied by a reduction in glomerular function, thence, quantity of urine voided and, consequently, oligohydramnios.[205,206] Another explanation is increased fetal plasma vasopressin and catecholamines as a result of stress with ensuing antidiuresis.[207] If diagnosed in the second trimester, the prognosis is extremely poor.[208–211] The importance of Doppler ultrasound in investigating anomalies of amniotic fluid is at two levels: search for and characterization of fetal anomalies in both oligo- and polyhydramnios, and visualization of the umbilical cord in oligohydramnios. In a recently published study[212] among 54 fetuses with polyhydramnios, 11 were found to have abnormal waveforms and 6 of these 11 had chromosomal anomalies, two had NIH, one had multiple congenital anomalies, and one had gastric atresia. Among 43 fetuses with normal waveforms, all had normal karyotypes, one had a tracheal anomaly, and one had NIH. In oligohydramnios, because of fetal crowding, it may be difficult to obtain an adequate view of the umbilical cord for Doppler sampling. The addition of color permits rapid identification of the umbilical vessels which, otherwise, could not be interrogated by Doppler. Doppler velocimetry has also been used in oligohydramnios for prediction of perinatal outcome. Patients with normal umbilical artery Doppler in the context of oligohydramnios had normal perinatal outcome. Abnormal Doppler was associated with IUGR.[213] In another study, IUGR was accompanied by abnormal flow-velocity waveforms, but normal velocimetric indices were obtained from the uterine and the umbilical arteries when the etiology of the oligohydramnios was renal anomalies or ruptured membranes.[214] In oligohydramnios secondary to ruptured membranes, Doppler velocimetry of the uterine or umbilical arteries is usually within normal range and, thus, ineffective in predicting complications.[215,216] As demonstrated above, Doppler velocimetry is an additional tool in the evaluation of the fetus for possible anomalies associated with derangements of AFV.

COMMENTS

It is very difficult to try to elucidate a common mechanism for decreased umbilical artery diastolic flow associated with congenital anomalies. One obvious explanation would be the presence of IUGR, in which case the abnormal velocimetry would not be an integral part of this anomaly itself, but rather, secondary to possible increased placental resistance.[217–219] However, not all fetuses with congenital anomalies demonstrate retarded growth secondary to placental insufficiency, but rather secondary to ''reduced growth potential.'' Furthermore, even among fetuses with normal growth, the incidence of abnormal Doppler studies is significantly higher, thus failing to point to IUGR as a direct etiology. A fetal mechanism may be responsible for the changes in the umbilical-placental circulation,[2] as placental flow may be regulated in part by the fetus.[220,221] Another explanation is the induction of placental vascular changes by whatever etiologic agent is involved in the fetal abnormality.[222] Although most fetal malformations occur in patients with no known risk factors, certain etiologic factors can be recognized: *genetic* (or Mendelian) in about 20 percent, *environmental* in about 10 percent, *chromosomal* in about 5 percent, and *multifactorial* in about 15 percent. No etiology can be invoked in the largest group (50 percent). In anomalies of unexplained origin, a possible speculation is that abnormal placentation is responsible for early anoxia and subsequent maldevelopment. Very severe abnormal placentation would induce a lethal anomaly. The placental pathology would also possibly involve vascular alterations and, as a consequence, abnormal Doppler studies. Milder placental pathology would be accompanied by fetal nonlethal sequelae. This does not explain the frequent presence of abnormal blood flow in chromosomal disorders, although, as noted earlier, placentas of karyotypically abnormal fetuses also tend to demonstrate vascular anomalies.[195,196]

As previously stated, no single large prospective study has demonstrated the value of Doppler ultrasound in the assessment of fetal anomalies. One study looked at predicting lethality in fetuses with various congenital defects,[4] and numerous case reports have been published, mostly on the anecdotal use of Doppler (color-coded or not) in otherwise diagnosed fetal anomalies. Some authors[223] have studied the value of umbilical artery pulsatility index in the prediction of fetal outcome in cases of structural heart diseases. They found that the index was elevated but not clinically helpful. Doppler can furnish additional information and, in some cases, will definitely nail down the diagnosis. Doubtless, its use in the next few years will grow and extend and is certainly a potential but also already a partial reality.[224]

ACKNOWLEDGMENT

The authors wish to thank Janet R. Gilley for editorial comments.

REFERENCES

1. Trudinger BJ, Cook CM: Umbilical and uterine artery flow velocity waveforms in pregnancy with major fetal abnormality. Br J Obstet Gynaecol 92:660–670, 1985.
2. Meizner I, Katz M, Lunenfeld E, Insler V: Umbilical and uterine flow velocity waveforms in pregnancies complicated by major fetal anomalies. Prenat Diagn 7:491–496, 1987.
3. Hsieh FJ, Chang FM, Ko TM, Chen HY, Chen YP: Umbilical artery flow velocity waveforms in fetuses dying with congenital anomalies. Br J Obstet Gynaecol 95:478–482, 1988.
4. Levy DL, Abramowicz JS, Kuhlmann RS: The umbilical artery S/D ratio in congenital anomalies: prediction of lethality. Society of Perinatal Obstetricians Ninth Annual Meeting, New Orleans, La., 1989, abstract 323.
5. DeVore GR, Clark SL: The association of increased Doppler umbilical artery resistance and abnormal fetal ultrasound findings. Society of Perinatal Obstetricians Ninth Annual Meeting, New Orleans, La., 1989, abstract 311.

6. Hata K, Hata T, Senoh D, Aoki S, Takamiya O, Kitao M: Umbilical artery blood flow velocity waveforms and associations with fetal abnormality. Gynecol Obstet Invest 27:179–182, 1989.

7. Rochelson B, Kaplan C, Trunea C, Schulman H, Guzman E, Fleischer A, Reed K: Doppler velocimetry in the fetus with abnormal karyotype. Echocardiography 6:271–275, 1989.

Cranial-Intracranial

8. Jaeger R, Forbes RP: Bilateral congenital arteriovenous communications (aneurysm) of the cerebral vessels. Arch Neurol Psychiat (Chicago) 55:591–599, 1946.

9. Litvak J, Yahr M, Ransohoff J: Aneurysms of the great vein of Galen and midline cerebral arteriovenous anomalies. J Neurosurg 17:945–954, 1960.

10. Johnson W, Berry JM, Einzig S, Bass JL: Doppler findings in nonimmune hydrops fetalis and cerebral arteriovenous malformation. Am Heart J 115:1138–1140, 1988.

11. Schranz D, Jungst BK, Golla G, Schuind A, Vogel K, Schmitt T, Zimmer B, Huth R, Stopfkuchen H: Kongestive Herzinsuffizienz bei einem Neugeborenen mit arteriovenoser Malformation der Vena Galeni: Diagnose mittels farbcodierter Doppler-Bild-Echographie (Congestive heart failure in a newborn infant with arteriovenous malformation of the vein of Galen: diagnosis using color-coded Doppler image echography). Monatsschr Kinderheilkd 136:47–49, 1988.

12. Saliba E, Santini JJ, Chantepie A, Pottier JM, Cheliakire C, Gold F, Bloc D, Laugier J: Cardiac and cerebral involvement in aneurysms of the ampulla of Galen: contributions of echography and cerebral Doppler flow meter in the neonatal period. Neuro-chirurgie 33:296–301, 1987.

13. Jeanty P, Depple D, Roussis P, Shah D: In utero detection of cardiac failure from an aneurysm of the vein of Galen. Am J Obstet Gynecol 163:50–51, 1990.

14. Cubberly DA, Jaffe RB, Nixon GW: Sonographic demonstration of galenic arteriovenous malformations in the neonate. Am J Neuroradiol 3:435, 1982.

15. Mansour H, Veyrac C, Couture A: Role of cerebral echography in the diagnosis of aneurysm of the vein of Galen. Neuro-chirurgie 33:345–348, 1987.

16. Mao K, Adams J: Antenatal diagnosis of intracranial arteriovenous fistula by ultrasonography—case report. Br J Obstet Gynaecol 90:872–873, 1983.

17. Vintzileos A, Eisenfeld L, Campbell W, Herson VC, DiLeo PE, Chomeides L: Prenatal ultrasonic diagnosis of arteriovenous malformation of the vein of Galen. Am J Perinatol 3:209–211, 1986.

18. Mizejewski GJ, Polansky S, Mondragon-Tiu Fe A, Ellman AM: Combined use of alpha-feto protein and ultrasound in the prenatal diagnosis of arteriovenous fistula in the brain. Obstet Gynecol 70:452–453, 1987.

19. Mendelsohn DB, Hertzanu Y, Butterworth A: In utero diagnosis of a vein of Galen aneurysm by ultrasound. Neuroradiology 26:417–418, 1984.

20. Reiter AA, Huhta JC, Carpenter RJ, Segall GK, Hawkins EP: Prenatal diagnosis of arteriovenous malformation of the vein of Galen J Clin Ultrasound 14:623–628, 1986.

21. Soto G, Daneman A, Hellman J: Doppler evaluation of cerebral arteries in a Galenic vein malformation. J Ultrasound Med 4:673–675, 1985.

22. Sivakoff M, Nouri S: Diagnosis of vein of Galen arteriovenous malformation by two-dimensional ultrasound and pulsed-Doppler method. Pediatrics 69:84–86, 1982.

23. Hirsch JH, Cyr D, Eberhardt H, Zunkel D: Ultrasonographic diagnosis of an aneurysm of the vein of Galen in utero by duplex scanning. J Ultrasound Med 2:231–233, 1983.

24. Rizzo G, Arduini D, Colosimo C, Boccolini MR, Mancuso S: Abnormal fetal cerebral blood flow velocity waveforms as a sign of an aneurysm of the vein of Galen. Fetal Ther 2:75–70, 1987.

25. Mardini MK, Lazarte R, Huntington D, Hilliard J, Kramer L, O'Connell R, Allen R, Hepner SI, Ziai M: Diagnosis of cerebral arteriovenous malformation by contrast two-dimensional and Doppler ultrasonography of the head after saline injection in the umbilical arterial line. Am Heart J 114:450–454, 1987.

26. Deeg KH, Scharf J: Colour Doppler imaging of arteriovenous malformation of the vein of Galen in a newborn. Neuroradiology 32:60–63, 1990.

27. Tessler FN, Dion J, Vinuela F, Perrella RR, Duckwiler G, Hall T, Boechat MI, Grant EG: Cranial arteriovenous malformation in neonates: color Doppler imaging with angiographic correlation. AJR 153:1027–1030, 1989.

28. Vaksmann G, Decoulx E, Mauran P, Jardin M, Rey C, Dupuis C: Evaluation of vein of Galen arteriovenous malformation in newborns by two-dimensional ultrasound, pulsed and colour Doppler method. Eur J Pediatr 148:510–512, 1989.

29. Ciricillo SF, Schmidt KG, Silverman NH, Hieshima GB, Higashida RT, Halbach W, Edwards MS: Serial ultrasonographic evaluation of neonatal vein of Galen malformations to assess the efficacy of interventional neuroradiological procedures. Neurosurgery 27:544–548, 1990.

30. Hata T, Hata K, Senoh D: Antenatal Doppler color flow mapping of arteriovenous malformation of the vein of Galen. J Cardiovasc Ultrasonogr 7:301–303, 1988.

31. Jellinger KJ: Vascular malformations of the central nervous system: morphological review. Neurosurg Rev 9:177–216, 1986.

32. Grant EG, White EM, Schellinger D: Cranial duplex sonography of the infant. Radiology 163:177–185, 1987.

33. Mitchell DG, Merton D, Needleman L, Kurtz AB, Goldberg BB, Levy D, Rifkin MD, Pennell RG, Vilaro M, Baltarowich O, Dahnert W, Graziani L, Desai H: Neonatal brain: color Doppler imaging, Part 1: Technique and vascular anatomy. Radiology 167:303–306, 1988.

34. Deeg KH: Colour flow imaging of the great intracranial arteries in infants. Neuroradiology 31:40–44, 1989.

35. Arbeille P, Montenegro N, Tranquart F, Berson M, Roncin A, Pourcelot L: Assessment of the main fetal cerebrovascular areas by ultrasound color-coded Doppler. Echocardiography 7:629–634, 1990.

36. Arbeille P, Tranquart F, Berson M, Roncin A, Saliba E, Pourcelot L: Visualization of the fetal circle of Willis and intra-cerebral arteries by color-coded Doppler. Eur J Obstet Gynecol Reprod Biol 32:195–198, 1989.

37. Chervenak FA, Berkowitz RL, Romero R, Tortora M, Mayden K, Duncan C, Mahoney MJ, Hobbins JC: The diagnosis of fetal hydrocephalus. Am J Obstet Gynecol 147:703–716, 1983.

38. Vintzileos AM, Ingardia CJ, Nochimson DJ: Congenital hydrocephalus: a review and protocol for perinatal management. Obstet Gynecol 62:539–549, 1983.

39. Benacerraf BR, Birnholz JC: The diagnosis of fetal hydrocephalus prior to 22 weeks. J Clin Ultrasound 15:531–536, 1987.

40. Nyberg DA, Mack LA, Hirsch J, Pagon RO, Shepard TH: Fetal hydrocephalus: sonographic detection and clinical significance of associated anomalies. Radiology 163:187–191, 1987.

41. Abramowicz JS, Jaffe R: Diagnosis and intrauterine management of enlargement of the cerebral ventricles. J Perinat Med 16:165–173, 1988.

42. Wladimiroff JW, Tonge HM, Stewart PA: Doppler ultrasound assessment of cerebral blood flow in the human fetus. Br J Obstet Gynaecol 93:471, 1986.

43. Arbeille P, Patat F, Tranquart F, Body G, Berson M, Roncin A, Saliba E, Magnin G, Berger C, Pourcelot L: Doppler examination of the umbilical and cerebral arterial circulation of the fetus. J Gynecol Obstet Biol Reprod 16:45–51, 1987.

44. Satoh S, Koyanagi T, Hara K, Shimokawa H, Nakano H: Developmental characteristics of blood flow in the middle cerebral artery in the human fetus in utero, assessed using the linear-array pulsed Doppler method. Early Hum Dev 17:195–203, 1988.

45. Mari G, Moise KJ, Jr., Deter RL, Kirshon B, Carpenter RJ, Jr., Huhta JC: Doppler assessment of the pulsatility index in the cerebral circulation of the human fetus. Am J Obstet Gynecol 160:698–703, 1989.

46. Meerman RJ, van Bel F, van Qwieten PH, Oepkes D, den Ouden L: Fetal and neonatal cerebral blood velocity in the normal fetus and neonate: a longitudinal Doppler ultrasound study. Early Hum Dev 24:209–217, 1990.

47. Veille JC, Cohen I: Middle cerebral artery flow in normal and growth-retarded fetuses. Am J Obstet Gynecol 162:391–396, 1990.

48. Hill A, Volpe JJ: Decrease in pulsatile flow in the anterior cerebral arteries in infantile hydrocephalus. Pediatrics 69:4–7, 1982.

49. Santini JJ, Saliba E, Arbeille P: Mesure non-invasive du flux sanguin cerebral chez le nouveauné hydrocéphale. Neuro-chirurgia 31:7–13, 1985.

50. Kirkinen P, Muller R, Baumann H, Briner J, Lang W, Huch R, Huch A: Cerebral blood flow velocity waveforms in hydrocephalic fetuses. J Clin Ultrasound 16:493–498, 1988.

51. van den Wijngaard JAGW, Reuss A, Wladimiroff JW: The blood flow velocity waveform in the fetal internal carotid artery in the presence of hydrocephaly. Early Hum Dev 18:95–99, 1988.

Face and Neck

52. Jones KL: *Smith's Recognizable Patterns of Human Malformation,* 4th ed. Philadelphia, WB Saunders, 1988, p 726.

53. Shprintzen RJ, Siegel-Sadewitz VL, Amato J, Goldberg RB: Anomalies associated with cleft lip, cleft palate, or both. Am J Med Genet 20:585–595, 1985.

54. Christ JE, Meininger MG: Ultrasound diagnosis of cleft lip and cleft palate before birth. Plast Reconst Surg 68:854–859, 1981.

55. Seeds JW, Cefalo RC: Technique of early sonographic diagnosis of bilateral cleft lip and palate. Obstet Gynecol 62:2s–7s, 1983.

56. Sherer DM, Hearn B, Abramowicz JS: Echogenic oral labial fissure; An aid to rule out fetal cleft lip. J Ultrasound Med 10:239, 1991.

57. Mahony BS, Hegge FN: "The face and neck," in Nyberg DA, Mahony BS, Pretorius DH (eds), *Diagnostic Ultrasound of Fetal Anomalies. Text and Atlas.* Chicago, Year Book Medical Publishers, 1990, pp 203–261.

58. Adam AH, Robinson HP, Aust F, Pont M, Hood VD, Gibson AAM: Prenatal diagnosis of fetal lymphatic system abnormalities by ultrasound. J Clin Ultrasound 7:361–364, 1979.

59. Frigoletto FD, Jr, Birnholz JC, Driscoll SG, Finberg WJ: Ultrasound diagnosis of cystic hygroma. Am J Obstet Gynecol 136:962–964, 1980.

60. Chervenak FA, Isaacson G, Blakemore KJ, Breg WR, Hobbins JC, Berkowitz RL, Tortora M, Mayden K, Mahoney KJ: Fetal cystic hygroma: cause and natural history. N Engl J Med 309:822–825, 1983.

61. Elejalde BR, Elejalde MM, Leno J: Nuchal cystic syndromes: etiology, pathogenesis and prenatal diagnosis. Am J Med Genet 21:417–432, 1985.

62. Garden AS, Benzie RJ, Miskin M, Gardner HA: Fetal cystic hygroma coli: antenatal diagnosis, significance and management. Am J Obstet Gynecol 154:224–225, 1986.

63. Abramowicz JS, Warsof SL, Doyle DL, Smith D, Levy DL: Congenital cystic hygroma of the neck diagnosed prenatally: outcome with normal and abnormal karyotype. Prenat Diagn 9:321–327, 1989.

64. McGahan JP, Schneider JM: Fetal neck hemangioendothelioma with secondary hydrops fetalis. Sonographic diagnosis. J Clin Ultrasound 14:384–388, 1986.

65. Pennell R, Baltarowich OH: Prenatal sonographic diagnosis of a fetal facial hemangioma. J Ultrasound Med 5:525–528, 1986.

66. Lasser D, Preis O, Dor N, Tancer ML: Antenatal diagnosis of giant cystic cavernous hemangioma by Doppler velocimetry. Obstet Gynecol 72:476–477, 1988.

67. Birnholz JC: Ultrasonic fetal ophthalmology. Early Hum Dev 12:199–209, 1985.

68. Birnholz JC, Farrell EE: Fetal hyaloid artery: timing of regression with US. Radiology 166:781–783, 1988.

Spine

69. Lemire RJ, Graham CB, Beckwith JB: Skin-covered sacrococcygeal masses in infants and children. J Pediatr 79:948–954, 1971.

70. Chervenak FA, Isaacson G, Touloukian R, Tortora M, Berkowitz RL, Hobbins JC: Diagnosis and management of fetal teratomas. Obstet Gynecol 66:666–671, 1985.

71. Holzgreve W, Mahony BS, Flick PL, Filly RA, Harrison MR, Delorimier AA, Holzgreve AC, Muller KM, Callen PW, Anderson RL, Golbus MS: Sonographic demonstration of fetal sacrococcygeal teratoma. Prenat Diagn 5:245–257, 1985.

72. Flake AW, Harrison MR, Adzick NS, Laberge IM, Warsof SL: Fetal sacrococcygeal teratoma. J Pediatr Surg 21:563–566, 1986.

73. Heloury Y, Vergnes P, Classe JM, Nomballais MF, Jehannin B, Weil D, Lopes P: Prenatal diagnosis of sacro-coccygeal teratomas. Chir Pediatr 31:202–206, 1990.

74. Holzgreve W, Flake AW, Langer JC: "The fetus with sacrococcygeal teratoma," in Harrison MR, Golbus MS, Filly RA (eds), *The Unborn Patient: Prenatal Diagnosis and Treatment.* Philadelphia, WB Saunders, 1990, pp 460–469.

75. Smith B, Passaro E, Clatworthy H: The vascular anatomy of sacrococcygeal teratomas. Its significance in surgical management. Surgery 49:534–539, 1961.

76. Smith WL, Stokka C, Franken EA: Arteriography of sacrococcygeal teratomas. Radiology 137:653–655, 1980.

77. Schmidt KG, Silverman NH, Harrison MR, Callen PW: High-output cardiac failure in fetuses with large sacrococcygeal teratoma: diagnosis by echocardiography and Doppler ultrasound. J Pediatr 114:1023–1028, 1989.

78. Bond SJ, Harrison MR, Schmidt KG, Silverman NH, Flake AW, Slotnick RN, Anderson RL, Warsof SL, Dyson DC: Death due to high output cardiac failure in fetal sacrococcygeal teratoma. J Pediatr Surg 12:1287–1291, 1990.

79. Gergely RZ, Eden R, Schifrin BS, Wade ME: Antenatal diagnosis of congenital sacral teratoma. J Reprod Med 24:229–231, 1980.

80. Hallgrimsson JTh: Sacro-coccygeal teratoma with acute hydramnios. Acta Obstet Gynecol Scand 60:517, 1981.

81. Kohga S, Nambu T, Tanaka K, Benirschke K, Feldman BH, Kishikawa T: Hypertrophy of the placenta and sacrococcygeal teratoma. A report of two cases. Virchows Arch A Path Anat Histol 386:223–229, 1980.

82. Cousins L, Bernirshke K, Porreco R, Resnik R: Placentomegaly due to congestive failure in a pregnancy with a sacrococcygeal teratoma. J Reprod Med 25:142–144, 1980.

83. Feige A, Gille J, von Maillot K: Praenatale diagnostik eine Steissbeinteratoms mit Hypertrophie der Plazenta. (Prenatal diagnosis of a sacrococcygeal teratoma with placental hypertrophy.) Geburtsh u Frauenheilk 42:20–23, 1982.

84. Kohler HG: Sacrococcygeal teratoma and "nonimmunological" hydrops fetalis. Br Med J 2:422, 1976.

85. Alter DN, Reed KL, Marx GR, Anderson CF, Shenker L: Prenatal diagnosis of congestive heart failure in a fetus with a sacrococcygeal teratoma. Obstet Gynecol 71:978–981, 1988.

86. Grisoni ER, Gauderer MWL, Wolfson RN: Antenatal diagnosis of sacrococcygeal teratomas: Prognostic features. Pediatr Surg Int 3:173, 1988.

87. Langer JC, Harrison MR, Schmidt KG, Silverman NH, Anderson RL, Goldberg JD, Filly RA, Crombleholme TM, Longaker MT, Golbus MS: Fetal hydrops and death from sacrococcygeal teratoma: rationale for fetal surgery. Am J Obstet Gynecol 160:1145–1150, 1989.

Thorax

88. Hilpert PL, Pretorius DH: "The thorax," in Nyberg DA, Mahony BS, Pretorius DH (eds), *Diagnostic Ultrasound of Fetal Anomalies. Text and Atlas.* Chicago, Year Book Medical Publishers, 1990, pp 262–299.

89. DiSessa TG, Emerson DS, Felker RE, Brown DL, Cartier MS, Becker JA: Anomalous systemic and pulmonary venous pathways diagnosed in utero by ultrasound. J Ultrasound Med 9:311–317, 1990.

90. Smith LG, Jr, Carpenter RJ Jr, Gonsoulin W, Mari G, Reiter AA, Greenberg F, Powell C:

Prenatal diagnosis of a chest wall mass with ultrasonography and Doppler velocimetry. A case report. Am J Obstet Gynecol 103:567–569, 1990.

91. Cullen ML, Klein MD, Philippart AI: Congenital diaphragmatic hernia. Surg Clin North Am 65:1115–1138, 1985.

92. Adzick NS, Harrison MR, Glick PL, Nakayama DK, Manning FA, deLorimier AA: Diaphragmatic hernia in the fetus: prenatal diagnosis and outcome in 94 cases. J Pediatr Surg 20:357–361, 1985.

93. Hobbins JC, Grannum PAT, Berkowitz RL, Silverman R, Mahoney MJ: Ultrasound in the diagnosis of congenital anomalies. Am J Obstet Gynecol 134:331–345, 1979.

94. Campbell S, Pearce JM: The prenatal diagnosis of fetal structural anomalies by ultrasound. Clin Obstet Gynaecol 10:475–483, 1983.

95. Aguero O, Zighelboim I: Intrauterine diagnosis of fetal diaphragmatic hernia by amniography. Am J Obstet Gynecol 107:971–972, 1970.

96. Bell MJ, Ternberg JL: Antenatal diagnosis of diaphragmatic hernia. Pediatrics 60:738–740, 1977.

97. Marwood RP, Davision OW: Antenatal diagnosis of diaphragmatic hernia: case report. Br J Obstet Gynaecol 88:71–72, 1981.

98. Chinn DH, Filly RA, Callen PW: Congenital diaphragmatic hernia diagnosed prenatally by ultrasound. *Radiology* 148:119–123, 1983.

99. Stehling MK, Mansfield P, Ordidge RJ, Coxon R, Chapman B, Blamire A, Gibbs P, Johnson IR, Symonds EM, Worthington BS, Coupland RE: Echo-planar magnetic resonance imaging in abnormal pregnancies. Lancet ii:157, 1989.

100. Harrison MR: "The fetus with a diaphragmatic hernia: pathophysiology, natural history and surgical management," in Harrison MR, Golbus MS, Filly RA (eds), *The Unborn Patient: Prenatal Diagnosis and Treatment*. Philadelphia, WB Saunders, 1990, pp 295–313.

101. Puri P, Gorman F: Lethal nonpulmonary anomalies associated with congenital diaphragmatic hernia: implications for early intra-uterine surgery. J Pediatr Surg 19:29–32, 1984.

102. Comstock CH: The antenatal diagnosis of diaphragmatic anomalies. J Ultrasound Med 5:391–396, 1986.

103. Steinberg I: Cardiovascular changes due to diaphragmatic hernia and cardiospasm. NY State J Med 67:2586, 1967.

104. Dibbins AW, Wiener ES: Mortality from neonatal diaphragmatic hernia. J Pediatr Surg 9:653–662, 1974.

105. Greenwood RD, Rosenthal A, Nadas AS: Cardiovascular abnormalities associated with congenital diaphragmatic hernia. Pediatrics 57:92–97, 1976.

106. Parker KJ, Huang SR, Musulin RA, Lerner RM: Tissue response to mechanical vibrations for "sonoelasticity imaging." Ultrasound Med Biol 16:241–246, 1990.

107. Lerner RM, Huang SR, Parker KJ: "Sonoelasticity" images derived from ultrasound signals in mechanically vibrated tissues. Ultrasound Med Biol 16:231–239, 1990.

108. Berman B, Lim HW: Concurrent cutaneous and hepatic hemangioma in infancy: Report of a case and review of the literature. J Dermatol Surg Oncol 4:869–873, 1978.

109. Nguyen L, Shardling B, Ein S, Stephens C: Hepatic hemangioma in childhood: medical management or surgical management? J Pediatr Surg 17:576–579, 1982.

110. Brunelle F, Chaumont P: Hepatic tumors in children: ultrasonic differentiation of malignant from benign lesions. Radiology 150:695–699, 1984.

111. Diakoumakis EE, Weinberg B, Seife B, Beck AR, Guttenberg ME: Infantile hemangioendothelioma of the liver. J Clin Ultrasound 14:137–139, 1986.

112. Nakamoto SK, Dreilinger A, Dattel B: The sonographic appearance of hepatic hemangioma in-utero. J Ultrasound Med 2:239–241, 1983.

113. Platt LD, DeVore GR, Benner P, Siassi B, Ralls PW, Mikity VG: Antenatal diagnosis of a fetal liver mass. J Ultrasound Med 2:521–522, 1983.

114. Moore TC: Gastroschisis and omphalocele: clinical differences. Surgery 82:561–568, 1977.

115. Schaffer RM, Barone C, Friedman AP: The ultrasonographic spectrum of fetal omphalocele. J Ultrasound Med 2:219, 1983.

116. Nakayama DK, Harrison MR, Gross BH, Callen PN, Filly RA, Golbus MS, Stephens JD, deLorimier AA: Management of the fetus with an abdominal wall defect. J Pediatr Surg 19:408–413, 1984.

117. Sermer M, Benzie RJ, Pitson L, Carr M, Skidmore M: Prenatal diagnosis and management of congenital defects of the anterior abdominal wall. Am J Obstet Gynecol 156:308, 1987.

118. Langer JC, Harrison MR: "The fetus with an abdominal wall defect," in Harrison MR, Golbus MS, Filly RA (eds), *The Unborn Patient: Prenatal Diagnosis and Treatment*. Philadelphia, WB Saunders, 1990, pp 453–459.

119. Touloukian RJ, Hobbins JC: Maternal ultrasonography in the antenatal diagnosis of surgically correctable fetal abnormalities. J Pediatr Surg 15:373–377, 1980.

120. Mann L, Ferguson-Smith MA, Desai M, Gibson AAM, Raine PAM: Prenatal assessment of anterior abdominal wall defects and their prognosis. Prenat Diagn 4:427–435, 1984.

121. Bair JH, Russ PD, Pretorius DH, Manchester D, Manco-Johnson ML: Fetal omphalocele and gastroschisis: A review of 24 cases. AJR 147:1047–1051, 1986.

122. Lindfors KK, McGahan JP, Walter JP: Fetal omphalocele and gastroschisis: pitfalls in sonographic diagnosis. AJR 147:797–800, 1986.

123. McCarthy SM, Filly RA, Start DD, Callen PW, Golbus MS, Hricak H: Magnetic resonance imaging of fetal anomalies in utero: Early experience. AJR 145:677–682, 1985.

124. Weinreb JC, Brown CEL: "Magnetic resonance imaging," in Eden RD, Boehm FH (eds), *Assessment and Care of the Fetus: Physiological, Clinical, and Medicolegal Principles*. Norwalk, Conn., Appleton and Lange, Norwalk, 1990, pp 307–315.

125. Duhamel B: Embryology of exomphalus and allied malformations. Arch Dis Child 38:142–147, 1968.

126. Godsen C, Brock DJH: Prenatal diagnosis of exstrophy of the cloaca. Am J Med Genet 8:95, 1981.

127. Mercer LJ, Petres RE, Smeltzer JS: Ultrasonic diagnosis of ectopia cordis. Obstet Gynecol 61:523–525, 1983.

128. Haynor DR, Shuman WP, Brewer DR: Imaging of fetal ectopia cordis: Role of sonography and computed sonography. J Ultrasound Med 3:25–28, 1984.

129. Meizner I, Bar-Ziv D: Prenatal ultrasonic diagnosis of cloacal exstrophy. Am J Obstet Gynecol 153:802, 1985.

130. Ghidini A, Sirtori M, Romero R, Hobbins JC: Prenatal diagnosis of pentalogy of Cantrell. J Ultrasound Med 7:567–572, 1988.

131. Gilbert WM, Nicolaides KH: Fetal omphalocele: associated malformations and chromosomal defects. Obstet Gynecol 70:633–635, 1987.

132. Mirk P, Calisti A, Fileni A: Prenatal sonographic diagnosis of bladder exstrophy. J Ultrasound Med 5:291, 1986.

133. Jaffe R, Schoenfeld A, Ovadia J: Sonographic findings in the prenatal diagnosis of bladder exstrophy. Am J Obstet Gynecol 102:675–678, 1990.

134. Van Bel F, Van Zwieten PH, Guit GL, Schipper J: Superior mesenteric artery blood flow velocity and estimated volume flow: duplex Doppler US study of preterm and term neonates. Radiology 174:165–169, 1990.

Genitourinary Tract

135. Helin I, Persson PH: Prenatal diagnosis of urinary tract abnormalities by ultrasound. Pediatrics 78:879–883, 1986.

136. Grannum PA: "The genitourinary tract," in Nyberg DA, Mahone BS, Pretorius DH (eds), *Diagnostic Ultrasound of Fetal Anomalies. Text and Atlas*. Chicago, Year Book Medical Publishers, 1990, pp 433–491.

137. Yared A, Barakat AY, Ichikawa I: "Fetal nephrology," in Eden RD, Boehn FH (eds), *As-*

sessment and Care of the Fetus: Physiological, Clinical, and Medicoligal Principles. Norwalk, Conn., Appleton and Lange, 1990, pp 69–91.

138. Hadlock FP, Deter RL, Carpenter R, Gonzalez ET, Park SK: Sonography of fetal urinary tract anomalies. AJR 137:261–267, 1981.

139. Chinn DH, Filly RA: Ultrasound diagnosis of fetal genitourinary tract anomalies. Urol Radiol 4:115, 1982.

140. Schmidt W, Kubli F: Early diagnosis of severe congenital malformations by ultrasonography. J Perinat Med 10:233–241, 1982.

141. Hobbins JC, Romero R, Grannum PA, Berkowitz RL, Cullen M, Mahony M: Antenatal diagnosis of renal anomalies with ultrasound. Am J Obstet Gynecol 148:868–877, 1984.

142. Quinlan RW, Cruz AL, Huddleston JF: Sonographic detection of fetal urinary tract anomalies. Obstet Gynecol 67:558–565, 1986.

143. Mahony BS, Filly RA: The genitourinary system in utero. Clin Diagn Ultrasound 18:1–21, 1986.

144. Jaffe R, Abramowicz JS, Fejgin M, Ben-Aderet N: Giant fetal abdominal cyst: Ultrasonic diagnosis and management. J Ultrasound Med 6:45–47, 1987.

145. Potter EL: Bilateral absence of ureters and kidneys. A report of 50 cases. Obstet Gynecol 25:3–12, 1965.

146. Dubbins PA, Kurtz AB, Wapner RJ, Goldberg BB: Renal agenesis: spectrum of in utero findings. J Clin Ultrasound 9:189–193, 1981.

147. Romero R, Cullen M, Grannum P, Jeanty P, Reece EA, Venus I, Hobbins JC: Antenatal diagnosis of renal anomalies with ultrasound III. Bilateral renal agenesis. Am J Obstet Gynecol 151:38–43, 1985.

148. Hoffman H, Chaoui R, Bollmann R, Halle H, Zienert A: Prenatal use of pulsed Doppler ultrasound within scope of the differential diagnosis of bilateral kidney abnormalities. Geburtshilfe Frauenheilk 50:203–206, 1990.

149. Campbell S, Vyas S: Color flow mapping in measurement of flow velocity in fetal renal arteries. First International Meeting. Fetal and neonatal color flow mapping. Dubrovnik, Yugoslavia, 1988.

150. Hecher K, Spernol R, Szalay S: Doppler blood flow velocity waveforms in the fetal renal artery. Arch Gynecol Obstet 246:133–137, 1989.

151. Vyas S, Nicolaides KH, Campbell S: Renal artery flow-velocity waveforms in normal and hypoxic fetuses. Am J Obstet Gynecol 161:168–172, 1989.

152. Veille JC, Kanaan C: Duplex Doppler ultrasonographic evaluation of the fetal renal artery in normal and abnormal fetuses. Am J Obstet Gynecol 161:1502–1507, 1989.

153. Hata R, Mari G, Reiter AA: Doppler velocity waveform of blood flow in the fetal renal artery in a case of Meckel syndrome. AJR 156:408, 1991.

Extremities

154. Hobbins JC, Bracken MB, Mahoney MJ: Diagnosis of fetal skeletal dysplasias with ultrasound. Am J Obstet Gynecol 142:306, 1982.

155. Jeanty P, Romero R: Fetal limbs: normal anatomy and congenital malformations. Semin Ultrasound, CT MR: 5:253–268, 1984.

156. Mahony BS, Filly RA: High resolution sonographic assessment of the fetal extremities. J Ultrasound Med 3:489–498, 1984.

157. Mari G: Arterial blood flow velocity waveforms of the pelvis and lower extremities in normal and growth-retarded fetuses. Am J Obstet Gynecol 165:143–151, 1991.

Nonimmune Hydrops

158. Warsof SL, Nicolaides KH, Rodeck KC: Immune and non-immune hydrops. Clin Obstet Gynecol 29:533–545, 1986.

159. Saltzman DH, Frigoletto FD, Harlow BL, Barss VA, Benacerraf BR: Sonographic evaluation of hydrops fetalis. Obstet Gynecol 74:106, 1989.

160. Holzgreve W: "The fetus with nonimmune hydrops," in Harrison MR, Golbus MS, Filly RA (eds), *The Unborn Patient: Prenatal Diagnosis and Treatment.* Philadelphia, WB Saunders, 1990, pp 228–245.

161. Poeschmann RP, Verheijen RHM, Van Dongen PWJ: Differential diagnosis and causes of nonimmunological hydrops fetalis: a review. Obstet Gynecol Surv 46:223–231, 1991.

162. Holzgreve W, Curry CJR, Golbus MS, Callen PW, Filly RA, Smith JC: Investigation of non-immune hydrops fetalis. Am J Obstet Gynecol 150:805–812, 1984.

163. Gudmundsson S, Huhta JC, Wood DC, Tulzer G, Cohen AW, Weiner S: Venous Doppler, ultrasonography in the fetus with non-immune hydrops. Am J Obstet Gynecol 164:33–37, 1991.

164. Kleinman CS, Donnerstein RL, DeVore GR, Jaffe CC, Lynch DC, Berkowitz RL, Talner NS, Hobbins JC: Fetal echocardiography for evaluation of in utero congestive heart failure. N Engl J Med 306:568–575, 1982.

165. Allan LD, Crawford DC, Sheridan R, Chapman MG: Aetiology of non-immune hydrops: The value of echocardiography. Br J Obstet Gynaecol 93:223–225, 1986.

166. Harrington JT, Kangos JJ, Sikka A, Spisso K, Natarajan N, Rosenfeld D, Leiman S, Korn D: Successful treatment of fetal congestive heart failure, secondary to tachycardia. N Engl J Med 304:1527–1529, 1981.

167. Abramowicz JS, Jaffe R, Altaras M, Ben Aderet N: Fetal supraventricular tachycardia: prenatal diagnosis and pharmacological reversal of associated hydrops fetalis. Gynecol Obstet Invest 20:109–112, 1985.

168. Hansmann M, Gembruch V, Bald R: New therapeutic aspects of nonimmune hydrops fetalis based on four hundred and two prenatally diagnosed cases. Fetal Ther 4:29–36, 1989.

169. Hsieh FJ, Chang FM, Huang HC, Lu CC, Ko TM, Chen HY: Umbilical vein blood flow measurement in non-immune hydrops fetalis. Obstet Gynecol 71:188–191, 1988.

Anomalies of Maternal Serum Alpha-Fetoprotein

170. Habib A: Maternal serum alpha-fetoprotein: its value in antenatal diagnosis of genetic disease and in obstetrical-gynecological care. Acta Obstet Gynecol Scand (Suppl) 61:1–72, 1977.

171. Simpson JS, Baum LD, Marder R, Elias S, Ober C, Martin AO: Maternal serum alpha-fetoprotein screening: low and high values for detection of genetic abnormalities. Am J Obstet Gynecol 155:593–597, 1986.

172. Salafia CM, Silberman L, Herrera NE, Mahoney MJ: Placental pathology at term associated with elevated midtrimester maternal serum alpha-fetoprotein concentration. Am J Obstet Gynecol 158:1064–1066, 1988.

173. Thomas RL, Blakemore KJ: Evaluation of elevations in maternal serum alpha-fetoprotein: a review. Obstet Gynecol Surv 45:269–283, 1990.

174. Merkatz IR, Nitowsky HM, Macri JN, Johnson WE: An association between low maternal serum alpha-fetoprotein and fetal chromosome abnormalities. Am J Obstet Gynecol 148:886–894, 1984.

175. Nelson LH, Burton BK, Sowers SG: Ultrasonography in patients with low maternal serum alpha-fetoprotein. J Ultrasound Med 6:59–61, 1987.

176. Richards DS, Seeds JW, Katz VL, Lingley LH, Albright SG, Cefalo RC: Elevated maternal serum alpha-fetoprotein with normal ultrasound. Is amniocentesis always appropriate? A review of 26069 screened patients. Obstet Gynecol 71:203–207, 1988.

177. Warsof SL, Abramowicz JS: Routine ultrasound. Obstet Gynecol Report 2:114–123, 1990.

178. Campbell S, Pearce JM, Hackett G, Cohen-Overbeek T, Hernandez C: Qualitative assessment of uteroplacental blood flow: early screening test for high-risk pregnancies. Obstet Gynecol 68:649–653, 1986.

179. Fleisher AC, Kurtz AB, Wapner RJ, Ruch D, Sacks GA, Jeanty P, Shah DM, Boehm FH: Elevated alpha-fetoprotein and a normal fetal sonogram: association with placental abnormalities. AJR 150–883, 1988.

Fetal Chromosomal Anomalies

180. Benacerraf BR, Gelman R, Frigoletto FD Jr: Sonographic identification of second trimester fetuses with Down's syndrome. N Engl J Med 317:1371–1376, 1987.
181. Perrella R, Duerinckx AJ, Grant EG, Tessler F, Tabsh K, Crandall BF: Second-trimester sonographic diagnosis of Down syndrome: role of femur length shortening and nuchal fold thickening. AJR 151:981–985, 1988.
182. Lockwood CJ, Lynch L, Berkowitz RL: Ultrasonographic screening for the Down syndrome fetus. Am J Obstet Gynecol 165:349–352, 1991.
183. Marchese CA, Carozzi F, Mosso R, Savin E, Campogrande M, Viora E, La Prova A, Dolfin GC, Carbonara AO: Fetal karyotype in malformations detected by ultrasound. Am J Hum Genet 37:A223, 1985.
184. Platt LD, DeVore GR, Lopez E, Herbert W, Falk R, Alfi O: Role of amniocentesis in ultrasound-detected fetal malformations. Obstet Gynecol 68:153–155, 1986.
185. Palmer CG, Miles JH, Howard-Peebles PN, Magenis RE, Patil S, Friedman J: Fetal karyotype following ascertainment of fetal anomalies by ultrasound. Prenat Diagn 7:551–555, 1987.
186. Berg KA, Clark EB, Aslemborsky JA, Boughman JA: Prenatal detection of cardiovascular malformations by echocardiography: an indication for cytogenetic evaluation. Am J Obstet Gynecol 159:477–481, 1988.
187. Al-Gazali W, Chapman MG, Chito SK, Crawford DC, Allan LD: Doppler assessment of umbilical artery blood flow for prediction of outcome in fetal cardiac abnormality. Br J Obstet Gynaecol 94:742–745, 1987.
188. McCowan LM, Erskine LA, Ritchie K: Umbilical artery Doppler blood flow studies in the preterm, small for gestational age fetus. Am J Obstet Gynecol 156:655–659, 1987.
189. Reed KL, Anderson CF, Shenker L: Changes in intracardiac Doppler blood flow velocities in fetuses with absent umbilical artery diastolic flow. Am J Obstet Gynecol 157:744, 1987.
190. Berkowitz GS, Mehalek KE, Chitkara U, Rosenberg J, Cogswell C, Berkowitz RL: Doppler umbilical velocimetry in the prediction of adverse outcome in pregnancies at risk of intrauterine growth retardation. Obstet Gynecol 71:742–746, 1988.
191. Gaziano EP, Knox GE, Wager GP, Bendel RP, Olson JD: Pulsed Doppler umbilical artery waveforms: significance of elevated umbilical artery systolic/diastolic ratios in the normally grown fetus. Obstet Gynecol 75:189–193, 1990.
192. Baton C, Bessis R, Papiernik E: Nul telediastolic flux. Prognostic value. J Gynecol Obstet Biol Reprod 17:615–623, 1988.
193. Brar HS, Platt LD: Reverse end-diastolic flow velocity on umbilical artery velocimetry in high-risk pregnancies: an ominous finding with adverse pregnancy outcome. Am J Obstet Gynecol 159:559–561, 1988.
194. Tonge HM, Wladimiroff JW, Noordam MJ, Van Kooten C: Blood flow velocity waveforms in the descending fetal aorta: comparison between normal and growth retarded pregnancy. Obstet Gynecol 67:851–855, 1986.
195. Kuhlmann RS, Werner AL, Abramowicz JS, Warsof SL, Arrington J, Levy DL: Placental histology in fetuses between 18 and 23 weeks' gestation with abnormal karyotype. Am J Obstet Gynecol 163:1264–1270, 1990.
196. Rochelson B, Kaplan C, Guzman E, Arato M, Hansen K, Trunca C: A quantitative analysis of placental vasculature in the third-trimester fetus with autosomal trisomy. Obstet Gynecol 75:59–63, 1990.

Abnormalities of Amniotic Fluid Volume

197. Cardwell MS: Polyhydramnios: A review. Obstet Gynecol Surv 42:612–617, 1987.
198. Peipert JF, Donnenfeld AE: Oligohydramnios: a review. Obstet Gynecol Surv 46:325–339, 1991.

199. Abramowich DR, Garden A, Jandial L, Page KR: Fetal swallowing and voiding in relation to hydramnios. Obstet Gynecol 54:15–20, 1979.
200. Hill LM: "Abnormalities in amniotic fluid," in Nyberg DA, Mahony BS, Pretorius DH (eds), *Diagnostic Ultrasound of Fetal Anomalies. Text and Atlas.* Chicago, Year Book Medical Publishers, 1990, pp 38–66.
201. Goldstein RB, Filly RA: Sonographic estimation of amniotic fluid volume: Subjective assessment versus pocket measurements. J Ultrasound Med 7:363–369, 1988.
202. Barkin SZ, Pretorius DH, Beckett MK, Manchester DK, Nelson TR, Manco-Johnson ML: Severe polyhydramnios: incidence of anomalies. AJR 148:155–159, 1987.
203. Hill LM, Breckle R, Thomas ML, Fries JK: Polyhydramnios: ultrasonically detected prevalence and neonatal outcome. Obstet Gynecol 69:21–25, 1987.
204. Seeds JW, Cefalo RC: Anomalies with hydramnios: diagnostic role of ultrasound. Contrib Gynecol Obstet 23:32–43, 1984.
205. Philipson EH, Sokol RJ, Williams T: Oligohydramnios: clinical associations and predictive value for intrauterine growth retardation. Am J Obstet Gynecol 146:271–275, 1983.
206. Deutinger J, Bartl W, Pfersmann C, Neumark J, Bernaschek G: Fetal urine volume production in cases of fetal growth retardation. J Perinat Med 15:307–315, 1987.
207. Ross MG: Mechanism of oligohydramnios. Am J Obstet Gynecol 159:271, 1988.
208. Hill LM, Breckle R, Wolfgram KR, O'Brien PC: Oligohydramnios: ultrasonically detected incidence and subsequent fetal outcome. Am J Obstet Gynecol 147:407–410, 1983.
209. Barss VA, Benacerraf BR, Frigoletto FD: Second trimester oligohydramnios, a predictor of poor fetal outcome. Obstet Gynecol 64:608–610, 1984.
210. Bastide A, Manning F, Harman C, Lange I, Morrison I: Ultrasound evaluation of amniotic fluid: outcome of pregnancies with severe oligohydramnios. Am J Obstet Gynecol 154:895–900, 1986.
211. Mercer LJ, Brown LG: Fetal outcome with oligohydramnios in the second trimester. Obstet Gynecol 67:840, 1986.
212. Rochelson B, Coury A, Schulman H, Dery C, Klotz M, Shmoys S: Doppler umbilical artery velocimetry in fetuses with polyhydramnios. Am J Perinat 7:340–342, 1990.
213. Lombardi SJ, Rosemond R, Ball R, Entman SS, Boehm FH: Umbilical artery velocimetry as a predictor of adverse outcome in pregnancies complicated by oligohydramnios. Obstet Gynecol 74:338–341, 1989.
214. Hackett GA, Nicolaides KH, Campbell S: Doppler ultrasound assessment of fetal and utero-placental circulation in severe second trimester oligohydramnios. Br J Obstet Gynaecol 94:1074, 1987.
215. Abramowicz JS, Sherer DM, Warsof SL, Levy DL: Feto-placental and utero-placental blood flow in premature rupture of membranes: a Doppler analysis. Am J Perinat 1992, in press.
216. Santolaya J, Sampson M, Nobles G, Font G, Ramakrishnan V, Warsof SL: Doppler evaluation of the fetoplacental circulation in the latent phase of preterm premature rupture of membranes. J Ultrasound Med 10:327–330, 1991.

Comments

217. Trudinger BJ, Giles WB, Cook C: Uteroplacental blood flow velocity time waveforms in normal and complicated pregnancy. Br J Obstet Gynaecol 92:39–45, 1985.
218. Rochelson B, Shulman H, Farmakides G, Bracero L, Ducey J, Fleischer A, Penny B, Winter D: The significance of absent end-diastolic velocity in umbilical artery velocity waveforms. Am J Obstet Gynecol 156:1213, 1987.
219. Jacobson SL, Imhof R, Manning N, Mannion V, Little D, Rey E, Redman C: The value of Doppler assessment of the uteroplacental circulation in predicting preeclampsia or intrauterine growth retardation. Am J Obstet Gynecol 162:110–114, 1990.
220. Nyland L, Lunell NO, Lewander R, Sarby B: Utero-placental blood flow index in intrauterine growth retardation of fetal or maternal origin. Br J Obstet Gynaecol 90:16–20, 1983.

221. Rankin JHG, McLaughlin MK: The regulation of the placental blood flows. J Dev Physiol 1:3–30, 1979.
222. Giles WB, Trudinger BJ, Baird PJ: Fetal umbilical artery flow velocity waveforms and placental resistance: pathological correlation. Br J Obstet Gynaecol 92:31–38, 1985.
223. Copel JA, Hobbins JC, Kleinman CS: Can umbilical artery pulsatility index predict the outcome of the fetuses with structural heart disease? J Ultrasound Med 10:323–326, 1991.
224. Grant EG: Maternal fetal Doppler sonography: potential or reality? Semin Roentgenol 26:75–86, 1991.

THIRTEEN

THE USE OF COLOR DOPPLER IMAGING IN INVASIVE OBSTETRICAL PROCEDURES

ABRAHAM LUDOMIRSKI
JOSEPH G. BELL

Prenatal diagnosis of congenital abnormalities has always been a major challenge for the perinatologist. With the constant growth in the number of conditions for which prenatal testing is available and the recent advances in ultrasound technology, abnormalities of almost all fetal organs can now be diagnosed.

The ability to detect genetic disorders prior to birth has improved immensely during the last 20 years. Recent advances in tissue culture technology has made possible the development of early invasive diagnostic modalities.

Direct access to the fetal circulation has always been the goal of the perinatologist. Cordocentesis has proven to be safe and efficient in experienced hands and has become the method of choice to access the fetal circulation.

This chapter describes the different techniques involved in invasive prenatal diagnosis and the application of color Doppler imaging in these procedures.

CHORIONIC VILLUS SAMPLING

Chorionic villus sampling (CVS) has become a widely utilized and well-accepted method of genetic diagnosis over the last 10 years. Several large clinical studies have demonstrated the efficacy and safety of CVS as an alternative to amniocentesis.[1–4] Pregnancy loss rates and diagnostic accuracy of CVS have proved to be comparable to those of amniocentesis.[5,6]

Transcervical CVS is usually performed at a gestational age of 9 to 12 weeks, although recent data have shown successful results at gestational ages younger than 9 weeks.[7] Precise sonographic imaging of the placental site is paramount to CVS safety and success. At earlier gestational ages, it is often difficult to delineate placental tissue from that of the surrounding decidua. Color Doppler imaging of the umbilical cord and its insertion allows exact localization of the placenta in these cases (Figs. 13-1 and 13-2).

Transabdominal CVS has also been recently advocated as an alternative method of prenatal diagnosis throughout the gestation.[5,8] Again, visualization of the umbilical cord insertion with the aid of color Doppler allows accurate placental identification. This is of great importance in transabdominal sampling of twin pregnancies. Brambati et al. have reported successful sampling of 13 twin gestations by this transabdominal method.[9] Individual placental cord insertions are identified and the needle tip directed into the placental tissue just below each insertion site for accurate localization and biopsy.

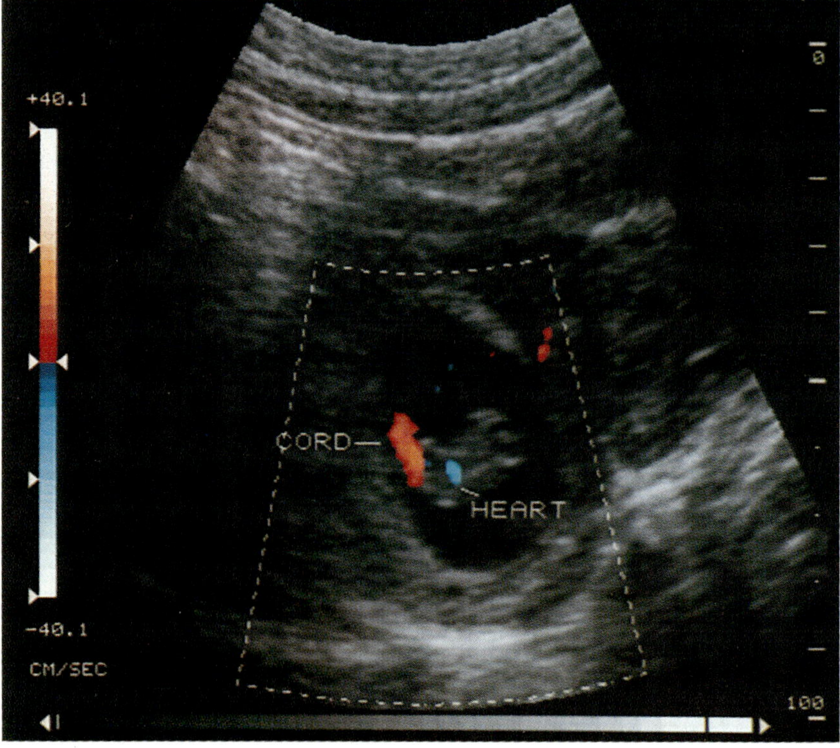

Figure 13-1 The direction of flow clearly visualized in an 8-week gestation.

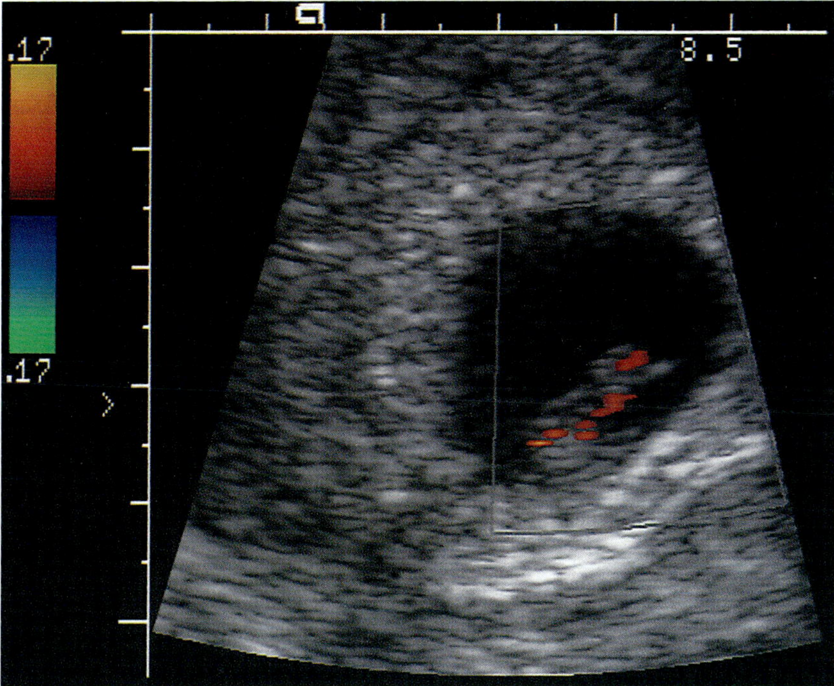

Figure 13-2   A second color image showing umbilical cord direction at 8 weeks gestation.

EARLY AMNIOCENTESIS

Early amniocentesis at 11 to 14 weeks gestation combined with a fast turnaround time is a viable alternative for chorionic villus sampling.

The earlier availability of chromosomal analysis, the decreased time a patient has to wait for the results, and the possibility of obtaining amniotic fluid alpha-fetoprotein (not available with CVS) are few of the advantages of early amniocentesis.

Early amniocentesis is performed with a 22-gauge spinal needle under direct ultrasound vision. The main technical problem regarding the procedure is tangling of the amniotic membranes by the tip of the needle causing sampling failure and an increased risk for postprocedure complications.

Color Doppler imaging is of major importance in the performance of early amniocentesis, as it assists in the identification of placental localization and the exact anatomic position of the umbilical cord. It is very important to avoid handling the umbilical cord during early amniocentesis (Figs. 13-1 and 13-2). Complications as a result of early amniocentesis include rupture of membranes, bleeding, infection, and fetal demise.

Different studies (although of small numbers) have quoted the fetal loss rate (pregnancy loss prior to 28 weeks) following this procedure to be 1.2 to 3.9 percent.[10–11] Genetic analysis of specimen from early amniocentesis carries a high percentage of mosaicism (2 to 3 percent), as does the chorionic villus sampling.[12]

The amniotic fluid volume aspirated is usually 1 cm^3 for every gestational week (13 cm^3 of amniotic fluid at 13 weeks gestation). This procedure is still being evaluated, and more studies of larger numbers are needed to reach a definitive answer regarding the clinical significance of this procedure.

SECOND TRIMESTER AMNIOCENTESIS

Second trimester genetic amniocentesis remains the most widely utilized and accepted method of prenatal diagnosis. Amniocentesis is usually performed at 16 to 18 weeks gestational age under ultrasound guidance. Sampling success rates are very high, and with able sonographic assistance it is a relatively simple procedure for the experienced obstetrician.

The addition of color Doppler imaging provides, in our experience, little added benefit to high-resolution gray-scale ultrasound in routine second trimester genetic amniocentesis.

AMNIOINFUSION

Severe oligohydramnios presents significant diagnostic difficulties to the obstetrician along with the likelihood of adverse fetal outcome. This is true especially when it occurs in the second trimester. The ability to visualize fetal anatomy, in particular the genitourinary system, is severely limited by marked oligohydramnios. In addition, prolonged and early oligohydramnios may result in fetal pulmonary hypoplasia, intrauterine growth retardation, musculoskeletal abnormalities, and facial deformities.[13–18] Several other reports have documented the poor perinatal outcome of pregnancies with this diagnosis as management options were limited until recently.[19,20]

The use of *amnioinfusion* has in recent years shown a great promise both in diagnosis and in potential in utero treatment of oligohydramnios. Installation of fluid into the uterine cavity via amnioinfusion often provides great improvement in visualization of fetal anatomy in patients with oligohydramnios. In addition, access to the uterine cavity during this procedure may offer more precise ultrasound imaging of the umbilical cord insertion for future cordocentesis and the opportunity for dye injection into the uterine cavity in cases of suspected rupture of membranes. Finally, by increasing amniotic fluid volume, umbilical cord compression can be relieved and fetal oxygenation could improve.

Recent works by several investigators have provided further possible diagnostic and treatment options through amnioinfusion. Using intrauterine manometry, Nicolini et al. have established that amniotic fluid pressures are decreased with severe oligohydramnios and that abnormal intrauterine pressure gradients may be responsible for the significant incidence of pulmonary hypoplasia in these fetuses.[21–23] By installing normal saline into the uterine cavity through amnioinfusion, they were able to restore normal amniotic fluid pressures and markedly improve anatomic diagnosis. Their efforts were also promising in demonstrating a reduction in the incidence of skeletal deformities, and possibly pulmonary hypoplasia, through serial amnioinfusions, by decreasing intrauterine crowding and increasing amniotic fluid pressure.[24] Amnioinfusion is commonly performed by inserting a 20-gauge spinal needle, under ultrasound visualization, into the uterine cavity and installing warmed normal saline or electrolyte solution into the intrauterine space.[23,25] We have utilized color Doppler imaging to identify the umbilical cord and to avoid the choosing of a cord-filled amniotic fluid pocket as the site for needle insertion and saline infusion (Figs. 13-3 and 13-4). With oligohydramnios, these pockets containing cord loops are often difficult to image without color Doppler imaging. As mentioned previously, the use of amnioinfusion in conjunction with color Doppler, may also improve optimal access to the placental cord insertion or free cord loops for cordocentesis to further aid in the diagnostic evaluation of oligohydramnios.

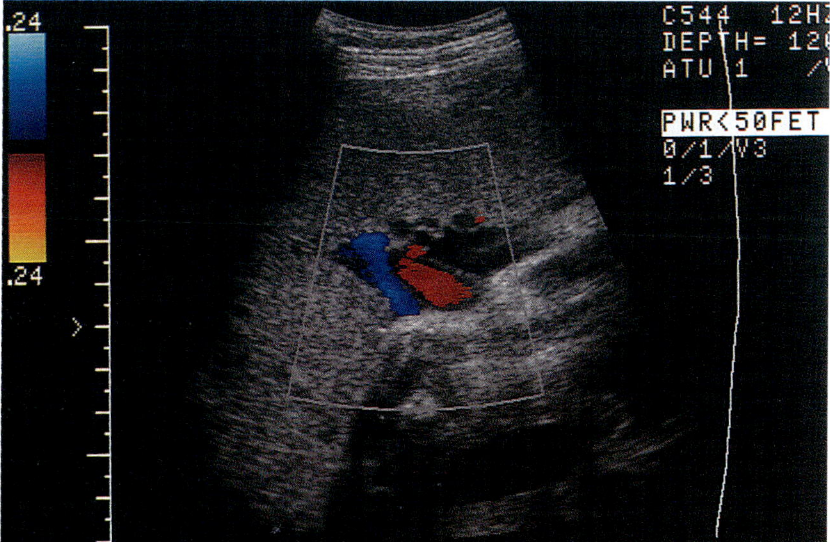

Figure 13-3   Umbilical cord insertion in severe oligohydramnios.

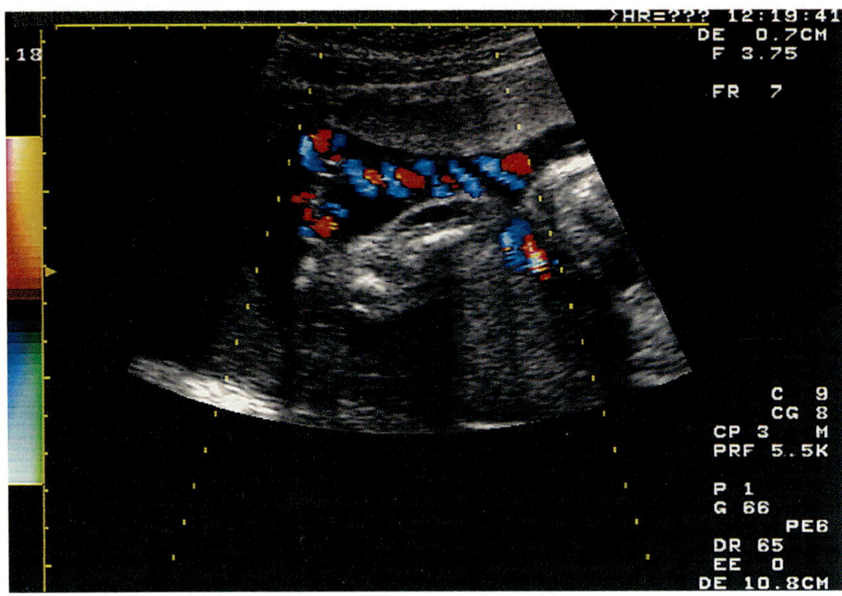

Figure 13-4 The cord clearly visualized by color Doppler imaging in oligohydramnios to avoid cord puncture.

CORDOCENTESIS

Direct access to the fetal circulation has long been a goal of the perinatologist to permit a greater understanding of fetal physiology and provide a direct approach to prenatal diagnosis and treatment.

Ultrasound-guided *fetal umbilical blood sampling* may offer a relatively safe technique by which fetal intravascular access can be obtained.

Historically, Valenti[26] first described fetal blood sampling in 1973 for the detection of hemoglobinopathies. During the following decade, several approaches to fetal blood sampling were described, and they all had severe limitations or involved a significant risk to the fetus. Placental aspiration with ultrasound guidance yielded a 78 percent rate of maternal blood contamination.[27] *Fetoscopy* was developed to observe the fetus for pathognomonic structural features[28,29] with a second channel in the fetoscopy permitting guidance of a thin needle into a fetal vessel on the placental surface. However, maternal blood and amniotic fluid contamination was common. This procedure can be readily performed only during a limited period in the second trimester with a risk of miscarriage of 2 to 5 percent.[30] A third technique, *fetal scalp blood sampling,* is feasible only when the uterine cervix is dilated and the membranes ruptured. These conditions limit the usefulness of fetal scalp blood sampling to patients in active labor.

Direct access to fetal circulation during the second and third trimester of pregnancy using an ultrasonographically guided needle insertion is now feasible, overcoming the limitations of earlier sampling techniques.[31–34]

Percutaneous umbilical blood sampling (PUBS), or cordocentesis, involves the insertion of a needle directly into a fetal umbilical vessel. Percutaneous umbilical blood sampling can be accomplished between 17 and 40 weeks of gestation, although there is one center in Italy that is performing cordocentesis at 12 to 13 weeks.[35] It has an acceptable low complication rate and promises a tremendous potential for fetal evaluation and intrauterine treatment.

FETAL BLOOD SAMPLING: TECHNIQUE

Direct access to the fetal circulation using real-time ultrasonographic guidance of a needle is achieved by placing the tip of the needle into an umbilical vessel (vein or artery) (Fig. 13-5), hepatic vein, or by direct intracardiac insertion of the needle. The most commonly used procedure is the insertion of the needle into an umbilical vessel. Prior to viability, the procedure can be performed in an outpatient facility. When fetal viability is achieved, the procedure must be

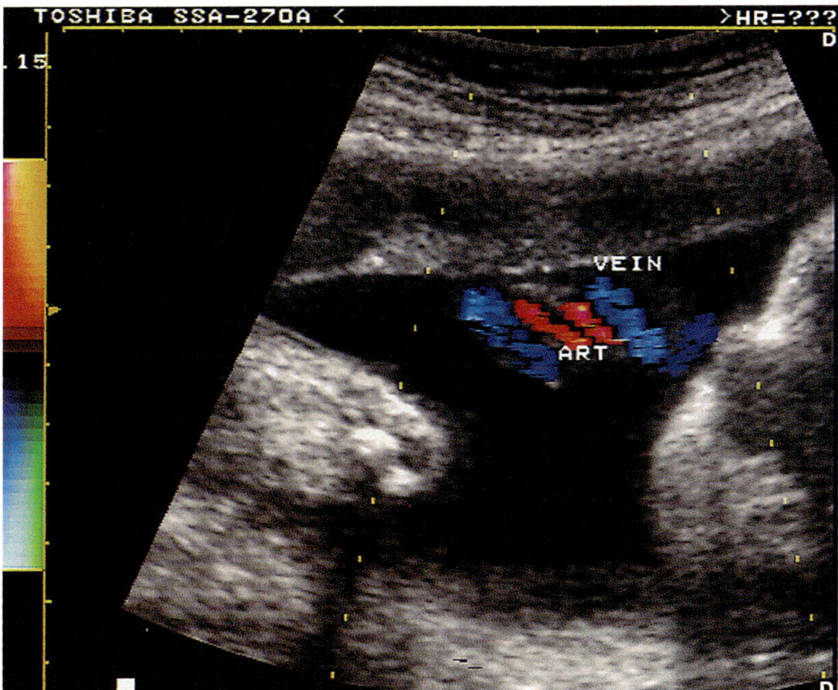

Figure 13-5   A color Doppler image of the umbilical cord clearly demonstrating the separate vein and arteries.

done near an operating room to be able to perform an emergency cesarean section if fetal distress develops. Basic ultrasonic measurements are performed to confirm gestational age, estimate fetal weight, and exclude fetal anatomic malformations. High-resolution real-time ultrasound using a 3- to 5-MHz linear or sector transducer is used to locate the umbilical cord insertion site on the placenta (Fig. 13-6). Color Doppler imaging can be helpful in difficult cases (Fig. 13-7).

The nonsterile gel is then removed from the maternal skin, and the patient is prepared as for an operative procedure. The performer wears a surgical hat, gloves, mask, and gown, and the maternal abdomen is prepared with povidone and sterile drapes. The ultrasound transducer is covered with a sterile cover, and sterile gel is placed on the patient's skin. Placental location and insertion site of the needle are again defined by the investigators. A freehand technique and a needle guiding device attached to the transducer are two ways to perform the procedure.

Local anesthesia is administered in the area where the needle will be inserted into the patient's abdominal wall.

The most common needles used for this procedure are 10 to 16-cm spinal needles, based on the measured distance from the skin surface to the targeted segment of the umbilical cord. The needles range from 20 to 25 gauge with the

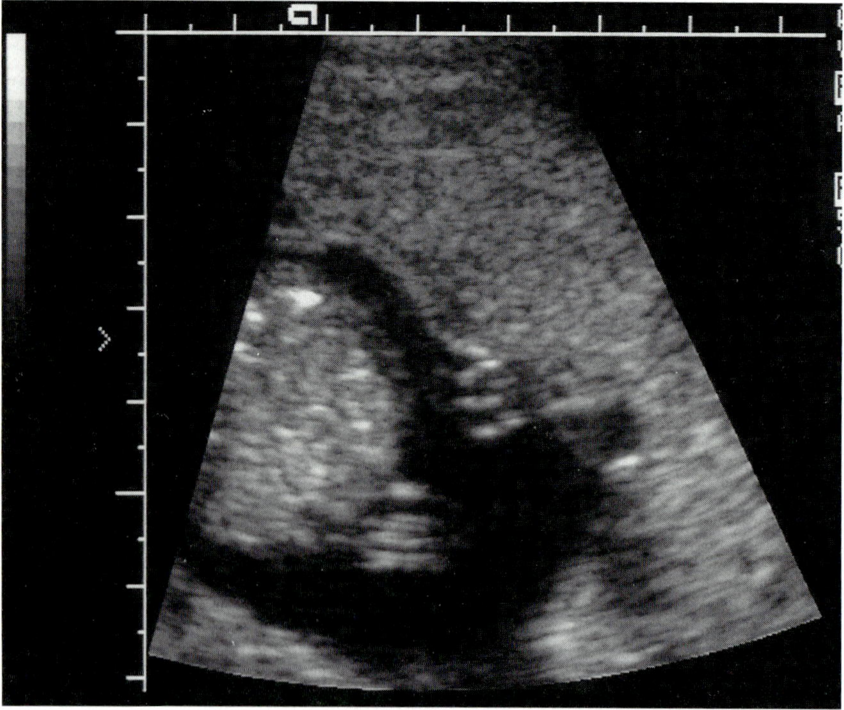

Figure 13-6 Cord insertion at placental site using sector a transducer.

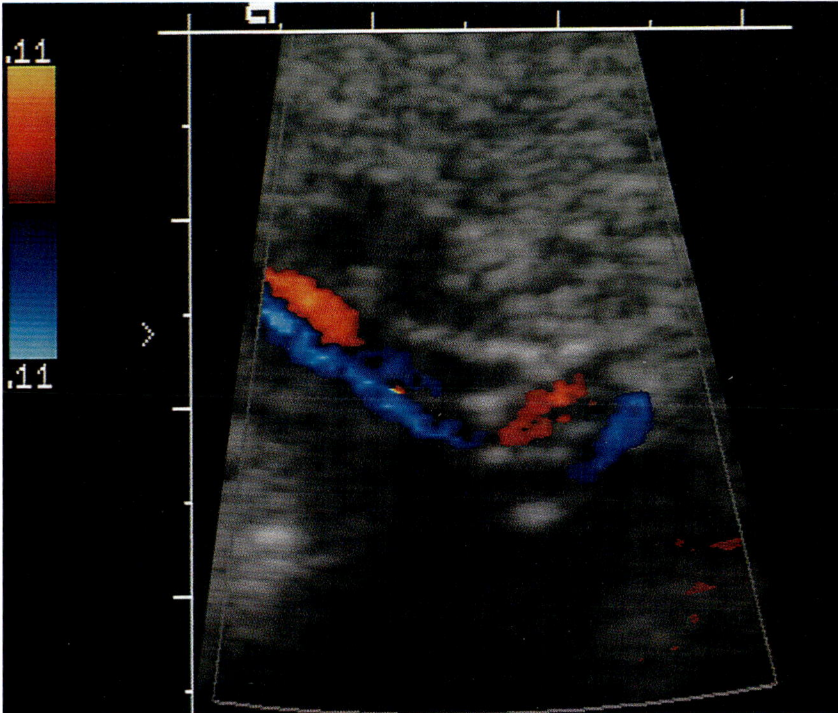

Figure 13-7   Improved visualization of umbilical cord direction using color Doppler imaging.

22-gauge needle most widely used. The needle is then inserted and followed by ultrasound guidance into the umbilical vessel. Ideally, the umbilical cord is punctured 1 to 2 cm from its placental insertion. At this point the cord is well anchored and will not move, and the risk of maternal blood contamination from the placenta is small. Either the umbilical vein or artery can be sampled with apparently equal success and safety, although there is some concern about vascular spasm and fetal bradycardia after arterial puncture. This is significant, especially in intrauterine growth retarded fetuses. If fetal therapy, i.e., transfusion, is contemplated, however, there might be some advantage to entering a fetal umbilical artery. Nevertheless, the vein is often more easily punctured because of its larger diameter, straighter course, and thinner vessel wall. When the needle tip has been inserted into the vessel lumen, the stylet is removed and 0.5 cm^3 of fetal blood is aspirated into a small heparinized syringe (citrate can also be used) and discarded to avoid maternal contamination. The diagnostic sample (0.5 to 3.0 cm^3 based on gestational age) is then aspirated into a new syringe and immediately labeled and transferred for analysis. The specimen must, of course, bc placcd in a test tube containing the appropriate medium for the specific biologic assay.

Placement of the needle tip in the vessel is best guided by ultrasound views that offer a cross section of the vessel and the middle shaft with the tip at the same time. If the position of the needle tip is uncertain, the injection of 3 mL of Ringer's lactate solution will demonstrate a typical ultrasound picture of intravascular turbulence if the needle is in place. In addition, if simultaneous two-dimensional and pulse Doppler information is available, placement of the Doppler sample at the needle tip may help confirm intravascular placement. This may also be used to monitor fetal heart rate during the procedure and eliminate the need for movement of the transducer to view the fetal heart, a procedure which might cause dislocation of the needle tip from the umbilical cord vessel.

If the placenta is implanted on the anterior wall of the uterus, the umbilical vessel may be entered directly through the placenta without traversing the amniotic cavity. Although this anatomic arrangement is technically easiest in most operators' hands, there is a concern that this approach may worsen maternal blood group sensitization. To overcome this problem, Nicolini et al.[36,37] proposed the fetal intrahepatic umbilical vein as an alternative to cord needling for prenatal diagnosis and therapy. With a posterior or fundal placenta, the cordocentesis needle is guided through the amniotic cavity to a point 1 to 2 cm from the cord insertion into the placenta. In cases of oligohydramnios or in a posterior insertion late in pregnancy when the insertion is not accessible, we accomplish fetal blood sampling by puncturing the free-floating loop and fixing the cord between the needle and the posterior wall of the uterus or the fetal body. When the sampling is completed, the needle is withdrawn and continuous real-time ultrasound visualization of the puncture site is performed to detect any blood leakage. Fetal heart rate monitoring is performed for 1 to 2 h if the fetus is deemed viable (gestational age of 24 weeks or more). A course of a broad-spectrum antibiotic for 3 to 5 days is administered to the patient following the procedure.

The employment of color Doppler imaging can be very helpful when performing cordocentesis in cases of severe oligohydramnios. In these situations, the absence of the "amniotic fluid window" does not permit easy identification of the umbilical cord insertion into the placenta and makes the procedure much more difficult. Color Doppler imaging enables the operator to insert the needle in the correct direction and angle to successfully achieve a blood sample.

REFERENCES

1. Rhoades GG, Jackson LG, Schlesselman SE, et al.: The safety and efficacy of chorionic villus sampling for early prenatal diagnosis of cytogenic abnormalities. N Engl J Med 320:609–617, 1989.
2. Ferguson JE, Vick DJ, Hogge JS, Hogge WA: Transcervical chorionic villus sampling and amniocentesis: a comparison of reliability, culture findings, and fetal outcome. Am J Obstet Gynecol 163:926–931, 1990.
3. Crane JP, Beaver HA, Cheung SW: First trimester chorionic villus sampling versus mid-trimester

genetic amniocentesis—preliminary results of a controlled prospective trial. Prenat Diagn 8:355–366, 1988.

4. Brambati B, Oldrini A, Ferrazzi E, Lanzani A: Chorionic villus sampling: an analysis of the obstetric experience of 1000 cases. Prenat Diagn 7:157–169, 1987.

5. Ledbetter DH, Martin AO, Verlinsky V, et al.: Cytogenetic results of chorionic villus sampling: high success rate and diagnostic accuracy in the United States, Collaborative study. Am J Obstet Gynecol 162:495–501, 1990.

6. Jahoda MGJ, Pijpers L, Reuss A, Lost FJ, Wladimiroff JW, Sacks ES: Evaluation of transcervical chorionic villus sampling with a completed follow-up of 1550 consecutive pregnancies. Prenat Diagn 9:621–628, 1989.

7. Brambati G, L Tulvi, G Simioni, M Travi: Genetic diagnosis before the eight gestational week. Obstet Gynecol 77:318–321, 1991.

8. Nicolaides KH, Rodeck CH, Soothill PW, et al.: Why confine chorionic villus (placental) biopsy to the first trimester? Lancet 1:543–544, 1986.

9. Brambati B, Lanzani A, Oldrini A: Transabdominal chorionic villus sampling. Clinical experience of 1159 cases. Prenat Diagn 8:609–617, 1988.

10. Godmilow L, Weiner S, Dunn L: Genetic amniocentesis performed between 12 and 14 weeks. Am J Hum Genet 41(suppl):A275, 1987.

11. Platt LD, DeVore GR, Gilmousky ML: Failed amniocentesis: the role of membrane testing. Am J Obstet Gynecol 144:479–480, 1982.

12. Benacerraf BR et al.: Early amniocentesis for prenatal cytogenetic evaluation. Radiology 169:709–710, 1988.

13. Thibeault DW, Beatty EC, Hall RT, Bowen SK, O'Neill DH: Neonatal pulmonary hypoplasia with premature rupture of fetal membranes and oligohydramnios. J Pediat 107:273–277, 1985.

14. Chamberlain PF, Manning FA, Morrison I, Harman CR, Lange IR: Ultrasound evaluation of amniotic fluid volume. Am J Obstet Gynecol 150:245–249, 1984.

15. Nimrod C, Varela-Gittings F, Machin G, Campbell D, Wesenberg R: The effect of very prolonged membrane rupture on fetal development. Am J Obstet Gynecol 148:540–543, 1984.

16. Potter EL: Bilateral absence of ureters and kidneys. Obstet Gynecol 25:3–12, 1965.

17. Adzick NS, Harrison MR, Glick PL, Villa RL, Finkbeiner W: Experimental pulmonary hypoplasia and oligohydramnios: relative contributions of lung fluid and fetal breathing movements. J Pediatr Surg 19:658–663, 1984.

18. Thomas IT, Smith DW: Oligohydramnios, cause of the nonrenal features of Potter's syndrome, including pulmonary hypoplasia. J Pediatr 84:811–814, 1974.

19. Barss VA, Benacerraf BR, Frigoletto FD: Second trimester oligohydramnios, a predictor of poor fetal outcome. Obstet Gynecol 64:608–610, 1984.

20. Koontz WL, Seeds JW, Adams NJ, Johnson AM, Cefalo RC: Elevated maternal serum alpha-feto-protein, second trimester oligohydramnios, and pregnancy outcome. Obstet Gynecol 62:301–304, 1983.

21. Nicolini U, Fisk NM, Rodeck CH, Talbert DG, Wigglesworth JS: Low amniotic pressure in oligohydramnios—is this the cause of pulmonary hypoplasia? Am J Obstet Gynecol 161:1098–1101, 1989.

22. Nicolini U, Fisk NM, Talbert DG, Rodeck CH, Kochemour NK, Greco P, Hubinot C, Santolaya J: Intrauterine manometry: technique and application to fetal pathology. Prenat Diagn 9:243–254, 1989.

23. Fisk NM, Tannirandorn Y, Nicolini U, Talbert DG, Rodeck CH: Amniotic pressure in disorders of amniotic fluid volume. Obstet Gynecol 76:210–214, 1990.

24. Fisk NM, Ronderos-Dumit D, Soliani A, Nicolini U, Vaugham J, Rodeck CH: Diagnostic and therapeutic transabdominal amnioinfusion in oligohydramnios. Obstet Gynecol 78:270–278, 1991.

25. Gembrunch U, Hansmann M: Artificial instillation of amniotic fluid as a new technique for the diagnostic evaluation of cases of oligohydramnios. Prenat Diagn 8:33–45, 1988.

26. Valenti C: Antenatal detection of hemoglobinopathies: a preliminary report. Am J Obstet Gynecol 115:851–853, 1973.
27. Cao A, Furbetta M, Angius A, et al.: Hematological and obstetrical aspects of antenatal diagnosis of beta thalassemia: Experience with 200 cases. J Med Genet 19:81–87, 1982.
28. Hobbins J, Mahoney MJ: Fetoscopy in continuing pregnancies. Am J Obstet Gynecol 129:440–442, 1977.
29. Rodeck CH, Campbell S: Umbilical cord insertion as a source of pure fetal blood for prenatal diagnosis. Lancet 1:1244–5, 1979.
30. Special report: The status of fetoscopy and fetal tissue sampling. Prenat Diagn 4:79–81, 1984.
31. Daffos F, Cappella-Pavlovsky M, Forestier F: Fetal blood sampling via the umbilical cord using a needle guided by ultrasound. Report of 66 cases. Prenat Diagn 3:271–277, 1983.
32. Daffos F, Cappella-Pavlovsky M, Forestier F: Fetal blood sampling during pregnancy with use of needle guided by ultrasound: a study of 606 consecutive cases. Am J Obstet Gynecol 153:655–660, 1985.
33. Weiner CP: Cordocentesis for diagnostic indications: two years' experience. Obstet Gynecol 70:664–668, 1987.
34. Ludomirski A, Weiner S: Percutaneous fetal umbilical blood sampling. Clin Obstet Gynecol 31:19–26, 1988.
35. Orlandi F, Damiani C, Jakil S, Lauricellar S, Bertolino O, Maggio A: The risks of early cordocentesis (12–21 weeks): Analysis of 500 procedures. Prenat Diagn 10:425–428, 1990.
36. Nicolini U, Santolaya J, Ojo OE, Fisk NM, Hubinot C, Tonge M, Rodeck CH: The fetal intrahepatic umbilical vein as an alternative to cord needling for prenatal diagnosis and therapy. Prenat Diagn 8:665–671, 1988.
37. Nicolini U, Kochenour NK, Creco P, Letshy EA, Johnson RD, Contreras M, Rodeck CH: Consequences of fetomaternal hemorrhage after intrauterine transfusion. Br Med J 297:1379–1381, 1988.

FOURTEEN

NORMAL AND ABNORMAL UTERINE PERFUSION

ASIM KURJAK
SANJA KUPESIC-UREK

Transvaginal color Doppler is a new technique that gives information related to the physiologic state of the pelvic circulation.[1–3]

The uterus has an extensive vascular network. The blood supply to the uterus is from the uterine artery, which is a branch of the hypogastric artery. The color Doppler signal from the main uterine vessels can be seen laterally to the cervix at the level of the cervicocorporeal junction of the uterus.[4] The arcuate vessels can be visualized in the outer third of the myometrium, and the uterine venous structures are more prominent than the arterial. There is no significant difference in uterine artery blood flow between both sides.[5,6] The uterine perfusion is largely dependent on the patient's age, phase of the menstrual cycle, and other specific conditions (e.g., pregnancy, tumor).[7]

The increase in blood flow to the uterus in response to estrogens during a normal menstrual cycle is well documented.[8,9] The decreased impedance to blood flow in the uterine artery is noticed during the week preceding spontaneous ovulation and during the secretory phase of the menstrual cycle.[10]

BENIGN UTERINE MASSES

Leiomyoma

Leiomyomas are common tumors consisting of smooth muscle and connective tissue. Actually, it is estimated that myomas are present in 20 percent of women over 35 years of age. Myomas usually develop in the myometrium of the upper contractile fundal and corporeal portions of the uterus. Only 3 percent is of the cervical region.

Leiomyomas can remain intramural, or they can extend into the uterine lumen to become submucosal or outward to become subserosal or pedunculated. Myomas are usually multiple and of various sizes. Since leiomyomas have a varying amount of smooth muscle and connective tissue, these benign uterine tumors also have a variety of sonographic features. The echogenicity of a fibroid depends on the relative ratio of fibrous tissue to smooth muscle, the presence and type of degeneration, and the vascular supply.[1,11–13]

The most common cause of calcification within the uterus is calcific degeneration within a fibroid. Other types of degeneration within myomas include cystic, myxomatous, and hyaline degeneration. In some cases vaginal sonography with high frequency and high-resolution capability is definitive in separating adnexal masses from uterine pathology.[14]

The addition of color flow imaging facilitates the measurement of blood flow impedance in small vascular branches and increases the reproducibility of mea-

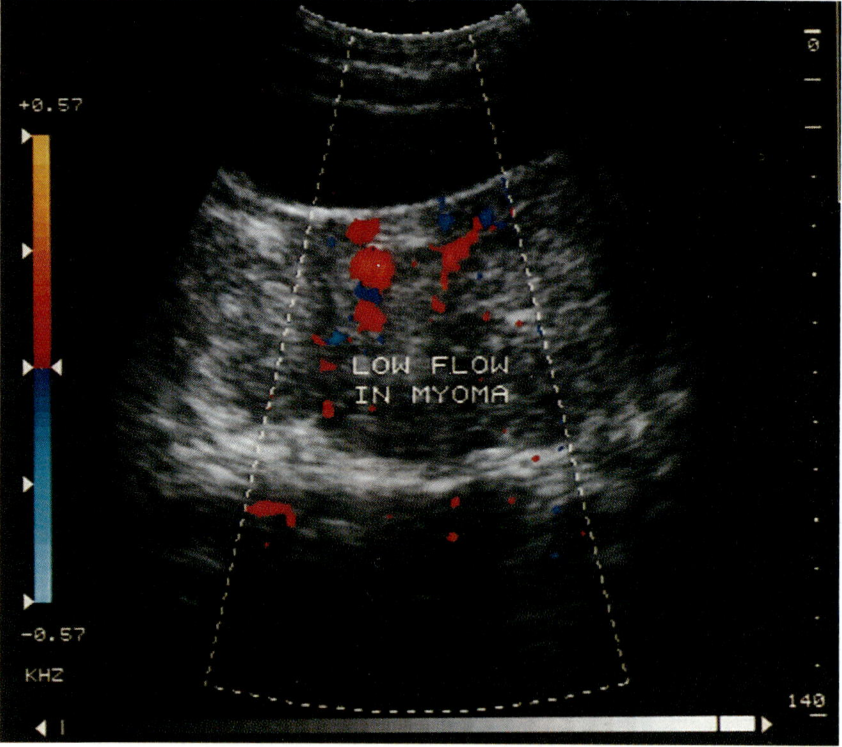

Figure 14-1 Color flow imaging of abundant small vessel blood flow within a fibroid uterus.

surements. Small vessels which feed growing tumor tissue can easily be detected by transvaginal color Doppler[2,3,12] (Fig. 14-1).

Transvaginal color Doppler is a noninvasive diagnostic tool that can be used for assessing the fibroid vascularity as well as physiologic and pathophysiologic characteristics of uterine artery blood flow.[1] This is an established technique in evaluation of the impedance to flow as measured by the resistance index (RI) and pulsatility index (PI) (Chap. 1).

The vascularization of benign uterine masses is supported by normally existing vessels: the myometrial vessels originating from terminal branches of the uterine artery. The Zagreb group studied fibroid arterial supply and uterine flow in 161 patients: 101 patients with palpable uterine fibroids and 60 women attending the clinic for annual checkups. The diastolic flow was always present in the tumors and was usually increased in comparison to that of the uterine artery. The mean Pourcelot resistance index of myometrial blood flow was 0.54 (Table 14-1) and the mean PI was 0.89. The vascularization of the benign uterine masses was largely dependent on the tumor size, its position, and the extent of secondary degenerative changes. Large and laterally positioned fibroids, and especially those with necrosis, degenerative, and inflammatory changes, showed increased diastolic flow and lower RI ($RI_{min} = 0.35$) (Fig. 14-2). Uterine artery flow velocity had a RI of 0.84 in the control group, whereas a decreased RI of 0.74 was noted

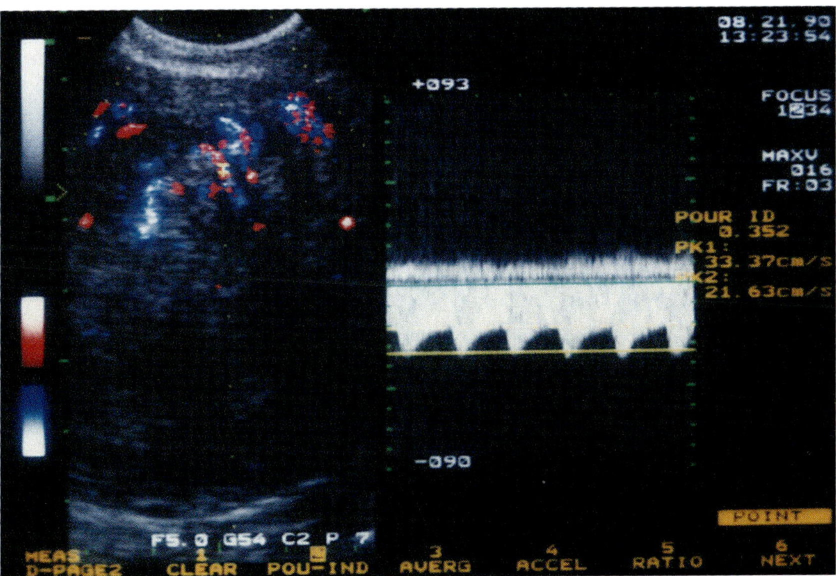

Figure 14-2 Transvaginal scan of the uterus with a uterine fibroid in the posterior wall and superimposed color Doppler (*left*). Waveform analysis (*left*) indicates high velocity and low resistance of the tumor blood flow (RI = 0.35). Necrosis and degenerative and inflammatory changes within the fibroid were confirmed by histopathology.

in the group with uterine fibroids. The difference in uterine artery blood flow between patients with fibroids and healthy volunteers was statistically significant and may have a predictable value in growth rate evaluation of benign uterine masses.

Adenomyosis

Adenomyosis, or internal endometriosis, is characterized by ingrowth of endometrium into the myometrium.[15,16] Histologically, glandular and stromal elements are observed among muscular fibers. Sonographically, there is a spectrum of different appearances: from a slightly enlarged uterus with small cystic structures affecting the uterine texture homogenicity to multiple adenomyomas.[17] This condition can be sonographically diagnosed to have a thickened and "swiss cheese" appearance due to areas of hemorrhage and clotting within the muscle.[18] Flow-velocity waveform analysis of the vessels observed in this condition showed a mean RI of 0.58 (Table 14-1). Intrauterine endometriotic cysts usually do not demonstrate increased vascularity.[12]

Endometrial Hyperplasia

Transvaginal sonography clearly depicts changes in the endometrial texture and thickness during the menstrual cycle.[19] In perimenopausal women an endometrial thickness greater than 12 mm is an indication for further investigation. The same is true for postmenopausal women with an endometrium thicker than 8 mm. The sonographic findings have to be interpreted in light of the patient's clinical presentation and laboratory findings. The peak incidence of adenomatous hyperplasia is between 40 and 50 years of age.[20] Some data indicate that lesions with malignant potential can be identified by cytologic atypia at the time of the initial diagnosis.[21] Medical evaluation and treatment of such patients have to be more aggressive and will often lead to hysterectomy. Color flow was always present on the border of the hyperplastic endometrium showing moderately high to very high RI (RI > 0.50) (Table 14-1).

Table 14-1   Transvaginal color Doppler assessment of benign uterine masses (n = 175)

Histopathology	Total n	Color flow n	%	RI (2 SD)
Leiomyoma	101	71	70.3	0.54 (0.09)
Adenomyosis	46	32	69.6	0.58 (0.12)
Endometriotic cyst	3	0	—	—
Endometrial hyperplasia	14	9	64.3	0.50 (0.07)
Endometrial polyps	11	5	45.5	0.48 (0.06)

Endometrial Polyp

Endometrial polyps develop as solitary or multiple soft, sessile, and pedunculated tumors often composed of hyperplastic endometrium.[22,23] The clinical picture is one of nonspecific abnormal uterine bleeding. Endometrial polyps differ in size and location, and most arise in the fundus or cornua of the uterus. Approximately two-thirds contain no functional endometrium, and they often display a microscopic picture of cystic hyperplasia. In such lesions color Doppler signals are usually not found (Fig. 14-3). Sometimes polyps are necrotic and inflamed, and in these cases it is possible to identify flow in thin vessels and analyze the velocity of blood flow through them. The diastolic flow is always present, and the RI is higher than 0.45 (Table 14-1).

Endometritis can produce increased echogenicity, thickness, and vascularity of the endometrium.[23] The waveforms in these cases always showed a moderately high RI (RI > 0.52).

MALIGNANT UTERINE MASSES

Endometrial Cancer

Malignant uterine tumors are difficult to distinguish from fibromas. Typical findings include uterine enlargement and nonhomogeneous tumor texture due to

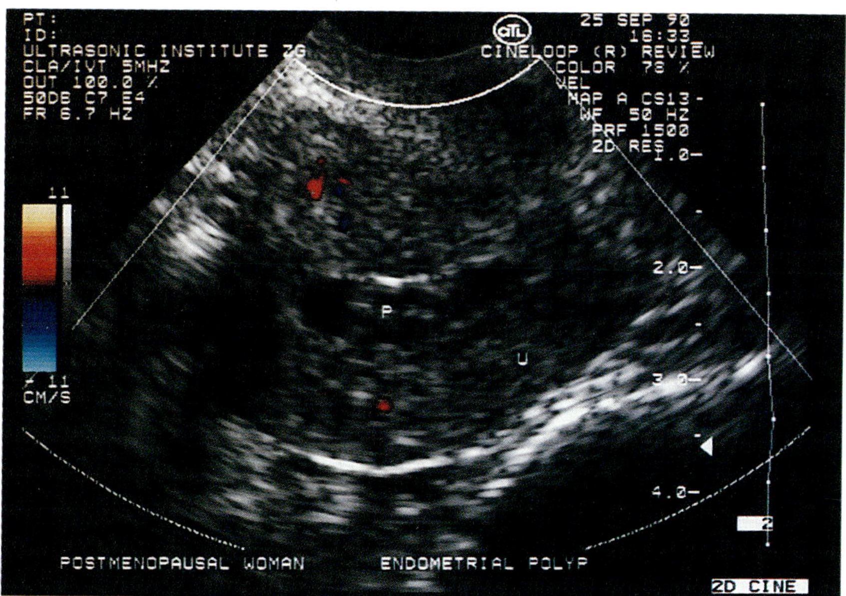

Figure 14-3 Transvaginal longitudinal scan of the uterus. In the uterine cavity an endometrial polyp is clearly visible (P) as a homogenous echogenic structure in the middle.

necrosis and other secondary changes. Pathologic proliferation of the endometrium may be visualized a long time before symptoms become apparent.[23] Advanced carcinomas of the endometrium always show a pathologically thickened endometrium with a typical "fuzzy," nonhomogeneous margins toward the myometrium and a typical echo-poor area of carcinoma invasion into the myometrium.[24,25] The depth of invasion of an endometrial carcinoma (superficial, intermediate, deep), its longitudinal dimension, and possible involvement of the cervix can be evaluated. More differentiated tumors tend to be more echogenic than the less differentiated. Our preliminary data show the great potential of transvaginal color Doppler ultrasonography in early and precise detection of malignant tumors. One of the major advantages of the color Doppler is rapid visualization of newly formed tumor vessels. Being very thin and randomly dispersed within the tissue, such vessels were difficult to find before the use of transvaginal color Doppler.[12] Sequential use of this technique to detect the vascularization and measure the impedance to blood flow in the uterus should allow early detection of malignant tumors. Based on our own experience, this technique is going to play the major role in noninvasive characterization of uterine malignancy and may so directly influence therapeutic procedures. An abnormal blood flow pattern has been noted in all cases of endometrial adenocarcinoma. The typical finding was the presence of thin, irregular, and randomly dispersed vessels. Pulsed Doppler demonstrated low velocity and low resistance to blood flow (mean RI = 0.35) in all these cases (Table 14-2 and Fig. 14-4A and B).

Leiomyosarcoma

Leiomyosarcomas are uncommon tumors of mixed origin containing stromal and müllerian elements.[1] Patients tend to be in their 50s and 60s and are postmenopausal. The uterus is usually enlarged two to three times the normal size and is filled with polypoid masses. This tumor can arise from a preexisting leiomyoma, muscle, connective tissue within the myometrium, or blood vessels.

Table 14-2 Transvaginal color Doppler in the assessment of malignant uterine masses (*n* = 18)

Histopathology	Total *n*	Color flow *n*	%	RI (2 SD)
Endometrial cancer	14	14	100	0.35 (0.05)
Leiomyosarcoma	3	3	100	0.31 (0.03)
Sarcoma botryoides	1	1	100	0.33

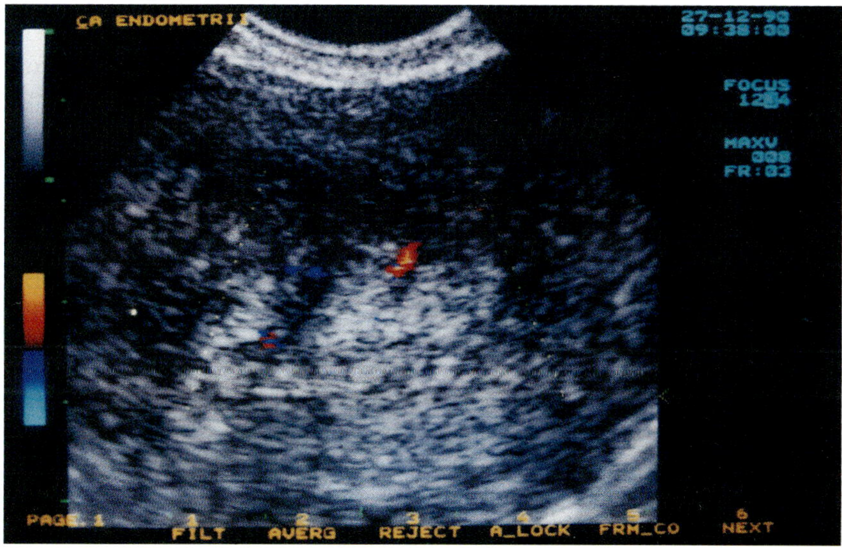

A

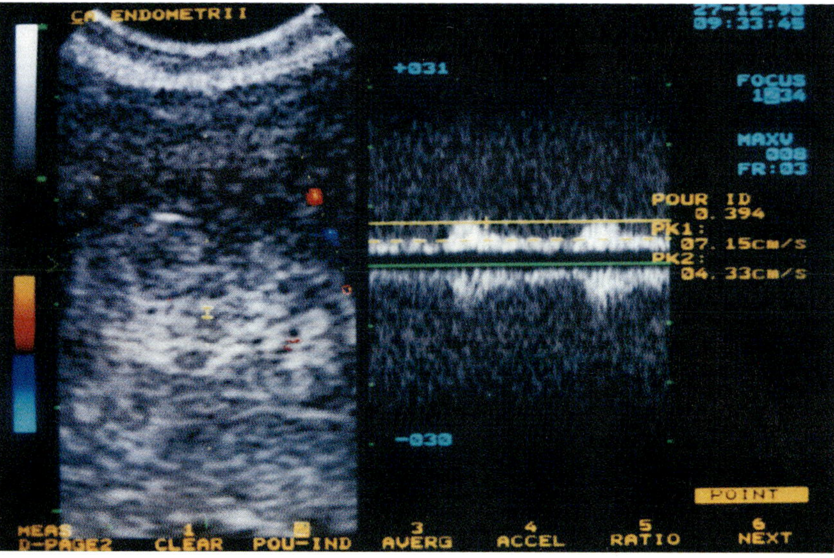

B

Figure 14-4   Color and pulsed Doppler ultrasound findings in a patient with endometrial cancer. *A.* Proliferation of the endometrium is clearly visible. *B.* Waveform analysis shows a very low resistance index (RI = 0.39), which is highly suggestive of an endometrial cancer.

Sarcoma Botryoides

Sarcoma botryoides is a rare tumor arising from the uterus in children.[26] Ultrasonographically, it appears as a complex, large, polypoid mass that deforms the uterine outline. Abundant color signals are obtained from these malignant uterine masses.[27] Waveform analysis of flow in thin vessels shows high velocity and very low resistance to flow (mean RI = 0.32) (Table 14-2). The amount of color corresponds with the number of vessels and blood flow through them.

INFERTILITY

Blood flow studies of the pelvic circulation represents the most recent development in the ultrasound assessment of infertile patients.[28] Because of the short distance between the probe and the vessels, improved resolution, and a patient's convenience, as a full bladder is not necessary, transvaginal color Doppler will become the technique of choice for the scanning of the pelvic circulation in fertility patients.[4–6]

The uterine artery blood flow can easily be seen just lateral to the cervix at the level of the cervicocorporeal junction. The use of blood flow studies in uterine arteries has shown that there is a small diastolic flow component in these arteries during the proliferative phase. The results of an interesting study carried out on 100 infertile women and compared with 150 women attending the clinic for annual checkup follows. Uterine artery flow velocity waveforms had a resistance index of 0.88 in the proliferative phase with a decline starting the day before ovulation. A nadir of 0.84 ± 0.04 was reached on day 18 and the RI remained at that level for the rest of the cycle. In unovulatory cycles these changes did not occur. Some women with primary infertility showed marked reduction in uterine artery flow velocities. It was also recognized that in some infertile patients end-diastolic flow was absent. A significant decline in the resistance index began prior to ovulation and persistently lower RIs were demonstrated until the onset of menstruation. Since the changes in uterine flow velocities began prior ovulation, they may involve angiogenesis as well as hormonal factors (Fig. 14-5).

Transvaginal color Doppler imaging facilitates the identification of small vascular branches. The accuracy of the measurements is increased because of better resolution and shorter examination time.[28] By using transvaginal color Doppler imaging, it is possible to observe intraovarian (follicular and luteal) blood flow and study the alterations of the radial and spiral arterial blood flows under physiologic and pathophysiologic conditions. The knowledge of the alterations of endometrial blood flow may play an important role in predicting the optimal time for implantation and embryo transfer.

Transvaginal color Doppler imaging may in the future give us the answers to some interesting questions: Do blood flow changes play a role in infertility, and is inadequate vascularization responsible for early pregnancy loss? This simple

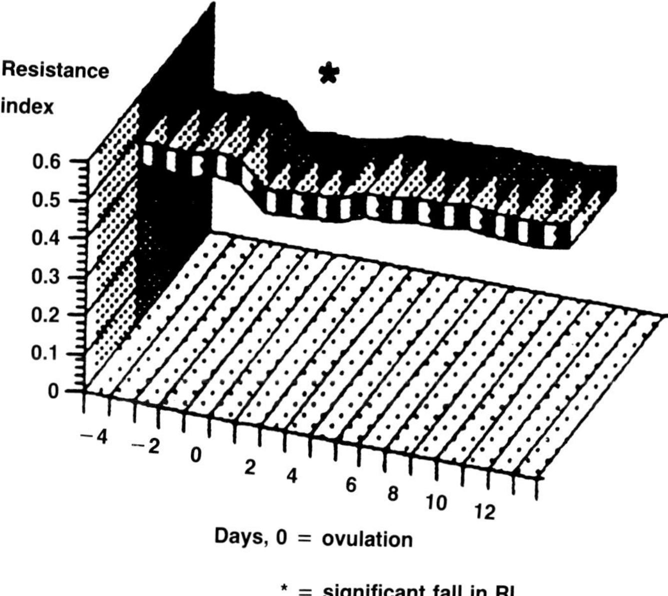

Figure 14-5 Ovarian flow velocity waveform RIs during a normal menstrual cycle. (From Kurjak A, Kupesic-Urek S, Schulman H, Zalud I: Transvaginal color flow Doppler in the assessment of ovarian and uterine blood flow in infertile women. *Fertil Steril* 56:870–873, 1991. Reproduced with permission of the publisher, The American Fertility Society.)

and noninvasive technique has so far proved to be very useful, and its continued employment promises exciting future developments.

REFERENCES

1. Kurjak A, Zalud I: "Uterine masses," in Kurjak A (ed), *Transvaginal Color Doppler*. Lancs, UK, Parthenon Publishers, 1991, pp 123–135.
2. Kurjak A, Zalud I, Jurkovic D, Alfirevic Z, Miljan M: Transvaginal color Doppler for the assessment of pelvic circulation. Acta Obstet Gynecol Scand 68:131, 1989.
3. Kurjak A, Jurkovic D, Alfirevic Z, Zalud I: Transvaginal color Doppler imaging. J Clin Ultrasound 18:227, 1990.
4. Kurjak A, Kupesic-Urek S, Schulman H, Zalud I: Transvaginal color flow Doppler in the assessment of ovarian and uterine blood flow in infertile women. Fertil Steril 56:870–873, 1991.
5. Goswamy RK, Williams G, Streptoe PC: Decreased uterine perfusion—a cause of infertility. Hum Reprod 33:955, 1988.
6. Goswamy RK, Streptoe PC: Doppler ultrasound studies of the uterine artery in spontaneous ovarian cycles. Hum Reprod 3:721, 1988.
7. Long MG, Boultbee JE, Hanson ME, Begent RHJ: Doppler time velocity waveform studies of the uterine artery and uterus. Br J Obstet Gynaecol 96:588–593, 1989.
8. Scholtes MCW, Wladimiroff JW, van Rijen HJM, Hop WCJ: Uterine and ovarian flow velocity

waveforms in the normal menstrual cycle: a transvaginal Doppler study. Fertil Steril 52:981–985, 1989.

9. Steer CV, Campbell S, Pampiglione JS, Kingsland CR, Mason BA, Collins WP: Transvaginal colour flow imaging of the uterine arteries during the ovarian and menstrual cycles. Hum Reprod 5:391, 1990.

10. Fleischer A: Ultrasound imaging 2000: assessment of utero-ovarian blood flow with transvaginal color Doppler sonography; potential clinical applications in infertility. Fertil Steril 55:684–691, 1991.

11. Hata T, Hata K, Senoch D, et al.: Transvaginal Doppler flow mapping. Gynecol Obstet Invest 27:217–218, 1990.

12. Kurjak A, Zalud I: The characterization of uterine tumors by transvaginal color Doppler. Ultrasound Obstet Gynecol 1:50–52, 1991.

13. Matta WM, Stabile I, Show RW, Campbell S: Doppler assessment of uterine blood flow changes in patients with fibroids receiving the gonadotropin-releasing hormone agonist Busereein. Fertil Steril 49:1083–1085, 1988.

14. Kurjak A, Zalud I: Transvaginal colour flow imaging and ovarian cancer. Br Med J 300:330, 1990.

15. Fleischer AC, Antman SS, Porrath SA, James AE: "Sonographic evaluation of uterine malformations and disorders," in Sanders RC (ed), *The Principles and Practice of Ultrasonography in Obstetrics and Gynecology*. Norwalk, Conn., Appleton-Century-Crofts, 1985, p 531.

16. Bowie J: Ultrasound of gynecologic pelvic masses: the indefinite uterus sizes and other patterns associated with diagnostic error. J Clin Ultrasound 5:323, 1977.

17. Timor-Trisch IE, Rottem S, Boldes R: "Scanning the uterus," in Timor-Trisch IE, Rottem S (eds), *Transvaginal Sonography*. New York, Elsevier, 1988, p 27.

18. Timor-Trisch IE, Rottem S, Thaler I: Review of transvaginal sonography: a description with clinical applications. Ultrasound Q 6:1, 1988.

19. Johnson M, Graham M, Cooperburg P: Abnormal endometrial echoes: sonographic spectrum of endometrial pathology. J Clin Ultrasound 1:181, 1982.

20. Ferenzy A: Endometrial hyperplasia and neoplasia: "A two-disease concept," in Berkowite RL, Cohen CJ, Kase NG (eds), *Obstetrics Ultrasonography/Gynecologic Oncology*. New York, Churchill-Livingstone, 1988, pp 197–213.

21. Osmers R, Volksen M, Schauer A: Vaginosonography for early detection of endometrial carcinoma. Lancet 335:1569–1571, 1990.

22. Lewit N, Thalet I, Rottem S: The uterus: a new look with transvaginal sonography. J Clin Ultrasound 18:331, 1990.

23. Fleischer AC, Gordon AN, Entman SS, Kepple DM: Transvaginal scanning of the endometrium. J Clin Ultrasound 18:337, 1990.

24. Fleischer AC, Dudley BS, Entman SS, Baxter JW, Kalemeris GC, James AE: Myometrial invasion by endometrial carcinoma: sonographic assessment. Radiology 162:303, 1987.

25. Cacciatore B, Lehtovitra P, Wahlstrom T: Preoperative sonographic evaluation of endometrial cancer. Am J Obstet Gynecol 160:133, 1989.

26. Woodring J, Halberg D, Daff D: Sarcoma botryoides of the uterus presenting as an abdominal mass: a case report. J Clin Ultrasound 10:347, 1982.

27. Folkman J: Anti-angiogenesis: new concept for therapy of solid tumors. Am Surg 175:183, 1972.

28. Kurjak A, Kupesic-Urek S: "Infertility," in Kurjak A (ed), *Transvaginal Color Doppler*. Lancs, UK, Parthenon Publishers, 1991, pp 33–41.

ULTRASOUND ASSESSMENT OF ADNEXAL MASSES

ASIM KURJAK
IVICA ZALUD

There are many clinical problems in differentiating benign and malignant adnexal masses in vivo. Known features that are characteristically different are the *mitotic index* and *pleomorphism,* but they cannot be detected by current imaging methods. However, many malignant tumors have bizarre vascular morphology with abnormal blood flow, which can be detected by Doppler ultrasound.

In general, tumor vasculature consists of (1) vessels recruited from the preexisting network of the host vasculature and (2) vessels recruited from the angiogenic response of host vessels to cancer cells.[1-3] Although the tumor vasculature originated from the host vasculature, its organization may be completely different depending on the tumor type, its growth rate and location. The architecture is different not only among various tumor types, but also between a spontaneous tumor and its transplants.[3] Macroscopically, the tumor vasculature can be studied in terms of two idealized categories: *peripheral* and *central* vasculatures. In tumors with peripheral vascularization, the centers are usually poorly perfused. In those with central vascularization, one would expect the opposite. In reality, a tumor may consist of many territories, each exhibiting one or the other of these two types of idealized vascular patterns.

NEOVASCULARIZATION

Great interest and study over the past few years have been focused on the process of *neovascularization (angiogenesis).* It is the process by which new blood vessels are induced, and it occurs in the corpus luteum, in embryogenesis, in tumors, and in wound healing. It is, therefore, a process of interest in relation to the application of Doppler ultrasound.

Solid tumor growth in animals and humans is accompanied by neovascularization. New capillary growth is elicited by a diffusible factor generated by malignant tumor cells. In the absence of neovascularization, most small tumors (2 to 3 mm in diameter) will become dormant.[4,5]

Folkman and collaborators have demonstrated that the development of an adequate vascular supply is critical to the growth and development of a cancer as well as its metastases.[6] When they injected cancer cells into the nonvascularized anterior chamber of a rabbit eye, nodules greater than 1 to 2 mm in diameter did not develop. However, the same cells introduced into a vascularized area of the eye developed a stromal blood supply and rapidly grew over the eye.[7] Thus, it is clear that tumor growth is dependent on blood supply. Often, primary tumors and their metastases outgrow their blood supply and undergo central ischemic necrosis, where the tumor cells are remote from the vascular supply of the normal surrounding tissue. Thus, with cancers, the primary lesions and their secondary implants may enlarge progressively while the central regions of necrosis expand.

The process of angiogenesis entails protease activity as well as cell differentiation, proliferation, and migration. The vascular morphology of one tumor differs from another and is determined to some extent by the growth pattern of cancer cells. Quantitative morphometric studies in induced animal tumors show that vascular volume, length, and surface area increase during the early stages of tumor growth and then decrease after the onset of necrosis. Frequency of large-diameter vessels increases in the later stages of growth.[8] New blood vessels and vascular channels in a tumor arise from older, preexisting vessels. Tumor vessels have a relative paucity of smooth muscle in their walls in comparison to their caliber. Since most of the resistance to flow resides at the level of the muscular arterioles, vessels deficient in these muscular elements present diminished resistance to flow and thereby receive a larger volume of flow than vessels with a high impedance. Obviously, microcirculation plays an important role in the growth, metastasis, detection, and treatment of tumors. Transabdominal pulsed Doppler imaging offers a view of the surrounding anatomy and evidence of blood flow in major pelvic vessels, but not in the microcirculation.[9,10] By contrast, transvaginal color Doppler offers a qualitative picture of blood flow in the vascular system in relation to surrounding anatomy.[11–14]

TISSUE CHARACTERIZATION BY PULSED AND COLOR DOPPLER

Wells et al.[15] and Burns et al.[16] documented the presence of abnormal flow spectra around the periphery of malignant tumors. These results were confirmed by several groups.[17–20] The abnormal flow signals consisted of an increase in signal amplitude when compared with the contralateral normal side (corresponding to a greater number of moving cells within the beam), an increase in peak systolic flow, and a characteristic distribution of the Doppler spectrum, showing a predominance of high power, low-frequency elements, and high-diastolic shift (in some tumors the systolic-diastolic variation is absent).

Color Doppler imaging is the latest addition to the many ultrasound techniques available to the clinician. It is best regarded as an extension of pulsed wave Doppler and conventional two-dimensional imaging. Taylor et al.[9] and Hata et al.[21] were the first to apply pulsed Doppler and transabdominal color Doppler in the study of the female pelvic circulation. In all cases of endometrial carcinoma, ovarian carcinoma, and trophoblastic disease, typically abnormal flows were observed by the Japanese team. However, all cases of cervical carcinoma with abnormal flows were stage IIb and above. They concluded that Doppler ultrasound is a pertinent diagnostic tool that can be used to observe changes in tumor vascularity in gynecologic malignancies before and after treatment.

Kurjak et al.[11–14,22,23] were the first to report that transvaginal color flow imaging can be used in the assessment of pelvic circulation and to differentiate between benign and malignant pelvic tumors. Using transvaginal color Doppler, Bourne et al.[24] showed that the absence of intratumoral neovascularization and a normal (high) pulsatility index can be used to exclude the presence of invasive primary ovarian cancer. The early recognition of ovarian cancer is the only approach to achieve a reduction in the mortality. Transvaginal color flow mapping may be used to identify potentially malignant ovarian masses and help elucidate the early stages of tumorigenesis. The routine application of this new technique will enable us to develop a screening program based on ultrasonography.

Intratumoral blood flow displayed on transvaginal color Doppler images indicates that flow is rapid enough to be detected. The presence of arteriovenous communications should be an important factor that produces sufficient velocity of flow, above the minimal threshold of color Doppler imaging. When tumoral blood flow is not visualized on transvaginal color Doppler examination, the following factors should be taken into consideration:

1. There is no blood flow owing to lack of newly formed vessels, a characteristic of malignant tumors.
2. The velocity of flow may be too slow to exceed the minimal threshold for measurement with current color Doppler systems.
3. Intratumoral blood flow is nonuniform and turbulent, and detectable blood flow on color Doppler imaging is distributed in certain regions of a tumor. It sometimes requires a considerable effort to obtain a good angle of insonation with the target for color flow imaging.

CLINICAL METHODS FOR DIFFERENTIATION OF OVARIAN MASSES

The standard evaluation for adnexal masses includes a *medical history, physical examination, CA 125 determination,* and *ultrasound.* Although few data are available regarding the accuracy of a physical examination to differentiate benign from malignant ovarian masses, it is generally agreed that clinical impression has little predictive value.

Pelvic examination is generally regarded as lacking sufficient sensitivity to be of any value in the early detection of ovarian cancer. The findings of MacFarlane et al.[25] are often quoted to support this view. They discovered only six ovarian cancers during a total of 18,753 pelvic examinations performed on 1319 women over a 15-year period (1938–1952). It is not possible to reach any conclusion concerning either the specificity or sensitivity of the pelvic examination from this study.

Some evidence to support the view that the vaginal examination lacks sensitivity for the detection of an adnexal mass (either benign or malignant) was provided by the study of Andolf et al.[26] Each patient recruited underwent a pelvic examination prior to ultrasonography. The pelvic examination was reported as normal in 18 of 24 benign ovarian cysts, in two borderline malignancies, and in one ovarian carcinoma.

Encouraging levels of specificity were achieved by the combination of CA 125 measurements with either a pelvic examination (100 percent) or ultrasound (99 percent). This multimodel approach does appear to provide acceptable levels of specificity.[27]

Ultrasound examination of the pelvis and abdomen has become the standard diagnostic test for evaluation of adnexal masses (Figs. 15-1 to 15-9). Its principal value in this setting involves the confirmation of the presence of a mass, differentiating ovarian from uterine or tubal origin, delineating the internal appearance of the mass, and defining any associated abdominal findings.

Whether ultrasound can differentiate between benign and malignant pelvic masses has been the subject of many studies. Meire et al.[28] first examined the accuracy of ultrasound in delineating a malignant ovarian mass based on size and appearance. In that study, fixed septa, tumor size exceeding 5 cm, and multiloculation were considered ominous for ovarian malignancy. Only 16 of 27 patients with such findings were found to have ovarian cancer. Furthermore, ultrasound has proved to be disappointing as a means of detection of diseases outside the pelvis. Thus, to determine whether the mass is benign or malignant, operative intervention is necessary.

The first systematic approach to the use of pelvic sonography as a screening procedure for early detection of ovarian neoplasms was done by Campbell and his group.[29] Initially, they showed that ovarian size and morphology as assessed by transabdominal ultrasound examination agreed well with results obtained by direct measurement and observation at laparotomy. Recently, the results of a prospective study of 5479 self-referred women without symptoms were described in terms of the ovarian masses detected, the value of the screening procedure over time, and the development of new screening strategies entailing the use of defined changes in ovarian volume.[30] Five primary ovarian cancers were detected at stage Ia or Ib, and evidence from a follow-up study at least 1 year after the

(*Text continues on page 273.*)

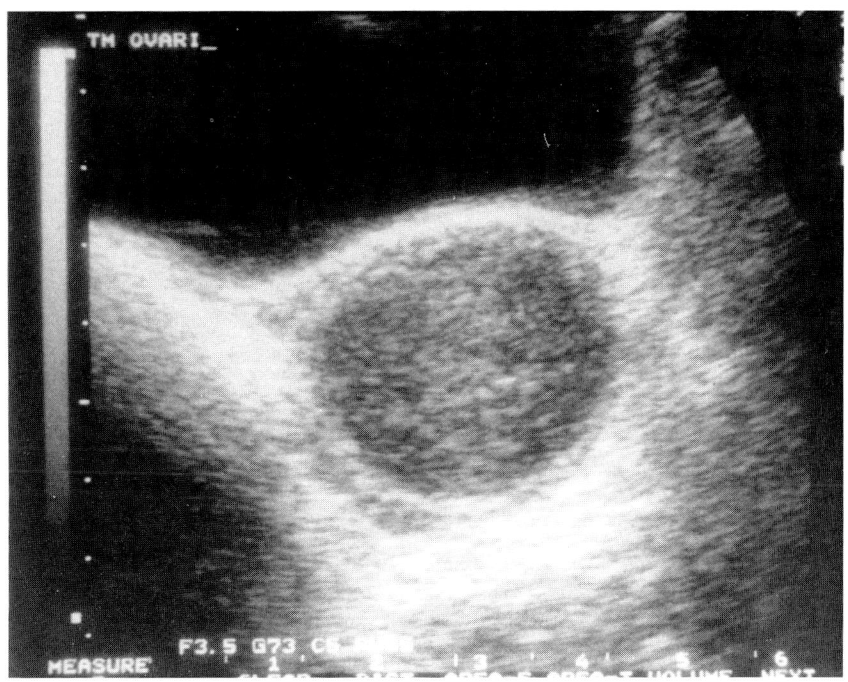

Figure 15-1 Enlarged ovaries diagnosed after hysterectomy.

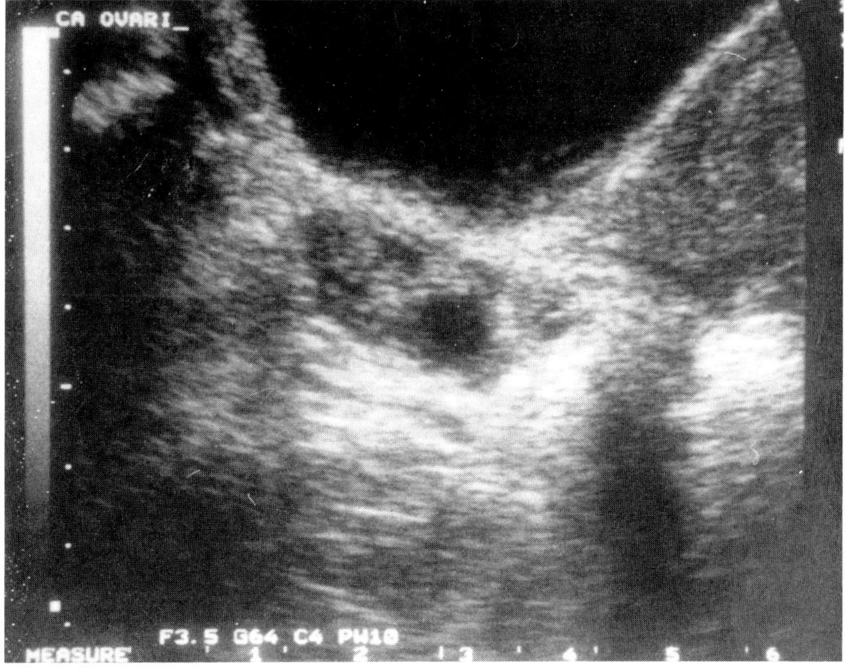

Figure 15-2 Slightly enlarged right ovary visualized by B-mode transabdominal ultrasound.

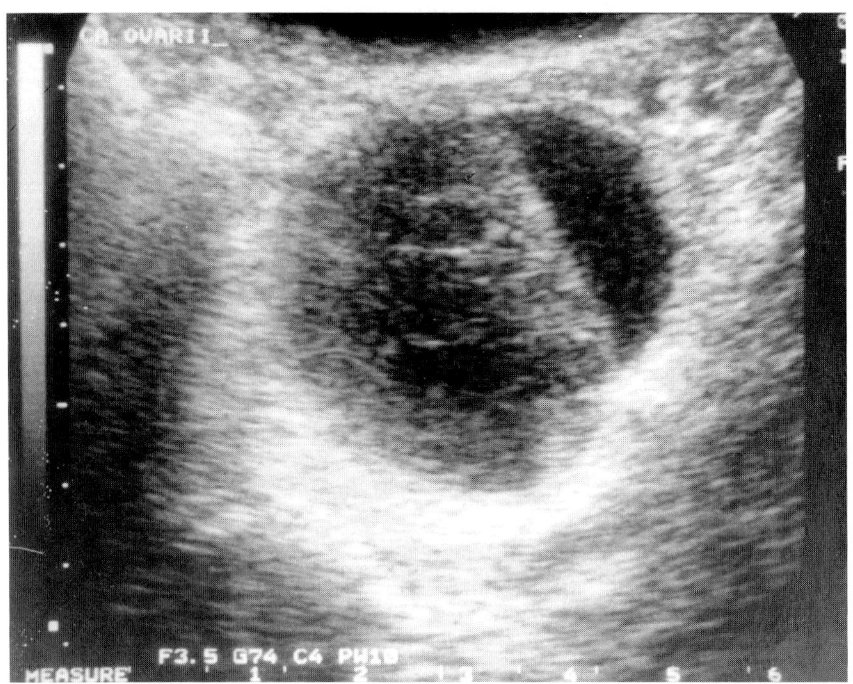

Figure 15-3 Complex, dominantly solid adnexal mass. Malignant tumor was confirmed after surgery.

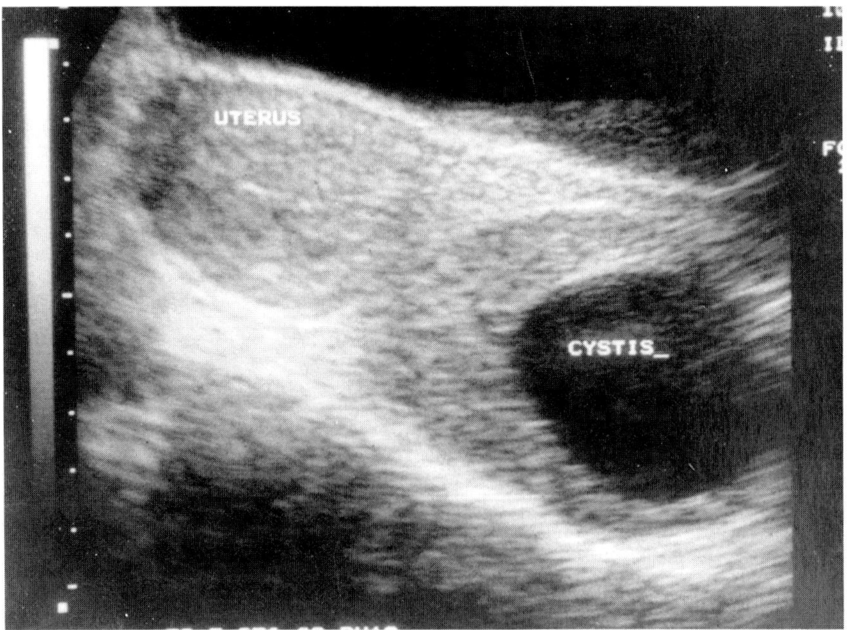

Figure 15-4 Unilocular ovarian cyst. Endometriotic cyst was found on the histopathologic examination.

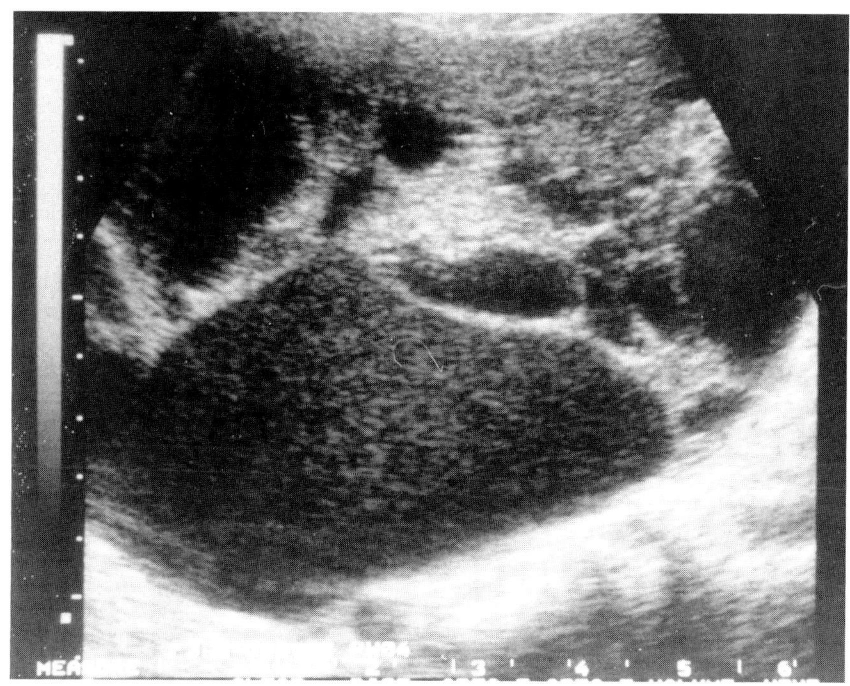

Figure 15-5 Bizarre ultrasonic finding in a case of ovarian cancer.

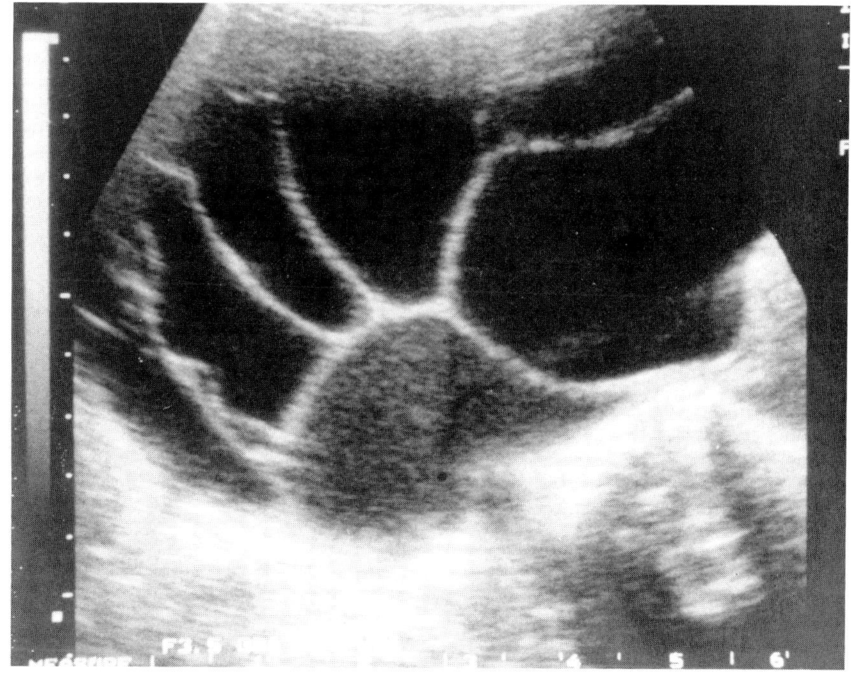

Figure 15-6 An additional scan of the same patient as in Fig. 15-5.

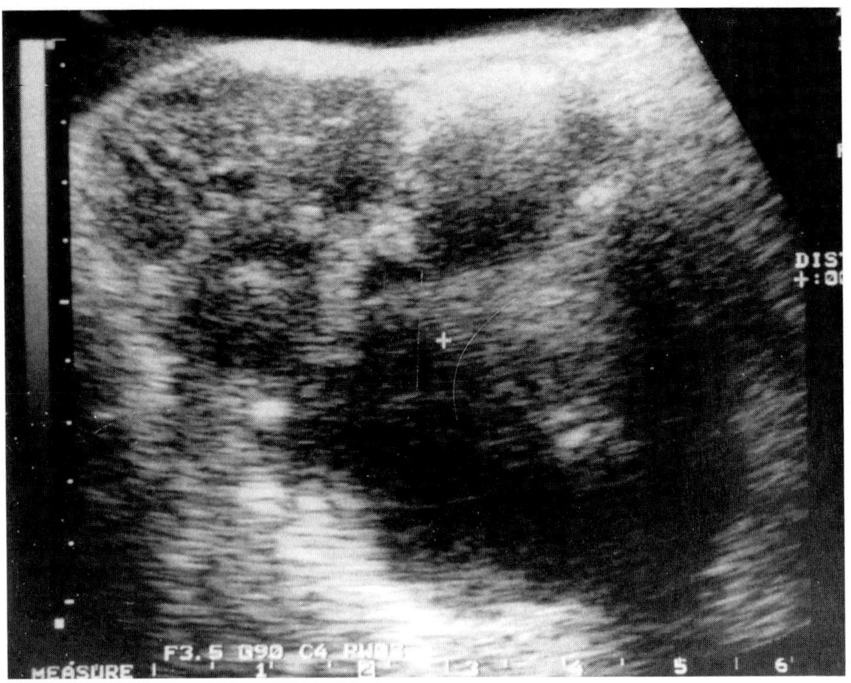

Figure 15-7 An example of a bizarre adnexal mass. Pelvic inflammatory disease was diagnosed on surgery.

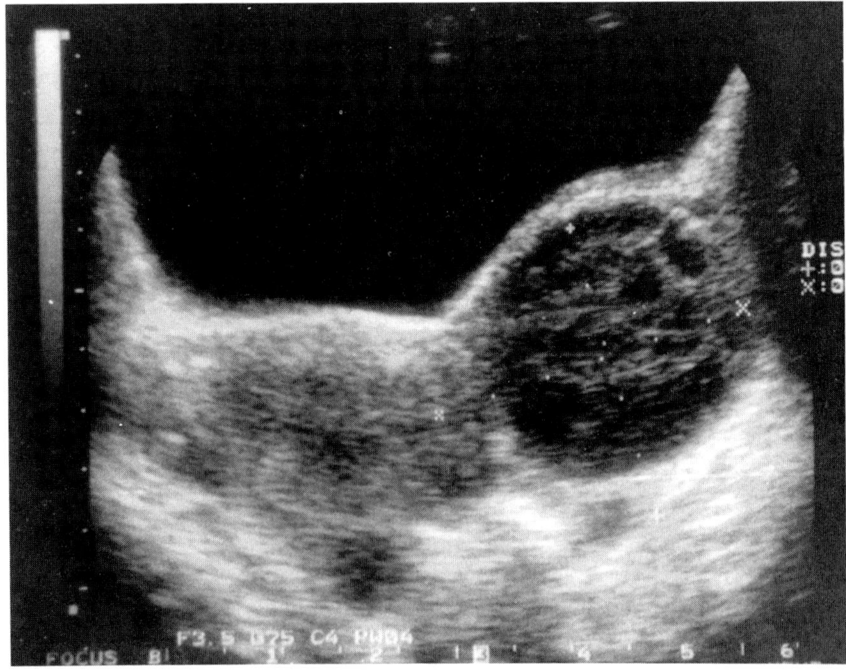

Figure 15-8 Enlarged left ovary. Ovarian cancer was diagnosed on histopathology.

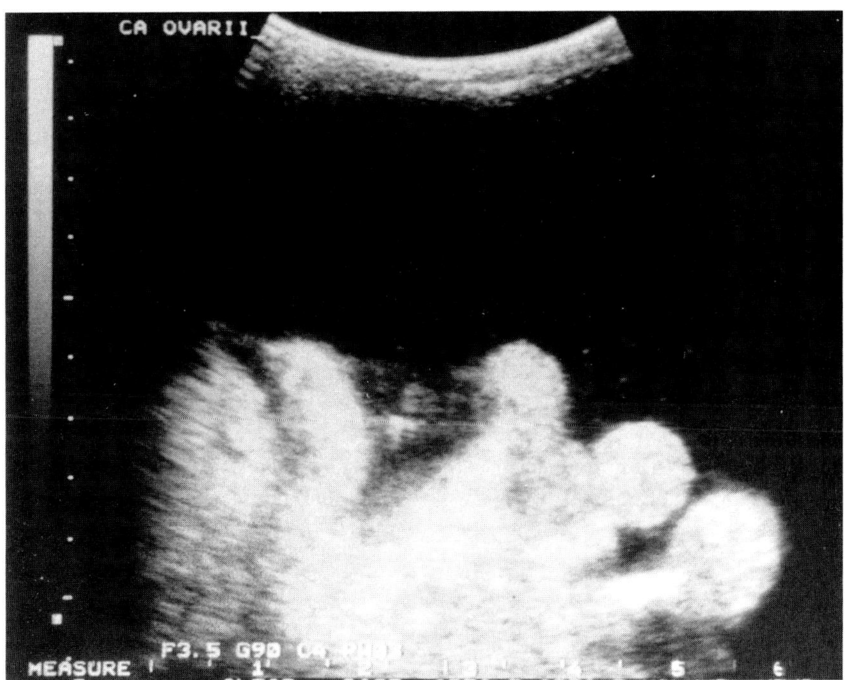

Figure 15-9 Advanced ovarian cancer with typical papillary projections.

last screening showed that the detection rate was 100 percent within the limitation of the study design. A screening procedure based on the presence of abnormal ovarian morphology at the first scan and a defined volume change on rescanning would have given a false-positive rate of 1.6 percent and a positive predictive value of 2.0 percent; that is, the odds against a positive screen result indicating the presence of primary ovarian cancer are 1:50. This odds ratio is mainly due to the difficulty of distinguishing malignant tumors from benign masses, tumorlike conditions or hydrosalpinges.

The value of routine ultrasound was examined by Andolf et al.[26] In their study, 805 women attending gynecologic outpatient clinics in Sweden were examined. Thirty-nine had surgery as a result of positive ultrasound findings, including one with malignant and two with borderline ovarian tumors as well as one with cancer of the cecum. Because the results were obtained from symptomatic women, it is difficult to know how to apply the findings to population screening. None of the four tumors detected by ultrasound were found on digital pelvic examination.

In a recent study, Bourne et al.[24] used transvaginal color Doppler to screen for ovarian cancer. Women were selected on the basis of their medical history and the result of a previous transvaginal ultrasound scan. Thirty women [10 premenopausal (scan performed on days 1 to 8 of the menstrual cycle) and 20 postmenopausal] had normal ovaries, and 20 had at least one ovary with abnormal morphology or volume, or both. Two women with a positive result on screening had hydrosalpinges, 10 a benign tumor or tumorlike condition, and 8 primary ovarian cancer. No areas of neovascularization were seen in the 30 women with morphologically normal ovaries or in the two patients with hydrosalpinges, and the pulsatility index ranged from 3.1 to 9.4 in these cases. Similarly, nine patients (10 affected ovaries) with a nonmalignant mass had no signs of neovascularization, and the pulsatility index ranged from 3.2 to 7.0. One patient with bilateral dermoid cysts containing nests of thyroidlike cells had vascular changes and pulsatility indices of 0.4 and 0.8. Seven patients (eight ovaries) with primary ovarian cancer (one stage IV, four stage III, and two stage Ia) showed clear evidence of neovascularization and pulsatility index values from 0.3 to 1.0. One patient with an intraepithelial serous cystadenocarcinoma in a small ovary (<5 mL volume) had no signs of any vascular changes, and the pulsatility index was 5.5. The authors concluded that transvaginal color flow imaging may be used to identify potentially malignant ovarian masses and help elucidate the early stages of tumorigenesis.

THE ZAGREB ULTRASOUND SCORING SYSTEM

Diagnosis of ovarian carcinoma at an early stage was very unusual before color Doppler ultrasound was introduced by us in 1987 for examination of the pelvic organs.[11] Color Doppler detects blood flow in small low-resistance vessels which form in neoplastic tissue. Pulsed Doppler is then used to quantify such color-coded flow using Pourcelot's resistance index. In this way ovarian malignancy is differentiated from other lesions which produce similar but not identical patterns of flow (Figs. 15-10 to 15-17).

In the first study we presented 14,317 asymptomatic or minimally symptomatic women who had been evaluated for ovarian carcinoma with color Doppler ultrasound and who had been followed up with this technique: 8620 asymptomatic women were referred by ''well woman'' or similar clinics for color Doppler examination; 5697 women were referred by gynecologists because of a suspected adnexal mass; 7495 (87 percent) of the women were premenopausal; and 1125 were postmenopausal. Every examination included abdominal B-mode and vaginal color Doppler scanning with pulsed Doppler examination. The equipment used was a SSD-680 ALOKA system with a 5-MHz transvaginal probe (Aloka Co., Japan). The uterus and individual adnexal organs were examined. The resistance index was calculated from at least five separate cardiac cycles, and the mean of these was recorded.[31] In premenopausal women the examinations were carried out at days 3 to 10 of the menstrual cycle to avoid false-positive results as a consequence of increased ovarian flow during the luteal phase.[32] Those who had a diagnosed adnexal mass had laparotomy within 6 weeks: all were carried out by the same surgeon. The same pathologist examined all spec-

(*Text continues on page 279.*)

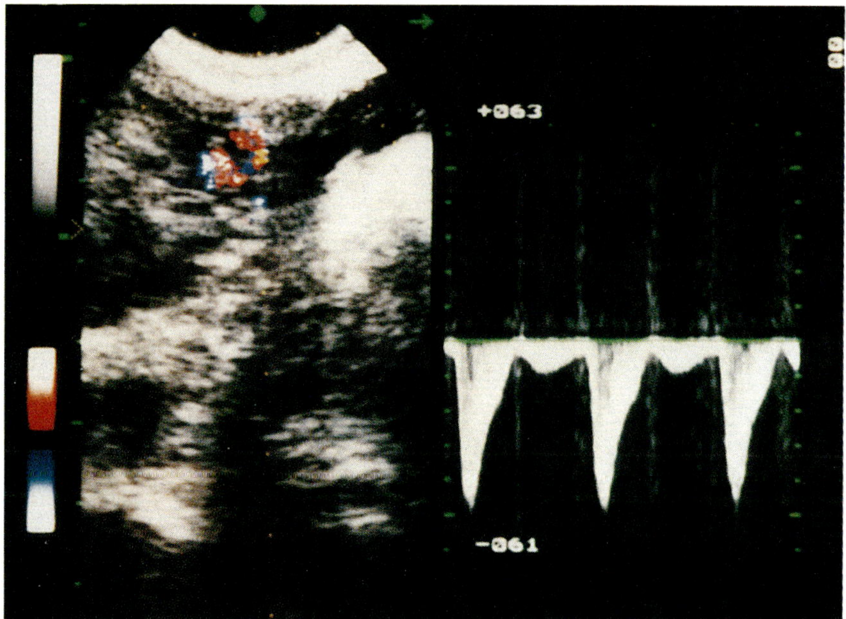

Figure 15-10 Transvaginal color Doppler shows blood flow in periphery of ovarian tissue. Pulsed Doppler waveforms (*right*) show high resistance and very low diastolic blood flow, which are normal findings.

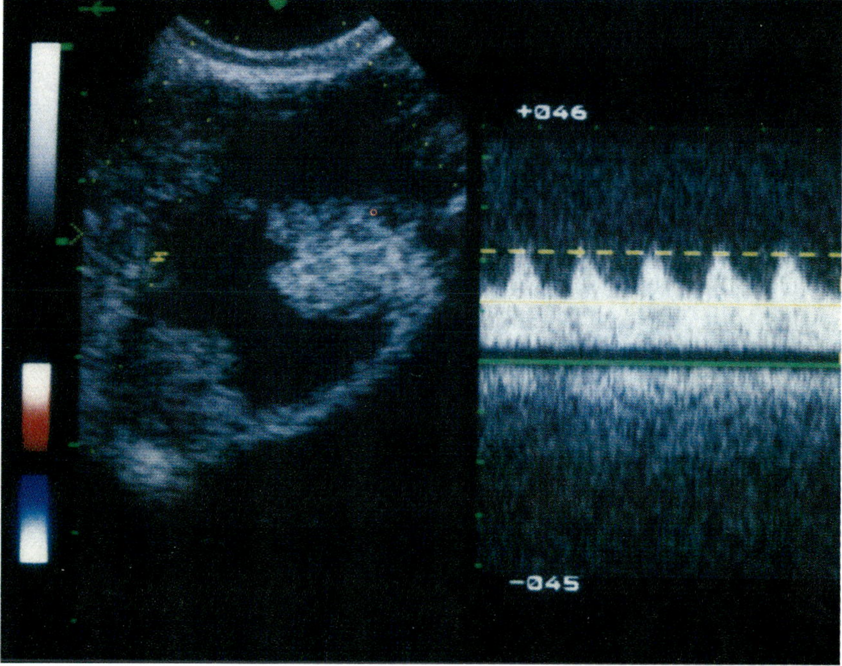

Figure 15-11 Enlarged, complex right ovary. Color Doppler demonstrates tumor blood flow. Pulsed Doppler (*right*) shows moderate resistance to flow (RI = 0.457). A benign tumor was confirmed by histopathology.

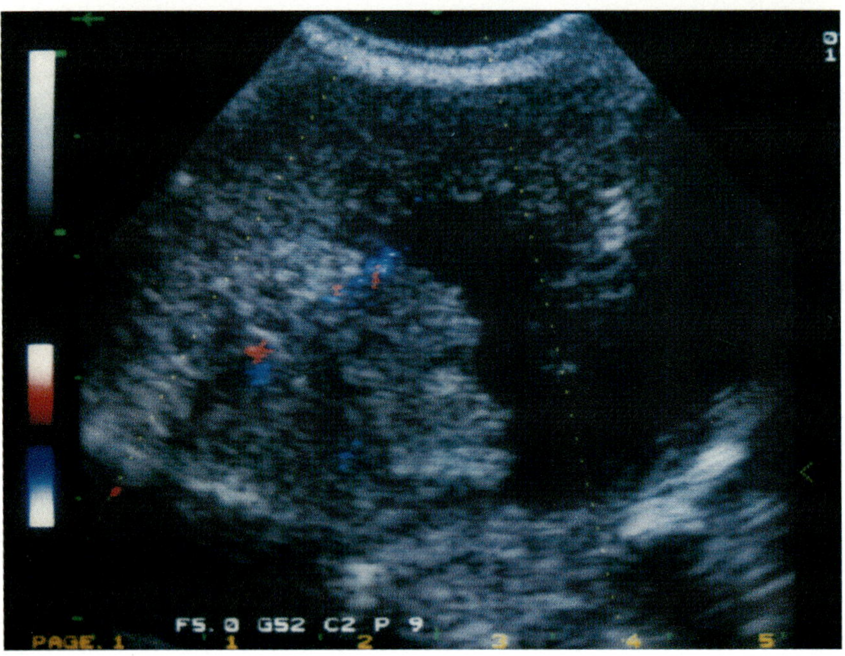

Figure 15-12 Color Doppler findings in the case of tuboovarian abscess. These findings may be a possible source of error in the diagnosis of ovarian malignancy.

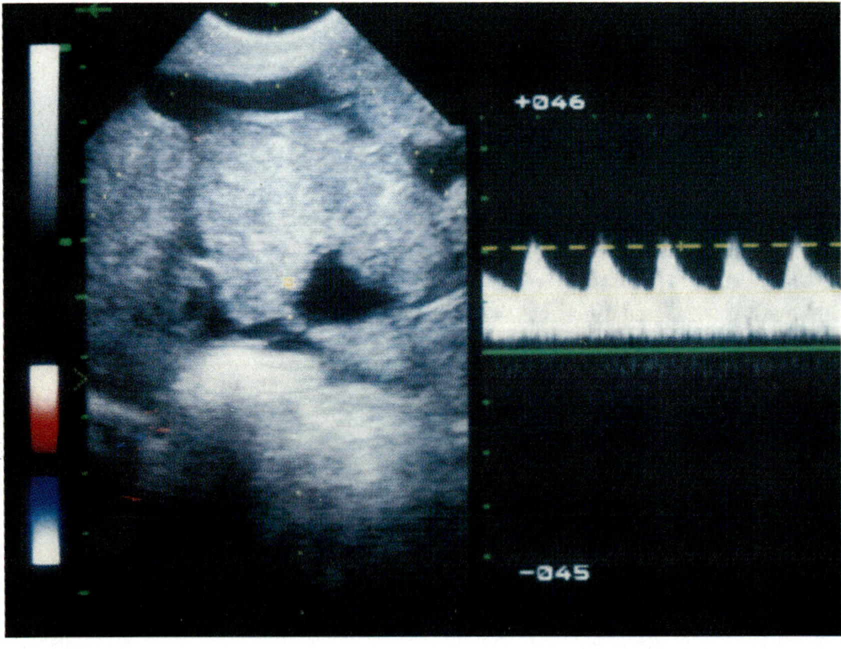

Figure 15-13 Large ovarian mass. Blood flow was detected on tumor periphery (RI = 0.470).

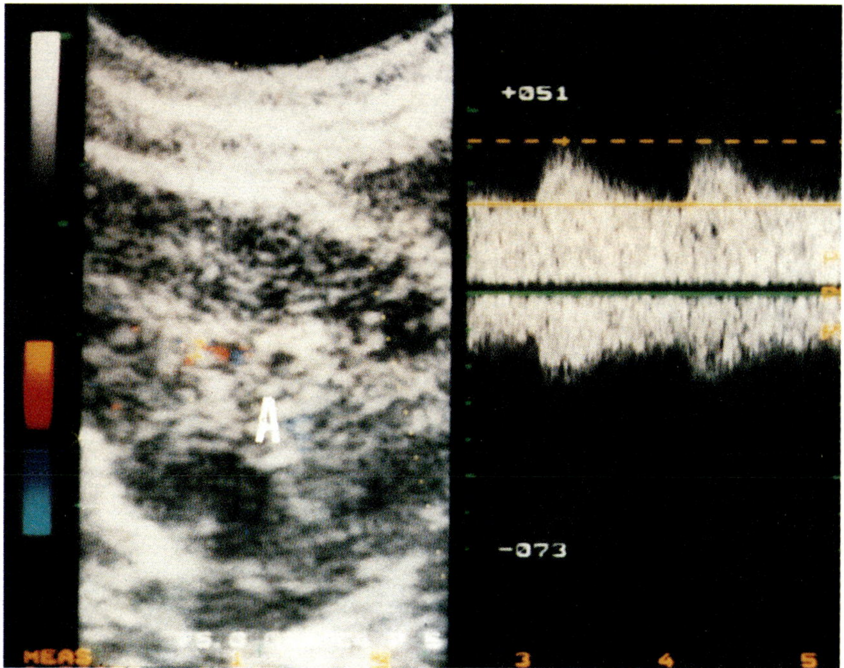

Figure 15-14 Solid adnexal mass. Blood flow was detected in the central part of the tumor. Pulsed Doppler (*right*) shows increased diastolic blood flow. The resistance index was borderline (RI = 0.426).

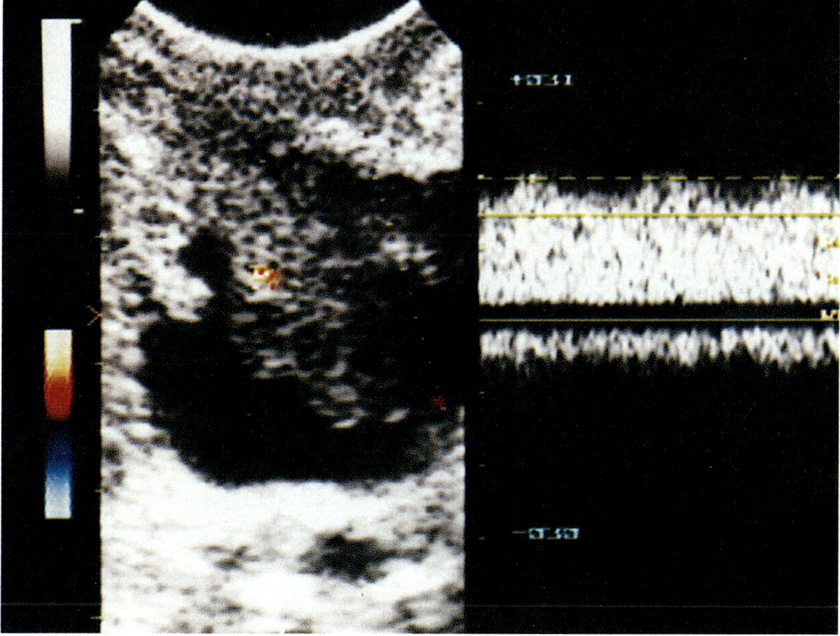

Figure 15-15 Complex ovarian mass. Blood flow was detected in the solid part of the tumor. Pulsed Doppler (*right*) shows very low resistance to flow (RI = 0.255). Typical finding in the case of ovarian malignancy.

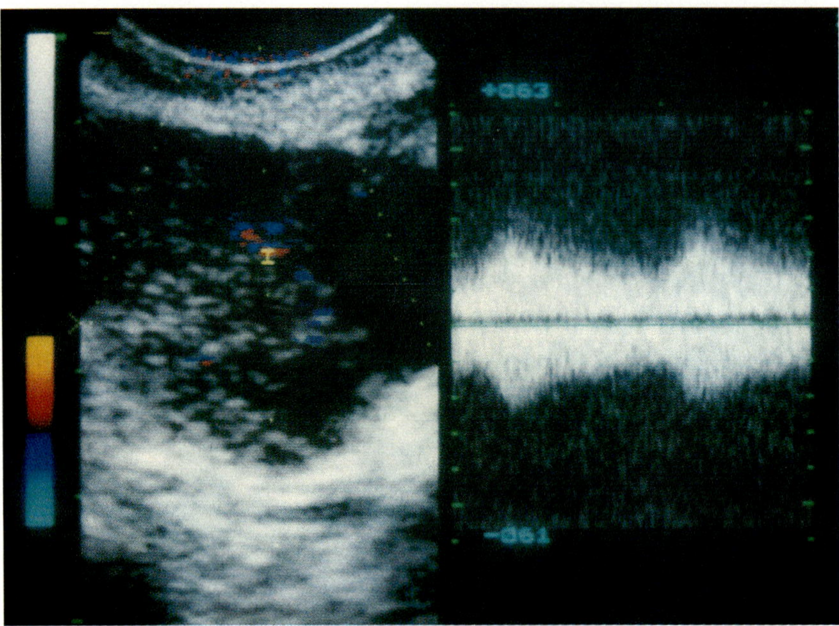

Figure 15-16 An additional example of a malignant ovarian mass diagnosed by transvaginal color Doppler.

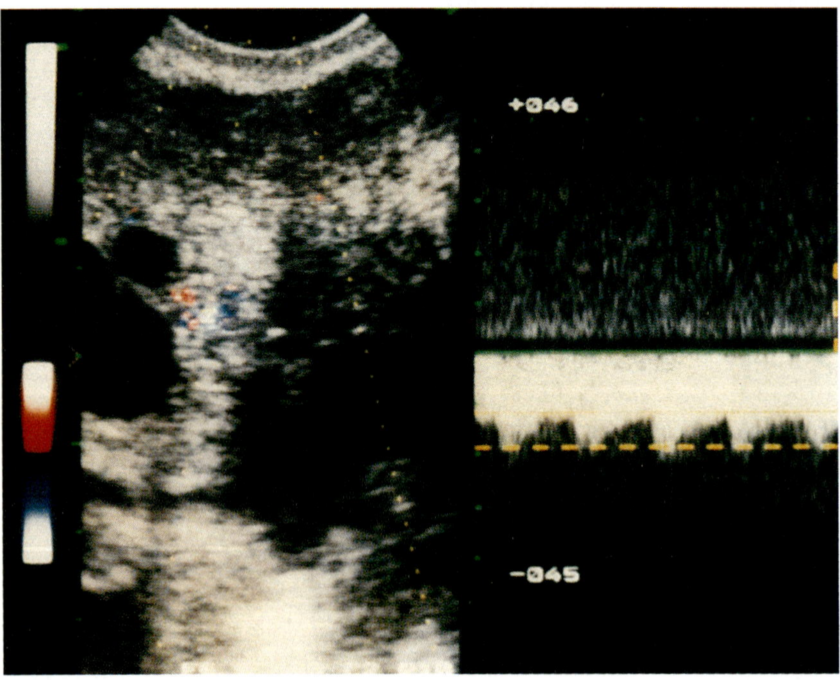

Figure 15-17 Color and pulsed Doppler findings in the case of an advanced stage of ovarian cancer.

imens. There were 624 benign adnexal tumors: in all these, with one exception, the RI was greater than 0.40. The exception was a chronic appendicitis with hydrosalpinx in which the RI was 0.39. Eleven primary and nine secondary stage I ovarian neoplasms were discovered. Five of the primary ovarian neoplasms were found in women known to have an adnexal mass, and six were in the asymptomatic group. Each of these tumors was stage I, between 3.5 and 5 cm in diameter. Neovascularization was found in 9 of the 11 primary neoplasms, and in these the RI was 0.32 to 0.40 (mean 0.36). Nine secondary ovarian neoplasms were found. The lesions were in the breast, thyroid, and rectum. Their mean diameter was 4.6 cm (range from 3.8 to 5.6 cm). In each of these the RI was 0.40 or less (mean 0.38; range from 0.28 to 0.40), and the color was not so prominent as in the primary lesions. In five of these nine cases clinical examination, transabdominal, or transvaginal ultrasound did not reveal any pelvic abnormality.

The remaining 40 malignant neoplasms were stage III and stage IV ovarian cancers with characteristic abnormal flow patterns in 39 cases. Three of them were found in the asymptomatic group. A secondary tumor from an endometrial cancer was not detected by means of color Doppler. However, sensitivity, specificity, and accuracy of this diagnostic method are acceptably high (Table 15-1).

The second stage included 1623 women studied by transvaginal color Doppler. B-mode, color, and pulsed Doppler findings were described according to our own scoring system (Table 15-2). Of these, 38 women were operated on for adnexal masses detected by ultrasound. Final diagnosis was made by a pathologist. Every patient was examined by transvaginal color Doppler 1 day before operation. Morphology and blood flow of adnexal masses were assessed according to our own scoring system.

Five ovarian cancers were diagnosed in these 1623 women. Two were at stage I, two at stage II, and one at stage III. When only the cutoff point of 0.4 resistance index was used to differentiate benign versus malignant ovarian masses,

Table 15-1   Transvaginal color Doppler in the detection of adnexal tumor malignancy (two-stage study)

Color flow present and RI ≤ 0.40	Histopathology		
	Malignant	Benign	Total
Yes	59	4	63
No	6	653	659
Total	65	657	722

Note: RI = resistance index; sensitivity = 90.8 percent; specificity = 99.4 percent; positive predictive value = 93.6 percent; negative predictive value = 99.1 percent; acuracy = 98.6 percent.

Table 15-2 The Zagreb ultrasound and Doppler scoring system for adnexal masses

Ovarian tumor ultrasound—Doppler classification
(Circle characteristics seen and add for score.)

Patient name ___________ Date ___________ Institution ___________

	Fluid		Internal borders		Size
Unilocular	Clear	(0)	Smooth	(0)	
	Internal echoes	(1)	Irregular	(2)	
Multilocular	Clear	(1)	Smooth	(1)	
	Internal echoes	(1)	Irregular	(2)	
Cystic-solid	Clear	(1)	Smooth	(1)	
	Internal echoes	(2)	Irregular	(2)	
Papillary projections	Suspicious	(1)	Definite	(2)	
Solid	Homogenous	(1)	Echogenic	(2)	
Peritoneal fluid	Absent	(0)	Present	(1)	

Color Doppler		RI (index)		Velocity
No vessels seen	(0)	(0)		
Regular separate vessels	(1)	>0.40	(1)	
Randomly dispersed vessels	(2)	<0.41	(2)	

If suspected corpus luteum, repeat in next menstrual cycle in proliferative phase.

Score	Ultrasound	Color
< 2	Benign	Benign
3–4	Questionable	Questionable
> 4	Suspicious	

Outcome
  Spontaneous resolution
  Surgery, type ___________
  Pathologic diagnosis ___________
  Complications ___________
  Follow-up, date, and status ___________

true positive diagnosis was done in two (40 percent) cases, false-negative diagnosis in three (60 percent) and false-positive diagnosis in another three cases (9 percent). When the scoring system (with a cutoff point of a score of 4) was used, true positive diagnosis was made in all five patients with ovarian cancer, false-positive diagnosis was done in four (12 percent) patients, and there was no false-negative diagnosis. With the employment of both previously mentioned criteria (RI and score), false-positive results were reduced to a minimal 7 percent, and there were no false-negative results. All cases of false-positive results had a final diagnosis of pelvic inflammatory disease or corpus luteum neovascularization.

CONCLUSION

Abdominal ultrasound is a useful tool to identify and delineate the characteristics of ovarian masses. Features of a mass which are of importance are unilocular or multilocular findings, opaque versus clear fluid, presence of solid components, presence of papillary projections, roughness of the internal lining, and presence of peritoneal fluid. Many of these features can help delineate benign from suspected malignant growths, although sensitivity beyond 70 percent has not yet been achieved. This figure is too low for a screening test.

Doppler ultrasound identifies the movement of erythrocytes in blood vessels. A signal is obtained and displayed on the monitor. From the display the contour and returned frequency can be calculated. We have learned from Doppler ultrasound that vessels with high resistance and low diastolic blood flow can be differentiated from those with low resistance and high diastolic blood flow. Normal pelvic vessels usually demonstrate high resistance and low diastolic flow. Malignant neoplasms may have low resistance and very high diastolic blood flow. When color is added to the Doppler system, the examiner is able to see many more vessels clearly, and particularly small vessels. In most cancers, there is a proliferation of vessels which were formerly identified in radiographic angiology as a tumor "blush." Doppler measurements can be made on these previously inaccessible vessels. We do believe that transvaginal color Doppler is a technology that will offer high sensitivity, specificity, and positive predictive values for the differentiation of ovarian masses, and consequently the early detection of ovarian cancer. Transvaginal ultrasound accurately identifies significant morphologic components of an ovarian enlargement. Color flow Doppler identifies the presence of abnormal blood vessels, and measurement of the systolic-diastolic components of this flow differentiates vessels into those of high- or low-velocity states. Our experience also stresses the importance of a thorough examination of the ovaries with color Doppler regardless of their B-mode ultrasound appearance and size.

REFERENCES

1. Gulino PM: "Extracellular compartments of solid tumors," in Becker H (ed), *Cancer*. New York, Plenum Press, 1975, pp 327–335.
2. Folkman J: Tumor angiogenesis. Adv Cancer Res 43:175–182, 1985.
3. Jain RK: Determination of tumor blood flow: a review. Cancer Res 48:2641–2645, 1988.
4. Jain RK: Transport of molecules across tumor vasculature. Cancer Metastasis Rev 6:559–563, 1987.
5. Jain RK, Baxter LT: Mechanisms of heterogeneous distribution of monoclonal antibodies and other macromolecules in tumors: significance of elevated interstitial pressure. Cancer Res 48:7022–7026, 1988.
6. Folkman J: Growth and metastasis of tumor in organ culture. Cancer 16:453–460, 1963.

7. Gimbrone MA: Tumor dormancy in vivo by prevention of neovascularization. J Exp Med 136:261–264, 1972.

8. Jain RK, Ward-Hartley KA: Dynamics of cancer cell interaction with microvasculature and interstitium. Biorheology 24:117–120, 1987.

9. Taylor KJW, Burns PN, Wells PNI, Conway DI: Ultrasound Doppler flow studies of the ovarian and uterine arteries. Br J Obstet Gynaecol 92:240–243, 1985.

10. Long MG, Boulbee JE, Hanson ME, Begent RHJ: Doppler time velocity waveform studies of the uterine artery and uterus. Br J Obstet Gynaecol 96:588–591, 1989.

11. Kurjak A, Zalud I, Jurkovic D, Alfirevic Z, Miljan M: Transvaginal color Doppler for the assessment of pelvic circulation. Acta Obstet Gynecol Scand 68:131–135, 1989.

12. Kurjak A, Zalud I, Alfirevic Z, Jurkovic D: The assessment of abnormal pelvic blood flow by transvaginal color Doppler. Ultrasound Med Biol 16:437–442, 1991.

13. Kurjak A, Jurkovic D, Alfirevic Z, Zalud I: Transvaginal color Doppler imaging. J Clin Ultrasound 18:227–234, 1990.

14. Kurjak A: *Transvaginal Color Doppler.* Carnforth, N.J., Parthenon Publishing, 1990.

15. Wells PNT, Halliwell M, Skidmore R, Webb AJ, Woodcock JP: Tumor detection by ultrasonic Doppler blood flow signals. Ultrasonics 15:231–235, 1977.

16. Burns PN, Halliwell M, Wells PNT, Webb AJ: Ultrasonic Doppler studies of the breast. Ultrasound Med Biol 8:127–130, 1987.

17. Srivastava A, Huges LE, Woodcock JP, Laider P: Vascularity in cutaneous melanoma detected by Doppler sonography and histology: correlation with tumor behavior. Br J Cancer 59:89–93, 1987.

18. Taylor KJW, Ramos I, Morse SS, Fortune K, Hammers L, Taylor CR: Focal liver masses: differential diagnosis with pulsed Doppler ultrasound. Radiology 164:643–646, 1987.

19. Taylor KJW, Morse SS: Doppler defects vascularity of some malignant tumors. Diagn Imaging 10:132–136, 1988.

20. Kujipers D, Jaspers R: Renal masses: differential diagnosis with pulsed Doppler ultrasound. Radiology 170:59–64, 1989.

21. Hata H, Hata K, Senoh D, Makihara K, Aoki S, Takamiya O, Kiato M: Doppler ultrasound assessment of tumor vascularity in gynecological disorders. J Ultrasound Med 8:309–312, 1989.

22. Kurjak A, Zalud I: "Transvaginal color Doppler sonography," in Timor-Tritsch IE, Rottem S (eds), *Transvaginal Sonography,* 2d ed. New York, Elsevier, 1991, pp 451–462.

23. Kurjak A, Zalud I: "Transvaginal color Doppler," in Kurjak A (ed), *Handbook of Ultrasound in Obstetrics and Gynecology.* Boca Raton, Fla., CRC Press, 1990, pp 447–452.

24. Bourne T, Campbell S, Steer C, Whitehead MI, Collins WP: Transvaginal colour flow imaging: a possible new screening technique for ovarian cancer. Br Med J 299:1367–1369, 1989.

25. MacFarlane C, Strugis MC, Fetterman FS: Results of an experiment in the control of cancer of the female pelvis organ and report of a fifteen year research. Am J Obstet Gynecol 69:294–297, 1955.

26. Andolf E, Svalenius E, Astedt B: Ultrasonography for early detection of ovarian carcinoma. Br J Obstet Gynaecol 93:1286–1289, 1986.

27. Jacobs IJ, Stabile I, Bridges J, et al.: Multimodal approach to screening for ovarian cancer. Lancet i:268–270, 1988.

28. Meire HB, Farrant P, Guha T: Distinction of benign from malignant ovarian cysts by ultrasound. Br J Obstet Gynecol 85:893–895, 1978.

29. Campbell S, Goessens L, Goswamy R, Whitehead MI: Real-time ultrasonography for the determination of ovarian morphology and volume. A possible early screening test for ovarian cancer. Lancet i:425–428, 1982.

30. Bhan V, Amso N, Whitehead MI, et al.: Characteristics of persistent ovarian masses in asymptomatic women. Br J Obstet Gynaecol 96:1384–1387, 1989.

31. Thompson RS, Trudinger BJ, Cook CM: Doppler ultrasound waveform indices: A/B ratio, pulsatility index and Pourcelot ratio. Br J Obstet Gynaecol 95:581–504, 1988.

32. Zalud I, Kurjak A: The assessment of luteal blood flow in pregnant and non-pregnant women by transvaginal color Doppler. J Perinat Med 18:215–221, 1990.

COLOR DOPPLER HYSTEROSALPINGOGRAPHY

ALBERT J. PETERS
J. JAROSLAV STERN
CAROLYN B. COULAM

Infertility, defined as the *inability to conceive after one year of unprotected intercourse,* is an increasing social and health concern.[1] This entity affects approximately 3 million couples in the United States annually,[2] and its significance is evidenced by the increasing number of office visits to physicians for infertility.[2] Of these 3 million couples affected by infertility, approximately 25 percent is secondary to some form of tubal blockage.[3,4] This chapter reviews the causes of infertility due to tubal disease and describes the procedures used to diagnose tubal occlusion. The focus of this chapter is to introduce and familiarize the reader with new techniques that employ the use of the Doppler effect through ultrasonography to evaluate fallopian tube patency. This new technique termed *color Doppler flow hysterosalpingography,* or simply ultrasound hysterosalpingography (US HSG), is compared with more traditional methods of fallopian tube assessment such as *x-ray hysterosalpingography* (X-RAY HSG) and *surgical chromopertubation* (CPT).

CAUSES OF OVIDUCTAL OBSTRUCTION

Oviductal disease is the cause of an estimated 25 percent of infertility.[3,4] The frequencies of the sites of obstruction of the fallopian tube among infertile women without a history of previous tubal ligation are shown in Table 16-1.

Distal occlusion accounts for 63 percent of oviductal obstructions, proximal

Table 16-1 The frequencies of sites of oviductal obstruction among infertile women

Site	No.	%
Distal only	100	63
Proximal only	27	17
Proximal and distal	31	20

occlusion for 17 percent, and proximal and distal tubal occlusion combine for 20 percent.[5–7] While previous infection or pelvic surgery and endometriosis have accounted for the majority of cases of distal tubal disease, histologic findings in the fallopian tubes of women demonstrating proximal occlusion have included salpingitis isthmica nodosa, chronic salpingitis, intratubal endometriosis, fibrous obliteration of the oviduct, and amorphous concretions.[5–8] The relative frequencies of each of these histologic findings in women with tubal obstruction are listed in Table 16-2.

The location of oviductal obstruction is important in prognosticating pregnancy success after correction of the occlusion. Table 16-3 summarizes the conception and live birth rate 2 years after microsurgical repair of tubal occlusion. The 65 percent pregnancy rate after surgical correction of proximal tubal occlusions is similar to the pregnancy rates reported after nonsurgical correction of proximal oviductal obstructions treated with transcervical balloon tuboplasty.[9] The probability of live births after 1, 2, and 3 years from the time of surgical repair of tubal obstruction is dependent on the site of occlusion and is summarized in Table 16-4.

While live birth rates of 35 to 53 percent are achieved after correction of

Table 16-2 Histologic diagnosis in patients with proximal and distal tubal obstruction

Diagnosis	Proximal only[6]		Proximal and distal[7]	
	No.	%	No.	%
Salpingitis isthmica nodosa	5	19	11	35
Chronic salpingitis	6	22	4	13
Intratubal endometriosis	1	4	3	10
Fibrous obliteration	2	7	13	42
Amorphous concretion	13	48	0	0
Total	27	100	31	100

Table 16-3   Conception and live birth rates 2 years after surgical repair of tubal occlusion

Site	Conceptions, %	Live birth, %
Distal only	51	33
Proximal only	65	47
Distal and promixal	12	0

proximal only and distal only obstructions, surgical repair of combined proximal and distal occlusions in the same patient have yielded no live births.[7] The poor surgical outcome in these patients suggest that in vitro fertilization and embryo transfer should be strongly considered as an option for primary treatment. It is, therefore, necessary to be able to document the site of tubal occlusion for counseling patients with tubal obstruction as a cause of infertility.

DIAGNOSIS OF TUBAL OBSTRUCTION

Traditionally, the diagnosis of tubal factor is made by insufflation of the fallopian tube. Early attempts at tubal evaluation were performed by Rubin in 1954.[10] In its original description, this technique employed the use of intrauterine carbon dioxide (CO_2), insufflation until the patient experienced shoulder discomfort which inferred intraperitoneal CO_2 extravasation, and diaphragmatic irritation. Over the course of the next seven to eight decades, other techniques have emerged as the more common tests. The most commonly used method is X-RAY HSG. If, however, the patient is undergoing laparoscopy, the preferred method is chromopertubation, where an aliquot of indigo carmine or methylene blue is insufflated transcervically and observed transabdominally for tubal spillage. Re-

Table 16-4   Cumulative probability of live birth after surgical repair of tubal obstruction

	% Live birth		
	Year		
Site	1	2	3
Distal only	22	33	35
Proximal only	27	47	53
Distal and proximal	0	0	0

cent reports have even employed radionuclide technology to evaluate patency.[11] These more modern methods have disadvantages such as dye exposure, radiation, general anesthesia, and/or surgical exposure. Herein, the technique of US HSG will be described.

Background for Use of Color Doppler Hysterosalpingography

The Doppler effect uses ultrasound to detect echoes from moving structures. Typically, the moving structure is blood flow; however, in US HSG, observed flow is sterile saline as it passes transcervically, through the uterine cavity into the fallopian tubes and subsequently spills in the posterior cul-de-sac (pouch of Douglas) (Fig. 16-1*A* and *B*).

Just as the Doppler effect occurs whenever there is relative motion between the source and the receiver of sound, a fixed transvaginal or transabdominal ultrasound transducer focuses on saline flowing through the uterine cavity and fallopian tubes and is reflected back to the transducer to produce an image which is interpreted as patency or occlusion. Color Doppler flow is observed at three sites: the uterine cavity (Fig. 16-2*A*), the fallopian tube (Fig. 16-2*B*), and the posterior cul-de-sac (Fig. 16-2*C*).

US HSG utilizes a combination two-dimensional technique of real-time ultrasound imaging with Doppler flow information superimposed. A color scale is used to represent flow velocity. Color seen passing through the fallopian tubes and into the cul-de-sac is interpreted as patent, and no color flow is interpreted as occlusion.

Materials and Techniques for Color Doppler Hysterosalpingography

Equipment needed to perform US HSG includes an ultrasound unit with color Doppler capability, and a 2-mm $\times$ 150-mm intrauterine catheter (H-S catheter) with a 1-mL distal balloon (Ackrad Labs., Inc., Cranford, N.J.) (Fig. 16-3). The technique is similar to standard X-RAY HSG. First, a pelvic ultrasound examination is performed giving particular attention to intrauterine anatomy. This will help identify anomalies such as fibroids, septa, other müllerian configurations, and uterine position. Next, the cervix is visualized and the H-S catheter is passed transcervically into the uterine cavity and the distal balloon inflated with 1 mL of air. Slight traction is placed on the catheter to prevent back leakage through the cervix. Approximately, 5 to 10 mL of sterile saline is instilled into the uterine cavity. Sonography can be either transvaginal or transabdominal, although transvaginal scanning is preferred by most patients because of the comfort of an empty bladder.

The first color Doppler observation is the uterine cavity to verify placement of the catheter (Fig. 16-4). The second observation is directed at either the left or right cornua to visualize the fallopian tube (Fig. 16-5). The third observation

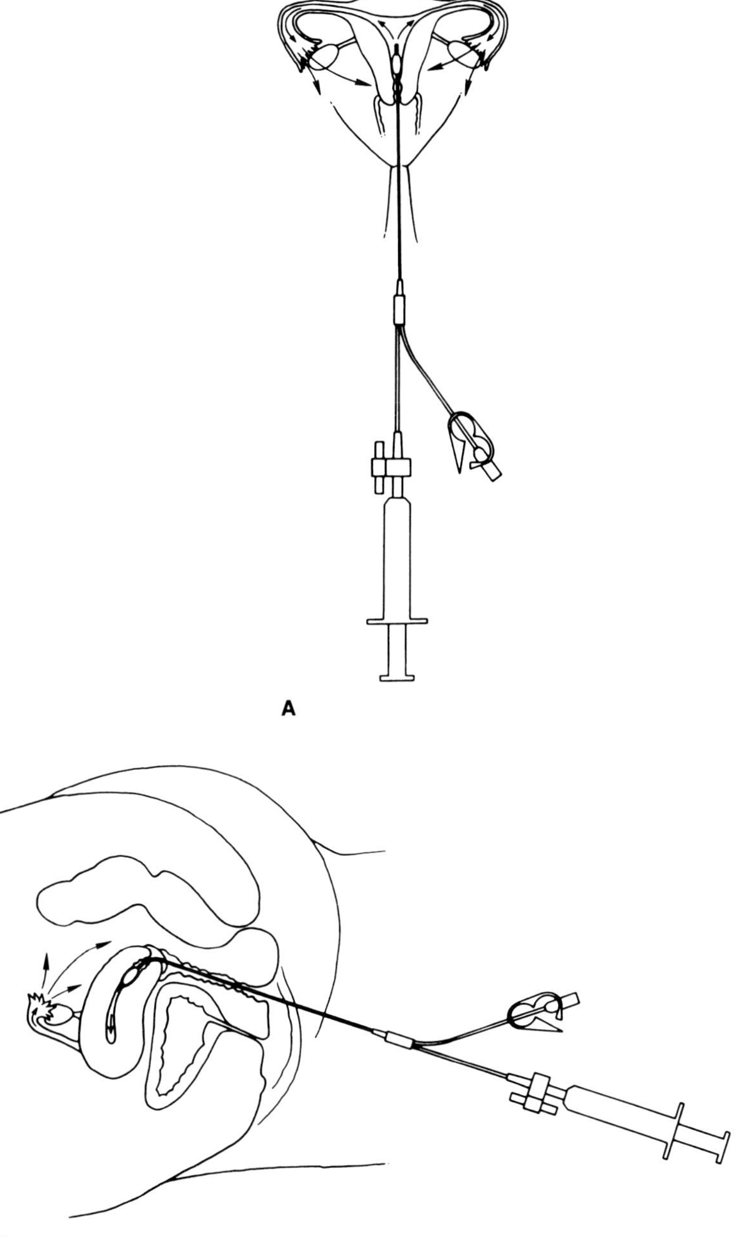

Figure 16-1   Illustration showing flow of sterile saline injected through the cervix into the reproductive tract. *A.* Demonstration of flow of saline through the cervix, into the fallopian tubes, out through the distal tube, and into the cul-de-sac. *B.* Sagittal view of saline flowing into cul-de-sac during US HSG procedure.

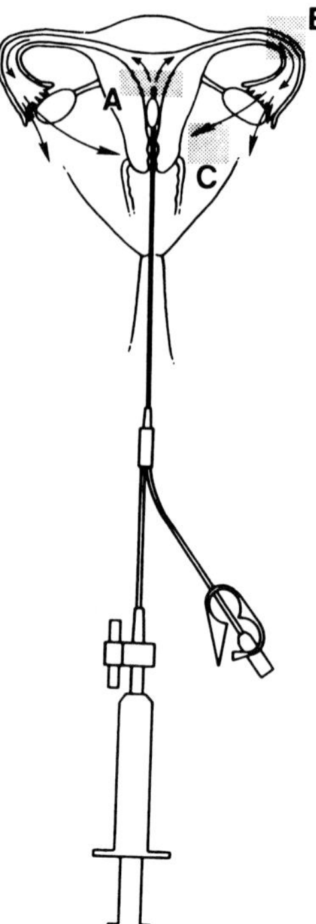

Figure 16-2   Illustration indicating sites of placement of color Doppler mapping for US HSG. Boxes indicate sites of observation of color Doppler flow for US HSG. Box A = saline flow in the uterine cavity; box B = saline flow in the fallopian tube; box C = saline flow into the posterior cul-de-sac.

is in the respective cul-de-sac to verify tubal patency observing spillage of fluid (Fig. 16-6).

The same procedure is repeated on the contralateral side. At the completion of the procedure the balloon is deflated and the H-S catheter is removed. Tubal occlusion can be observed if no flow is seen passing through the fallopian tube. This can be noted at the proximal (Fig. 16-7) or distal segments (Fig. 16-8).

In over 200 procedures performed, no antibiotic prophylaxis was used and no pelvic infections occurred. However, the same precautions should apply for US HSG as for X-RAY HSG. Therefore, the procedure should not be performed on patients with active pelvic infections, and antibiotic prophylaxis should be used for patients with a history of pelvic inflammatory disease.

Evaluation of Color Doppler Hysterosalpingography

Interpretation of the test is based on the appearance of color flow passing through the fallopian tube and in the respective cul-de-sac. Lack of color flow at any point in the tube or lack of flow in the cul-de-sac is designated as obstruction. As in X-RAY HSG, obstruction can be observed at any point along the course of the tube.

In a recent study by the authors,[12] 193 patients were evaluated by US HSG.

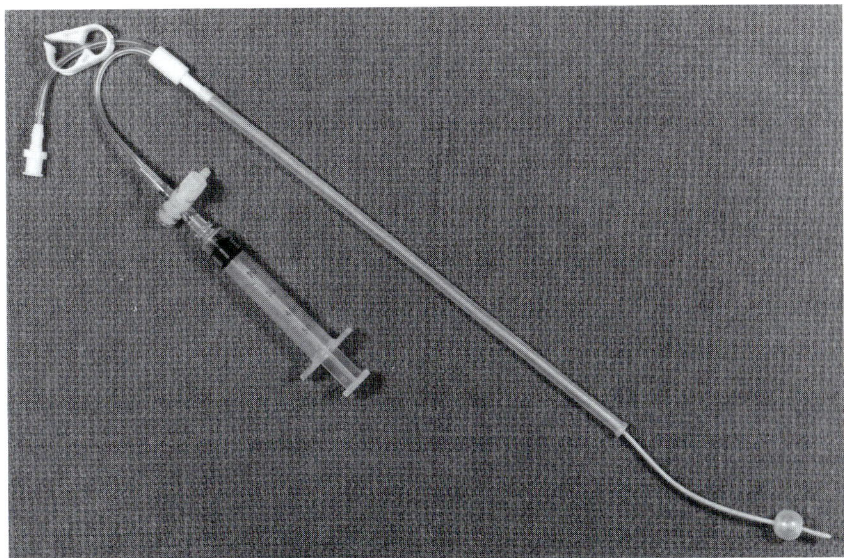

Figure 16-3   H-S catheter used to perform US HSG. Note the 1-mL intrauterine balloon which prevents saline backflow through the cervix.

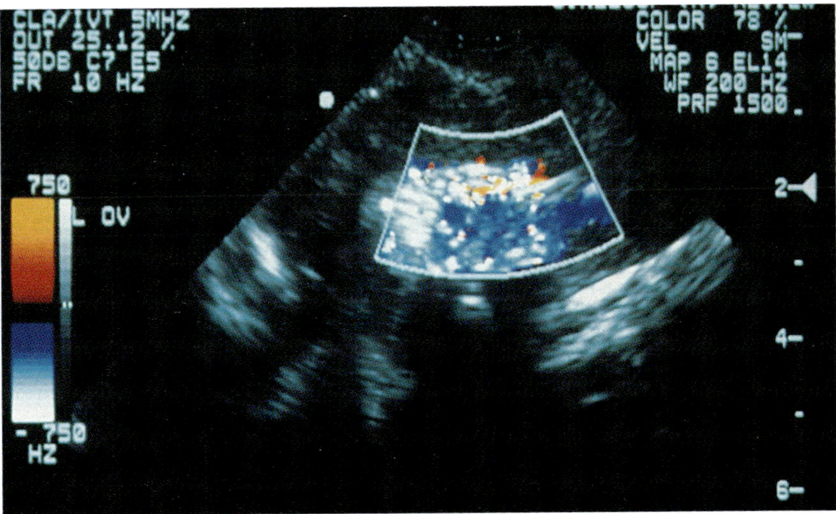

Figure 16-4   Color Doppler flow of saline passing into uterine cavity.

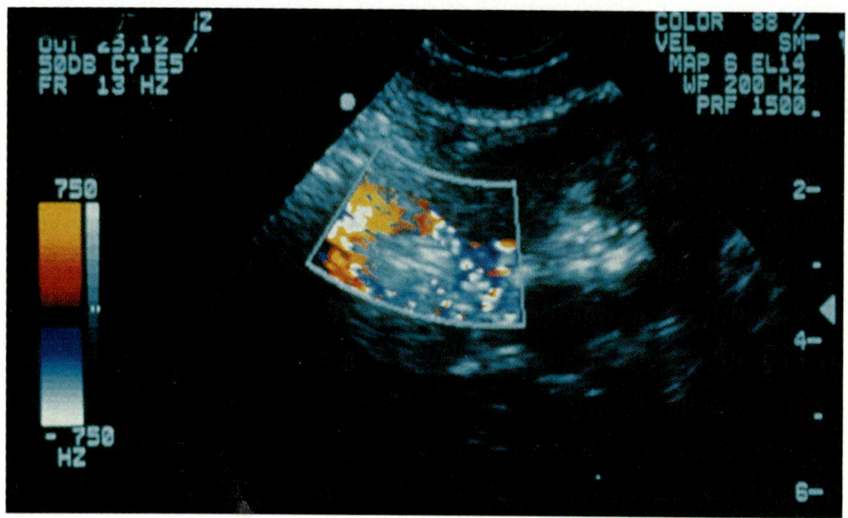

Figure 16-5 Color Doppler flow of saline passing through fallopian tube.

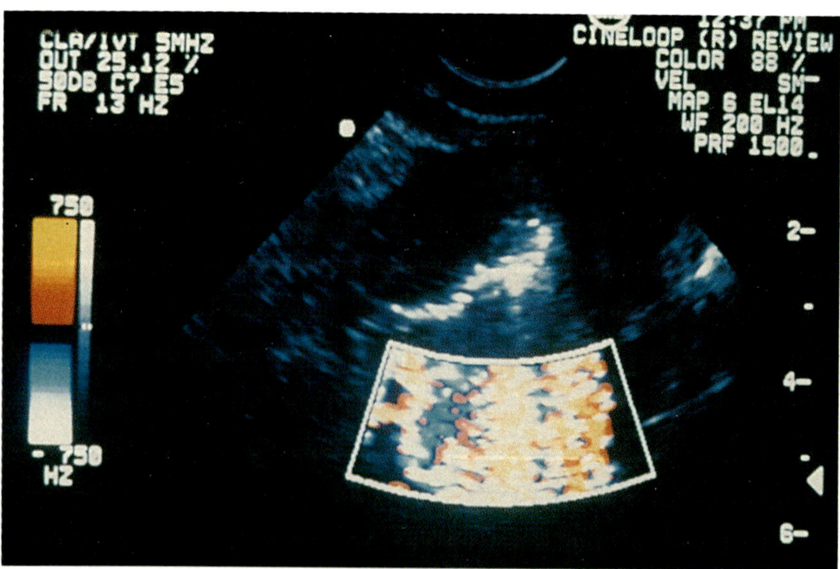

Figure 16-6 Color Doppler flow of saline passing into posterior cul-de-sac.

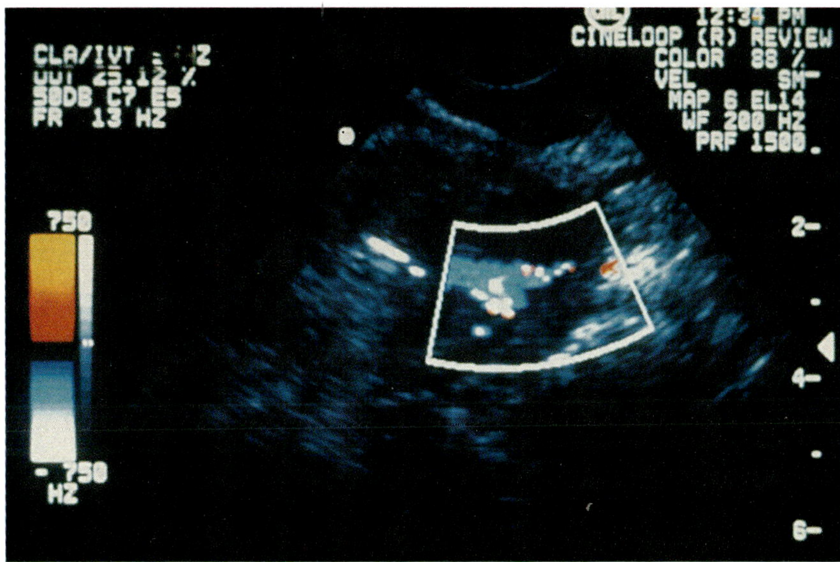

Figure 16-7   Proximal (or cornual) tubual occlusion as seen by color Doppler flow. Flow of saline abruptly stops at uterotubal junction.

Of the 193 patients, 94 patients also had laparoscopy with CPT and 57 had X-RAY HSG. US HSG correlated with CPT in 79 percent of the procedures, and X-RAY HSG correlated with CPT in 63 percent of the procedures. The specificity and sensitivity of US HSG when compared with CPT using chi square analysis was 89 and 76 percent, respectively. Twenty-one percent of the US HSG studies did not correlate with CPT, compared with 37 percent of X-RAY HSGs. It should be noted that most of the noncorrelations involved discrepancies of unilateral patency.[13] Therefore, we recommend repeating the US HSG if unilateral occlusion is diagnosed. As with any of the tubal insufflation procedures, spasm may account for a false-positive result. Another area of difficulty in interpretation is in the case of dilated hydrosalpinges. Due to turbulence of saline in the distal tube, a false interpretation of patency may occur (Fig. 16-8). However, similar false-negative results can occur using X-RAY HSG.

SUMMARY

US HSG represents another method to evaluate fallopian tube patency. According to our investigation, US HSG correlates with CPT 79 percent of the time for a sensitivity and specificity which is equal to or greater than that for X-RAY HSG.

Several advantages exist when using US HSG. These include no exposure to contrast dyes or radiation. Cost to the patient for US HSG is less than for

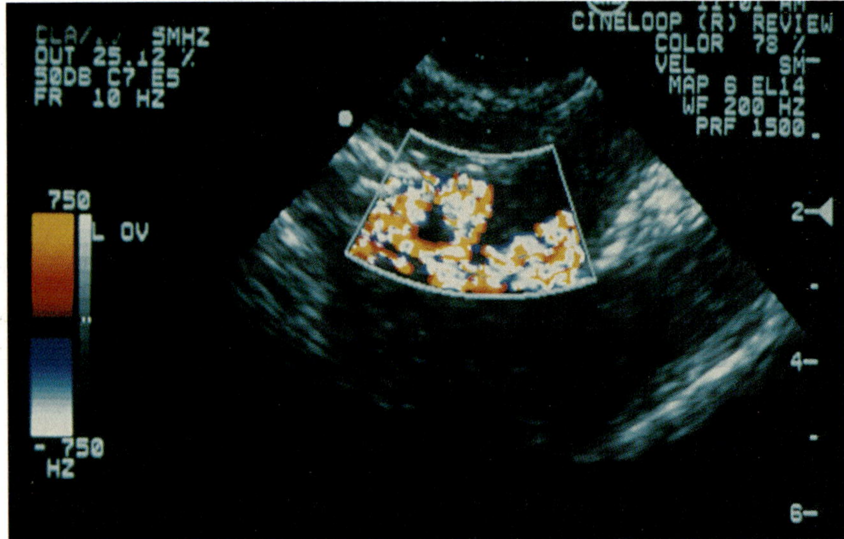

A

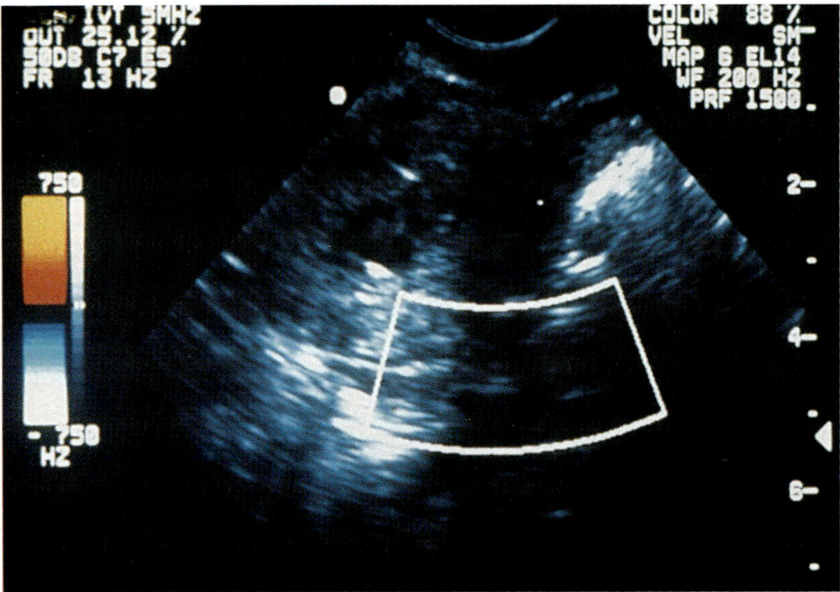

B

Figure 16-8   Distal tubal occlusion as seen by color Doppler flow. *A*. Fluid is seen collecting in the distal (infundibular) aspect of the clubbed fallopian tube. *B*. No cul-de-sac flow is observed.

X-RAY HSG. The procedure can easily be done in the office, saving the patient the inconvenience of having the test done at another location and allowing the physician to know the results immediately. Additionally, sonographic examination of the pelvis provides an advantage over X-RAY HSG. While false-positive and false-negative results do exist with US HSG, they are at no greater incidence than with X-RAY HSG.

The future for US HSG holds even more promise. New echodense liquid materials are currently being developed which may improve the resolution of this technique. However, at the present time US HSG using color Doppler flow seems to be a safe and efficacious method of evaluating fallopian tube patency.

REFERENCES

1. U.S. Congress, Office of Technology Assessment: Infertility, Medical and Social Choices, OTA-BA 358. Washington, D.C., U.S. Government Printing Office, May 1988.
2. Mosher WD, Pratt WF: Fecundity, infertility and reproductive health in the United States, 1982. Vital and Health Statistics Series 23, No 14. National Center for Health Statistics, Public Health Service, Washington, D.C., U.S. Government Printing Office, 1987, p 27.
3. Page H: Estimation of the prevalence and incidence of infertility in a population: a pilot study. Fertil Steril 71:571–577, 1989.
4. Davajan V, Mishell D: "Evaluation of the infertile couple," in Mishell D, Davajan V (eds), *Infertility, Contraception and Reproductive Endocrinology,* 2d ed. Oradell, N.J., Medical Economics Books, 1986, p 381.
5. Thie JL, Williams TJ, Coulam CB: Repeat tuboplasty compared with primary microsurgery for postinflammatory tubal disease. Fertil Steril 45:784–787, 1986.
6. Patton PE, Williams TJ, Coulam CB: Microsurgical reconstruction of the proximal oviduct. Fertil Steril 47:35–39, 1986.
7. Patton PE, Williams TJ, Coulam CB: Results of microsurgical reconstruction in patients with combined proximal and distal tubal occlusion: double obstruction. Fertil Steril 48:670–674, 1987.
8. Sulak PJ, Letterie GS, Coddington CC, Hayslip CC, Woodward JE, Klein TA: Histology of proximal tubal occlusion. Fertil Steril 48:437–440, 1987.
9. Confino E, Tur-Kaspa I, DeCherney A, Corfman R, Coulam C, Robinson E, Haas G, Katz E, Vermesh M, Gleicher N: Transcervical balloon tuboplasty. A multicenter study. JAMA 264:2079–2082, 1990.
10. Rubin I: Difference between the uterus and tubes as a cause of oscillations recorded during uterotubal insufflation. Fertil Steril 5:147, 1954.
11. McCalley M, Braunstein P, Stone S, Henderson P, Egbeat R: Radionuclide hysterosalpingography for evaluation of fallopian tube patency. J Nucl Med 26:868–874, 1985.
12. Peters AJ, Stern JJ, Coulam CB: Hysterosalpingography using color Doppler sonography. J Ultrasound Med 10:S37–S58, 1991.
13. Peters AJ, Coulam CB: Hysterosalpingography using color Doppler sonography. Am J Obstet Gynecol 164:1530–1534, 1991.

INDEX

P15RJG